Nutrition for Sport, Exercise, and Performance

Nutrition for Sport, Exercise, and Performance offers a clear, practical, and accessible guide to building a comprehensive understanding of sport and exercise nutrition from leading experts in nutrition and exercise science. Nutrition before, during, and after training or a sporting event can improve the comfort, energy, and performance of athletes of all levels, from elite to recreational, as well as providing long-term health benefits. As such, nutrition is a key element of an athlete's health and performance strategy, whether competing recreationally or at an elite level.

Split into three parts, this new and revised edition of **Nutrition for Sport, Exercise, and Performance** provides an evidence-based introduction to nutrition for sport, exercise, and performance. Part I focusses on nutrition and sport science by explaining key principles underpinning sports nutrition science, including energy systems, exercise physiology and metabolism, and the digestion and absorption of macronutrients and micronutrients essential for performance and discusses factors influencing dietary intake, energy availability, and the process of dietary assessment. Part II is focussed on nutrition for exercise, pre- and post-training, hydration, supplements, and body composition measurement and modification. The final part (Part III) focusses on applied sports nutrition for a range of sports and athletes. This second edition delivers new insights into working with female athletes, occupational athletes, and athletes in contemporary sports including sport climbing, surfing, skateboarding, and breaking.

Featuring contributions from a range of sport and exercise nutrition professionals with practical sports nutrition strategies and the latest evidence and practice guidelines, this is a core reference for undergraduate students, sports professionals, and aspiring athletes alike.

Adrienne Forsyth is an Associate Professor and Research Lead in Nutrition and Dietetics at Australian Catholic University, Australia. She is an Advanced Accredited Practising Dietitian, Advanced Accredited Sports Dietitian, and Accredited Exercise Physiologist with over two decades of experience in teaching, practice, and research. Adrienne leads community-based interventions that address nutrition-related chronic disease and facilitate healthy participation in sport and recreation as well as innovations in health professional education.

Evangeline Mantzioris is the Program Director of the Nutrition and Food Sciences Degree at the University of South Australia. She is a Senior Lecturer, Accredited Practicing Dietitian, and Accredited Sports Dietitian with over three decades of experience in research, university teaching, clinical dietetics, and clinical teaching at major teaching hospitals and in private practice. Evangeline's research interests include sports nutrition, fats, fatty acids, Mediterranean Diet, and the environment–food nexus.

Regina Belski is a Professor and Discipline Lead for Food, Nutrition and Dietetics at La Trobe University, Australia. Regina is an Advanced Accredited Practising Dietitian and Advanced Sports Dietitian. Regina specialises in a personalised nutrition approach for health and performance, this entails exploring factors which impact individuals' dietary intakes and health outcomes, including modifiable factors such as nutrition knowledge, behaviour, and more advanced fields such as nutrigenomics and variation of gene expression via dietary means as well as functional foods for human health and the microbiome. In her professional capacity as an Accredited Practising Dietitian, Regina has worked with clients including Olympic athletes and elite football and soccer players.

Nutrition for Sport, Exercise, and Performance

Science and Application

Second Edition

Edited by Adrienne Forsyth, Evangeline Mantzioris, and Regina Belski

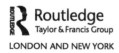

Routledge
Taylor & Francis Group

LONDON AND NEW YORK

Designed cover image: Getty Images

Second edition published 2024
by Routledge
605 Third Avenue, New York, NY 10158

and by Routledge
4 Park Square, Milton Park, Abingdon, Oxon, OX14 4RN

Routledge is an imprint of the Taylor & Francis Group, an informa business

First edition published by Allen & Unwin 2019

ISBN: 978-1-032-34274-0 (hbk)
ISBN: 978-1-032-34271-9 (pbk)
ISBN: 978-1-003-32128-6 (ebk)

DOI: 10.4324/9781003321286

Typeset in Sabon
by SPi Technologies India Pvt Ltd (Straive)

Contents

Figures

Tables

Boxes

Contributors

Rebekah Alcock is an Advanced Sports Dietitian and Accredited Practicing Dietitian at La Trobe University, Australia. Rebekah completed her PhD at the Australian Institute of Sport on nutrition support for connective tissue injuries. Rebekah has led sports nutrition roles in elite team sports and is currently at Essendon Football Club.

Bradley Baker is an Accredited Sports Dietitian and works as a dietitian-nutritionist and researcher within the Australian Department of Defence, Australia. He is currently undertaking a work-based PhD in collaboration with Swinburne University and La Trobe University, investigating strategies to improve the dietary intakes, health, and performance of infantry trainees.

Regina Belski is a Professor and Discipline Lead for Food, Nutrition and Dietetics at La Trobe University, Australia. Regina is an Advanced Accredited Practising Dietitian and Advanced Sports Dietitian. She is a highly regarded researcher and experienced clinician in sports dietetics.

Martyn Binnie is a Performance Scientist based out of the Western Australian Institute of Sport (WAIS), Australia. Martyn completed his PhD with WAIS in 2013 and has provided applied physiology support across a range of Olympic sport programs, including rowing, sprint kayak, cycling, sailing, hockey, netball, and water polo.

Elizabeth Broad has been a sports dietitian for 30 years and has worked with elite athletes in Australia, Scotland, and the United States. Liz holds a PhD, has specialised in working with Paralympic athletes, and runs the Para Sports Nutrition podcast.

Louise M Burke, OAM, is a Professor at Australian Catholic University, Australia. This follows a 30-year career at the Australian Institute of Sport and attendance at six summer Olympic Games. Louise has published more than 400 peer-reviewed papers and book chapters and is a director of the IOC Diploma of Sports Nutrition.

Mikaeli Carmichael is a PhD candidate in the School of Allied Health, Human Services and Sport at La Trobe University, Australia, focusing on female athlete physiology and supporting female athletes.

Anthea C Clarke is a Senior Lecturer in the School of Allied Health, Human Services and Sport at La Trobe University, Australia. Anthea holds a PhD and specialises in the areas of exercise physiology and applied sport science, with research interests around female athlete in sport.

Erin Colebatch is an Accredited Practicing Dietitian and Sports Dietitian in Australia. Erin assists distance runners in her private practice to optimise their nutrition. Erin is also completing a master's degree at the University of South Australia on the relationship between diet, lifestyle, and running-related injuries in masters-aged distance runners.

Matthew Cooke is a Professor of Food and Nutrition at La Trobe University, Australia. He is a registered nutritionist and integrative physiologist who has published more than 130 papers and abstracts. Matthew's work explores the impact of nutrition on health, performance, and the mechanisms that underpin such effects from molecular to the gut microbiome.

Michelle Cort is the Lead Sports Performance Dietitian for Cricket Australia. She is an Advanced Sports Dietitian with over 20 years' experience as part of high-performance units with Olympic and professional sports.

Gregory Cox is an Associate Professor at Bond University, Australia, and is a Fellow of Sports Dietitians Australia. He has 30 years' experience supporting endurance athletes at all levels, from Olympic and world champions to recreational athletes. His research interests are sports nutrition strategies to optimise performance, health, and wellbeing.

Joel C Craddock is a Lecturer at the University of Wollongong, Australia. He holds a PhD and has worked with recreational athletes all the way up to Olympians to optimise their dietary intake. His research focuses on the influence of plant-based dietary patterns on health and exercise.

Ben Desbrow is a Professor, Accredited Practicing Dietitian, Fellow of Sports Dietitians Australia, and Head of Performance Nutrition at the Gold Coast Titans, Australia. Ben conducts research investigating the optimisation of diet, supplements, and food delivery systems to enhance human health and cognitive and physical performance.

Brooke L Devlin is an Advanced Sports Dietitian and Lecturer in Nutrition and Dietetics at the University of Queensland, Australia. Brooke holds a PhD and is an active researcher and educator focusing on the value nutrition can provide to athletic performance and overall health and wellbeing.

Matthew Driller is an Associate Professor at La Trobe University, Australia. He has more than 15 years of academic and industry experience in elite sport. Matt has published over 150 peer-reviewed papers and book chapters, with the majority on sleep and recovery in athletes.

Adrienne Forsyth is an Associate Professor and Research Lead for Nutrition and Dietetics at Australian Catholic University, Australia. As an Advanced Accredited Sports Dietitian and Accredited Exercise Physiologist, she works with students, health, and sporting organisations to implement interventions that address nutrition-related chronic disease and facilitate participation in sport and recreation.

Stephanie K Gaskell is an Advanced Sports Dietitian in Australia and former national competitive ultra-endurance runner working in gastrointestinal nutrition private practice for over a decade with athletes of all levels, from recreational to elite. She holds a PhD in exercise-induced gastrointestinal syndrome: exacerbation factors and translation into practice.

Kate Gemmell is an Accredited Practicing Dietitian and Advanced Sports Dietitian in Australia who has worked with elite and recreational athletes for the past decade. Kate's interests are in extreme sports as they are relatively understudied in nutrition and pose interesting nutritional challenges, often combined with relaxed attitudes from athletes.

Janelle Gifford is a Senior Lecturer in the Discipline of Exercise and Sport Science at the University of Sydney, Australia. She is an Advanced Accredited Practising Dietitian and Fellow of Sports Dietitians Australia and holds a PhD. Her main research interests include masters athlete sports nutrition and nutrition knowledge.

Andrew Govus is a Senior Lecturer in the School of Allied Health, Human Services and Sport at La Trobe University, Australia. Andrew holds a PhD and specialises in sports physiology with research interests in iron metabolism and sports metabolomics.

Rebecca Hall is an Advanced Accredited Sport Dietitian working with the Olympic Winter Institute of Australia and at Australian Catholic University, Australia. Prior to her current role, she completed a sport nutrition fellowship at the Australian Institute of Sport and worked at the Canadian Sports Institute Pacific.

Shona L Halson is a Professor and Deputy Director of the SPRINT Research Centre at Australian Catholic University, Australia. Shona's research focuses on sleep, recovery, and fatigue, and she has published over 170 peer-reviewed articles and multiple book chapters.

Patria Anne Hume is Professor of Human Performance and Director of the SPRINZ J.E. Lindsay Carter Kinanthropometry Clinic and Archive, New Zealand. Patria's research focuses on improving sport performance and reducing injury risk via sports biomechanics, anthropometry, and epidemiology analyses. Patria is an International Society for Biomechanics in Sports Geoffrey Dyson awardee.

Christopher Irwin is an Accredited Practicing Dietitian and Senior Lecturer at Griffith University, Australia. Christopher holds a PhD and conducts research focused on the impact of nutrition-related factors on human behaviour and performance, including the effects of hydration and factors influencing the effectiveness of fluid restoration following exercise-induced dehydration.

Nikki A Jeacocke is an Accredited Practicing Dietitian, Fellow of Sports Dietitians Australia, and Credentialed Eating Disorder Clinician at the Australian Institute of Sport, Australia. Nikki has extensive experience working with Olympic and professional sports to maximise performance and health outcomes and the prevention and management of eating disorders in sports.

Sarah L Jenner is an Advanced Sports Dietitian and Lead Performance Nutritionist for Bath Rugby, UK. Sarah previously worked with a range of team-based sports, including Australian Football. Sarah's PhD research explored the intake and nutrition knowledge of male and female Australian Football athletes and the factors that influence food choice.

Stephen J Keenan is a Sports Dietitian and Lecturer in Dietetics at Swinburne University of Technology, Australia. He has supported elite Australian soccer players in optimising their nutrition and his PhD research focussed on the impact of timing of energy intake on body composition in active individuals.

Annie-Claude M Lassemillante is an Accredited Practicing Dietitian and Senior Lecturer at La Trobe University, Australia. She holds a PhD and brings together her passion for food and understanding of human physiology and her drive to help people achieve a healthier life through evidence-based strategies.

Dana M Lis is an internationally recognised Performance Dietitian, USA, with research experience across a variety of areas and elite sports. Her seminal PhD work established the fundamentals for the application of FODMAP modification for athletic populations. Dana now investigates practical nutrition strategies to improve athletes' connective tissue health and injury recovery.

Bronwen Lundy is an Advanced Sports Dietitian and Accredited Practising Dietitian in Australia with extensive experience in sports nutrition. She is primarily a clinician but with a strong interest in research to support practice and recently completed a PhD examining energy availability and bone injury in rowing.

Evangeline Mantzioris is a Senior Lecturer at the University of South Australia, Australia, and an Accredited Practicing Dietitian and Sports Dietitian. Evangeline holds a PhD, and her research interests include fats and fatty acids, the Mediterranean diet across the lifespan, the environment–food nexus, and sports nutrition.

Alan McCubbin is a Researcher and Senior Teaching Fellow at Monash University, Australia. He holds a PhD and studies the impact of dietary interventions on athlete health and performance in extreme environments. Alan also consults to endurance and ultra-endurance athletes across a variety of sports, from recreational to professional and Olympic athletes.

Anthony Meade is an Accredited Sports Dietitian from Adelaide, Australia, with 25 years' experience working with both elite national-level teams and in private practice consulting to individual athletes of all ages and abilities.

Marisa Michael holds a position on the USA Climbing Medical Committee and owns a private practice in Oregon, USA. She has completed the International Olympic Committee's Diploma in Sports Nutrition.

Kane Middleton is a Senior Lecturer in the School of Allied Health, Human Services and Sport at La Trobe University, Australia. Kane holds a PhD and specialises in sport and occupational biomechanics. His main research interests are the enhancement of human performance and the reduction of injury risk in both the sporting and occupational contexts.

Michelle Minehan is a sports dietitian and currently holds an academic position at the University of Canberra, Australia, where she teaches and conducts research in sports nutrition. She holds a PhD and has worked with elite Paralympic athletes throughout her career since 1999.

Lachlan Mitchell is an Accredited Sports Dietitian, Lecturer, and researcher at Australian Catholic University, Australia. Lachlan holds a PhD, and his research interests are in the manipulation of diet and exercise for performance and body composition change in athletes.

Aimee Morabito is an Accredited Practicing Dietitian, Accredited Sports Dietitian, and PhD candidate at Australian Catholic University, Australian Institute of Sport, Australia. Aimee is passionate about working with extreme and lifestyle sport athletes, and recently presented at Surfing Medicine International's (SMI) World Conference.

Helen O'Connor was an Associate Professor at the University of Sydney and a Fellow and the inaugural President of Sports Dietitians Australia. Helen was a pioneer of the profession in Australia, initiating performance nutrition services for professional teams and awarded the Australian Sports Medal for her services to sports nutrition in 2000.

Craig Patch is the CEO and cofounder of Vernx Pty Ltd, 5iv Pty Ltd and cofounder of NeuroSports Labs Pty Ltd, Australia, who develop diagnostics and therapeutics for concussion. Craig holds a PhD, is a dietitian and biotechnology entrepreneur, and his interests include the effects of omega-3 fats in infant development and concussion management.

Alan J Pearce is a neurophysiologist and Professor at La Trobe University, Australia. His research interests are brain injuries in sports and nutritional interventions following concussion. He was the first to publish longitudinal studies on chronic outcomes of repetitive brain injuries in retired professional Australian rules football and rugby league players.

Yasmine C Probst is an Associate Professor at the University of Wollongong and a Research Fellow at the Illawarra Health and Medical Research Institute, Australia. Yasmine is an Advanced Accredited Practising Dietitian and Fellow of the Australasian Institute for Digital Health. Her research has focussed on the application of food composition data to practice including dietary assessment methodology.

Georgia Romyn is a PhD Scholar at the Australian Institute of Sport and Central Queensland University, Australia, with over 10 years' experience working in high-performance sport with elite athletes. Her research focusses on the impact of sleep, napping, and travel on athletic performance.

Greg Shaw is the Head of Performance Support for Swimming Australia and is a Fellow of Sports Dietitians Australia and Accredited Practicing Dietitian in Australia. Greg holds a PhD, and his research interest area is the use of nutrition and supplemental interventions to improve sporting performance.

Gary Slater is an Associate Professor at the University of the Sunshine Coast, Australia. He is an Advanced Accredited Sports Dietitian and the National Performance Nutrition Network Lead at the AIS. He has authored more than 100 peer-reviewed manuscripts. Gary supported the Australian Olympic team during the 2020 Tokyo Olympic Games.

Stephen Smith is a performance nutritionist working in elite sport, including motorsport (MotoGP, Formula 1), America's Cup sailing and several endurance sports across the world. Stephen gained his PhD from Liverpool John Moores University, examining gastrointestinal permeability in response to exercise.

Rachel Stentiford is an Advanced Sports Dietitian, Australia. She has supported the nutrition demands of athletes from pathway level through to Olympic, Paralympic, and World Champions at High Performance Sports Institutes in Scotland, Ireland, New Zealand, and most recently Australia, at the Victorian Institute of Sport.

Ryan Tam is a Lecturer in Nutrition and Dietetics at Australian Catholic University, Australia. He is an Accredited Sports Dietitian and exercise scientist with previous experience in elite sports and private practice. He holds a PhD, and his research interests are in understanding how nutrition knowledge can influence dietary habits in athletes.

Gina Trakman is a Senior Lecturer in Dietetics and Human Nutrition at La Trobe University, Australia. Gina is an Accredited Practising Dietitian and a Sports Dietitian with clinical and community experience. She holds a PhD, and her research interests include dietary questionnaire development and interventions to improve nutrition knowledge, and the role of diet in inflammatory bowel disease.

Sam SX Wu is a Lecturer at Swinburne University, Australia. He holds a PhD, and his research interest is in exercise and performance physiology in endurance sports and the effects of ergogenic aids on health and exercise performance. Sam is dedicated to practical and feasible outcomes for the athletic, ageing, and general populations.

Preface

As academics teaching sports nutrition, we designed this textbook to provide a single source of evidence-based scientific information written at just the right level for our undergraduate students. The chapters in this book are written by sports nutrition experts who understand the science behind nutrition recommendations and the challenges encountered in implementing these recommendations in practice. They share the most up-to-date sports nutrition guidelines and explain how they can be practically implemented, making this textbook a great resource for athletes and developing sports and nutrition professionals as well as students.

This book has been developed in three parts:

Part I (Chapters 1–8): The science of nutrition and sport
The chapters contained in this part will help you to develop the underlying knowledge in physiology, nutrition, and assessment required to understand and apply concepts in sports nutrition. Some of these chapters may serve as review or reference material for students who have completed previous study in nutrition and exercise physiology.

Part II (Chapters 9–16): Nutrition for exercise
These chapters will provide you with evidence-based recommendations for foods and fluids to consume before, during, and after exercise, and explore special considerations for specific contexts such as injury management and rehabilitation, gastrointestinal disturbances, and environmental considerations.

Part III (Chapters 17–28): Applied sports nutrition
This part includes chapters that describe the nutrition requirements of athletes participating in a range of sports, and the unique nutrition needs of athletes at different developmental stages and with other special needs. The final chapter describes the art of sports nutrition practice and practising sports nutrition professionals share practical strategies for working with athletes and providing nutrition support in challenging circumstances.

It is important to remember that sports nutrition research is constantly growing and that practice changes as new evidence emerges. The information presented in this book reflects the evidence available at the time of writing, so it is a contemporary resource for the mid-2020s.

We trust that you will find this textbook to be a source of reliable nutrition information that is easy to understand and apply in sports settings.

Adrienne Forsyth
Evangeline Mantzioris
Regina Belski

Part I

The science of nutrition and sport

1 Introduction to sport and exercise

Kane Middleton, Andrew Govus and Anthea C Clarke

This book has been written for athletes, people working with athletes, and those who would like to work with athletes in the future. A good understanding of the practical and physiological impacts of physical activity, exercise, and sport is needed to be able to provide appropriate nutrition advice to athletes. This chapter will provide an overview of key concepts related to sport, exercise, and performance, and outline the body's responses and adaptations to exercise.

Learning outcomes

This chapter will:

- define physical activity, exercise, and sport;
- describe different types of sport and exercise, and relate these to differing physiological processes and adaptations;
- explain how to measure exercise performance and intensity;
- outline the principles of exercise prescription;
- describe muscle types and actions;
- describe the body's physiological response and chronic adaptations to exercise;
- outline how the body recovers from exercise.

Physical activity, exercise, and sport

Although often used interchangeably, there are distinct conceptual differences between physical activity, exercise, and sport. **Physical activity** is any movement performed by the body that expends energy. The simplest categorisation of physical activity is based on proportioning activities in daily life—namely, sleep, work, and leisure. The energy expenditure during sleep is very small, whereas the energy expenditure during work would depend on the type of employment. A nurse who spends a lot of time walking around a hospital ward would expend much more energy than an office worker who spends most of their workday sitting down. Humans typically perform leisure-time physical activity incidentally (e.g., walking to buy groceries), in the household (e.g., gardening), or during exercise and sport.

DOI: 10.4324/9781003321286-2

Physical activity

Any bodily movement produced by skeletal muscles that results in energy expenditure.

Exercise

Physical activity that is planned, structured, repetitive, and purposeful with the aim to improve or maintain one or more components of physical fitness.

Exercise is a subcategory of physical activity. Although it still includes body movements that result in energy expenditure, it is different to physical activity in that it is planned, structured, and repetitive. The purpose of exercise is to improve or maintain components of physical fitness, including:

- aerobic and anaerobic capacity (described later in this chapter);
- muscular endurance, strength, and power;
- body composition;
- flexibility;
- balance.

Aerobic capacity

The ability of the body to take in and distribute oxygen to the working muscles during exercise.

Examples of structured exercise include a running program to promote fat loss and/or increase **aerobic capacity**, a conditioning program to increase muscular strength, or a stretching program to increase joint flexibility. Such programs are most effective when planned before beginning. The plan would incorporate purposeful exercise and progress the exerciser through mental stages of readiness to change. The program would be delivered in a structured, repetitive manner, considering the concepts of periodisation and progressive overload (this is discussed in more detail later in this chapter under **Chronic Adaptations to Exercise**).

It has been difficult to develop a universally approved definition of sport. The Global Association of International Sports Federations states that the following criteria must be met for a sport to become a member of the Association:[1]

- the sport proposed should include an element of competition;
- the sport should not rely on any element of 'luck' specifically integrated into the sport;
- the sport should not be judged to pose an undue risk to the health and safety of its athletes or participants;

- the sport proposed should in no way be harmful to any living creature;
- the sport should not rely on equipment that is provided by a single supplier.

Types of sport

Due to the variety of sports in existence, the Global Association of International Sports Federations has developed categories of sports. These categories are based on the primary (not exclusive) type of activities that make up the sport and include physical, mental, motorised, coordination, and animal-supported. Note that many sports may belong to multiple categories.

Physical sports are the most common and best known, and nutrition is an important consideration for these types of sports. Whether a sport is individual or team-based, the physical requirements of that sport will lie somewhere on an endurance–power continuum. Sports such as marathon running and triathlon are on the endurance end of the continuum, where repeated movement cycles are performed over a sustained period. In contrast, power lifting and track and field throws are on the power end of the continuum, where a single movement is performed at high intensity and often at high speed. To complicate this, sports often have different physical requirements for the disciplines within the sport or playing positions within a team. In track and field, a 100-metre sprinter has a different physical requirement than a 10,000-metre runner. In American Football, a defensive tackle is usually the biggest and strongest player on the team, whereas running backs tend to be smaller but fast and agile. These discipline- and position-specific differences result in discipline- and position-specific nutritional requirements.

Aerobic exercise

Exercise performed at an intensity that is low enough to allow the body's need for oxygen (to break down macronutrients) to be matched to the oxygen supply available.

Anaerobic exercise

Exercise performed at an intensity where the body's demand for oxygen is greater than the oxygen delivery rate, therefore resulting in the production of lactate and pyruvate.

Sporting activities are also sometimes categorised as **aerobic** or **anaerobic**. Endurance sports, which are performed at a lower intensity over a long period, are predominantly aerobic, meaning that the body can deliver oxygen at a rate that supports the breakdown of energy substrates to fuel metabolic processes and skeletal muscle activity. Power sports are performed at a high intensity and thus require an immediate energy source, hence the breakdown of energy substrates by oxidative processes is too slow. As such, the energy required to fuel skeletal muscle contraction and metabolic processes is provided by anaerobic energy pathways instead.

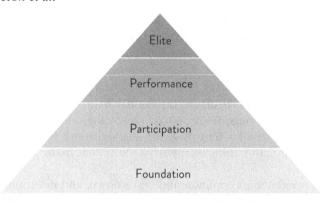

Figure 1.1 Levels of sports participation.

Levels of sports participation and competition

Sports participation can be thought of as a pyramid (Figure 1.1) that represents an inverse relationship between competition level and participation rate.[2] The foundation level of competitive sport most often occurs at a young age, when people are first introduced to a sport. An introduction to physical activity would typically occur during physical education classes. Sporting organisations and recreation centres also contribute to the foundation level by offering introductory programs, such as Kids' Athletics or Little League Baseball, which focus on developing the fundamental motor skills of those sports.

Once someone advances from an introduction to a sport to regularly engaging with that sport, they enter the participation level. As many people are introduced to various sports at the foundation level, there is an inevitable decline in numbers reaching the participation level. The engagement at this level is generally recreational, such as social sport; and although competition is present, i.e., there is a winner and a loser, the main aim of participating is enjoying the activity itself rather than the outcome.

The aim of competition changes from enjoyment to winning at the performance level. Whereas the skill level of people at the participation level is not overly important, performance athletes are often selected in teams or for competition based on their performance. They will often represent a club or team in these competitions, which are administered by official sporting organisations with standard rules and regulations. Representative sport will generally start in high school and continue through to adult competition. The critical development period from 18 to 23 years of age coincides with tertiary education for many high-achieving athletes. In Australia, the progress of these athletes is supported by national sporting organisations and state-based academies and institutes of sport. In the United Kingdom and New Zealand, it is through clubs and their respective national institutes of sport. The United States of America has established a college-based sports system, regulated by organisations such as the National Collegiate Athletic Association, and organised and funded by the colleges themselves.

The peak of sports participation is the elite level. This is like the performance level but only includes the very best representatives of a sport, meaning that this level has the fewest athletes of all the levels of the sports participation pyramid. The delineation of elite athletes from other high-performing athletes is difficult, but elite athletes often compete at the national or international level. Although the Olympic Games is still the pinnacle of elite amateur sport around the world, the evolution of elite sport has coincided with growing professionalism due to the resources dedicated to preparation, training, and competition. The large investments in professional sport make winning 'big business' and, given that the performance differential between athletes at the elite level is very small, nutritional interventions such as supplementation can have a large impact on performance and competition outcomes (see Chapter 12 for more information on this topic).

Monitoring exercise

Exercise can be categorised into **cardiorespiratory exercise** and **resistance exercise**. Whereas cardiorespiratory exercise involves predominantly whole-body, dynamic exercise involving a large skeletal muscle mass, resistance exercise aims to develop **physiological, neurological**, and **biomechanical** properties of skeletal muscle. Cardiorespiratory exercise is predominantly aerobic, while resistance exercise is predominantly anaerobic.

Cardiorespiratory exercise

Whole-body, dynamic exercise that involves predominantly the cardiovascular and respiratory systems, such as running, cycling, and swimming.

Resistance exercise

Exercise that predominantly involves the musculoskeletal system.

Skeletal muscle

Voluntary muscle attached to bones that move a part of the skeleton when stimulated with a nerve impulse.

Physiological

Pertaining to biological functions and body systems of living organisms.

Neurological

Pertaining to the nervous system, including the brain, spinal cord, and nerves.

Biomechanical

Pertaining to the mechanical nature of the body's biological processes, such as movements of the skeleton and muscles.

The intensity of cardiorespiratory and resistance exercise can be expressed in either absolute or relative terms. Absolute exercise intensity refers to the total amount of energy expended (expressed in **kilojoules** or **kilocalories**) to produce mechanical work, in the form of skeletal muscle contraction. See Chapter 2 for a more detailed discussion of energy, work, and power.

Kilojoules

A unit of energy equal to 1000 joules. A joule is a unit of energy equal to the amount of work done by a force of 1 Newton (the force required to accelerate 1 kilogram of mass at the rate of 1 metre per second squared in the direction of the applied force) to move an object 1 metre.

The internationally agreed decimal system of measurement (metric system) uses kilojoules (kJ), although kilocalories (kcal), commonly referred to simply as calories, are still commonly used to measure and refer to energy in many parts of the world (1 kcal = 4.18 kJ).

Kilocalories

A unit of energy equal to 1000 calories. A calorie is the energy required to increase the temperature of 1 gram of water by 1°C. The term 'calories', is commonly used to mean 'kilocalories'.

Absolute exercise intensity can also be expressed in **metabolic equivalents** (METs), which describe exercise intensity as a multiple of the amount of energy required by the body at rest. One MET is approximately equivalent to an oxygen uptake of 3.5 mL·kg^{-1}·min^{-1}, although the exact value will vary between individuals and should be measured directly (see Chapter 2 for more information about measurement of energy expenditure). For example, the oxygen consumption for a 70 kg (~154 pounds) male exercising at an absolute exercise intensity of five METs for 30 minutes would be calculated as:

$$\text{Oxygen consumption}\left(\dot{V}O_2\right) = 5 \times 3.5\text{mL} \cdot \text{kg}^{-1} \cdot \text{min}^{-1} = 17.5\text{mL} \cdot \text{kg}^{-1} \cdot \text{min}^{-1}O_2$$

$$\text{Oxygen consumption}\left(\dot{V}O_2\right) = 17.5\text{mL} \cdot \text{kg}^{-1} \cdot \text{min}^{-1} \times 70\text{kg} = 1225\text{mL} \cdot \text{min}^{-1}O_2$$

Oxygen consumption $\left(\dot{V}O_2\right) = 1225\text{mL} \cdot \text{min}^{-1} \times 30\text{min} = 36750\text{mLO}_2$

Oxygen consumption $\left(\dot{V}O_2\right) = \dfrac{36750\text{mL}}{1000} = 36.75\text{L O}_2$

From the estimated oxygen consumption, one can calculate the energy expenditure during exercise since each litre of oxygen yields ~20.9 kJ (~5 kcal) (see Chapter 2 for a detailed explanation). Therefore, the estimated energy expenditure for the example above is:

Energy expenditure $\left(\text{kcal}\right) = 36.75\text{LO}_2 \times 5\text{kcal} = 183.75\text{kcal}$

To convert kilocalories to kilojoules $\left(\text{kJ}\right) = 183.75\text{kcal} \times \dfrac{4.18\text{kJ}}{\text{kcal}} = \sim 768\text{kJ}$

In comparison, relative exercise intensity refers to exercise that is expressed relative to an individual's maximal capacity for a given task or activity. The intensity of cardiorespiratory exercise is commonly expressed as a percentage of an individual's **maximum aerobic power (VO$_2$max)**, heart rate (HRmax), or rating of perceived exertion (RPE).

Maximum aerobic power (VO$_2$max)

The maximum amount of oxygen an individual can use per minute during dynamic exercise using large muscle groups.

Oxygen reserve (%VO$_2$R)

The difference between resting oxygen consumption and maximal oxygen consumption.

The most accurate method of monitoring the intensity of submaximal exercise is by expressing the exercise intensity as a percentage of the individual's maximal oxygen uptake (%VO$_2$max) or **oxygen reserve (%VO$_2$R)**.

Percent maximal oxygen uptake $\left(\%\dot{V}O_2\ \text{max}\right) = \dot{V}O_2\ \text{max} \times \text{intensity}\ (\%)$

Percent oxygen reserve $\left(\%\dot{V}O_2R\right) = \left[(\dot{V}O_2\ \text{max} - \dot{V}O_2\text{rest}) \times \text{intensity}(\%)\right] + \dot{V}O_2\text{rest}$

A linear relationship exists between heart rate and oxygen uptake during incremental exercise (Figure 1.2). An individual's heart rate, rather than their oxygen uptake, is more regularly used to monitor exercise intensity since heart rate monitoring is both cheaper and less invasive than measuring oxygen consumption.

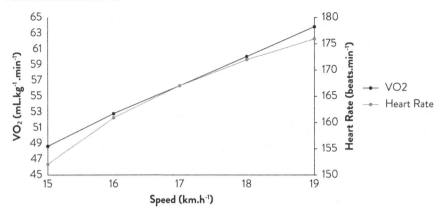

Figure 1.2 The relationship between oxygen uptake (VO$_2$) and heart rate during treadmill running.

Several different equations exist to estimate an individual's HRmax and the equation used should be appropriate for the population being measured. One common formula is that of Gellish et al.:[3]

$$\text{Maximum heart rate (HRmax)} = 207 - \left[0.70 \times \text{Age (years)} \right]$$

Another method of estimating exercise intensity using heart rate methods is by calculating the percentage of **heart rate reserve (%HRR)**. Heart rate reserve is often known as the Karvonen formula.[4] The HRR and %HRR are calculated using the equations below.

Percent heart rate reserve (%HRR)

Heart rate reserve multiplied by the desired percentage of exercise intensity.

$$\text{Heart rate reserve (HRR)} = \text{HRmax} - \text{HRrest}$$

$$\text{Percent heart rate reserve (\%HRR)} = \left[(\text{HRmax} - \text{HRrest}) \times \text{intensity}(\%) \right] + \text{HRrest}$$

The advantages and disadvantages of using heart rate-based methods to monitor the intensity of cardiorespiratory exercise are summarised in Table 1.1.

Table 1.1 Advantages and disadvantages of measuring exercise intensity using heart rate monitoring.

Advantages	*Disadvantages*
Objective measurement	Need to know (or accurately estimate) maximum heart rate for effective exercise prescription
Easy to use in daily training	Average heart rate for a workout can be misleading if exercise intensity varies within a session
Heart rate and blood lactate response remain stable over time	Limited usefulness for very high-intensity intervals performed above the maximum heart rate

Table 1.2 The Borg 6–20 scale of perceived exertion

Rating	Descriptor
6	No exertion at all
7	Extremely light
8	-
9	Very light
10	-
11	Light
12	-
13	Somewhat hard
14	-
15	Heavy
16	-
17	Very hard
18	-
19	Extremely hard
20	Maximal

Source: Borg, G. (1970). Perceived exertion as an indicator of somatic stress. Scandinavian Journal of Rehabilitation Medicine, 2(2), 92–98.

In addition to measuring oxygen consumption or heart rate, exercise intensity can be expressed as an individual's current level of effort or exertion, relative to their perceived maximal exertion. The most common method of measuring an individual's perceptual response to exercise is by using visual analogue scales such as Borg's 6–20 scale of perceived exertion[5] (Table 1.2) or Foster's Category Ratio (CR) 10-point scale.[6]

In comparison, resistance exercise may be expressed relative to the maximum amount of mass that a particular muscle group can move successfully for one repetition, which is known as the one repetition maximum (1 RM), or by using perceptual methods such as RPE or repetitions in reserve. Exercise intensity for resistance training can then be expressed as a percentage of an individual's 1 RM. For example, an athlete with a 1 RM for the back-squat exercise of 120 kg (~264.6 pounds) wishes to develop their muscular strength, and so should lift ~85% of their 1 RM in training. The mass they should lift in training can be calculated as follows:

$$85\%\,1\,RM = 0.85 \times 120\,kg = 102\,kg$$

Exercise intensity is stratified into categories related to the level of challenge experienced. The intensity of the stimulus applied during a training session (e.g., the amount of weight lifted, or the speed of running) determines the physiological and mechanical loads placed upon the body during training and, consequently, the physiological adaptations that occur. Consistent with the principle of progressive overload (discussed later in this chapter), exercise intensity is one exercise prescription variable that can be manipulated to overload the body. Physiological and perceptual methods of monitoring exercise intensity include HRR/VO_2R, % VO_2max, % HRmax, and RPE (6–20).[5] The American College of Sports Medicine[7] stratifies exercise intensity as follows:

- very light intensity: HRR/VO_2R <30, <37% VO_2max, <57% HR max, RPE (6–20)[5] <9;
- light intensity: HRR/VO_2R 30–39, 37–45% VO_2max, 57–63% HR max, RPE (6–20)[5] 9–11;

- moderate intensity: HRR/VO$_2$R 40–59, 46–63% VO$_2$max, 64–76% HR max, RPE (6–20)[5] 12–13;
- vigorous intensity: HRR/VO$_2$R 60–89, 64–90% VO$_2$max, 77–95% HR max, RPE (6–20)[5] 14–17;
- near maximal intensity: HRR/VO$_2$R ≥90, ≥91% VO$_2$max, ≥96% HR max, RPE (6–20)[5] ≥18.

Acute responses to cardiorespiratory exercise

Acute exercise stresses several of the body's physiological systems, including the cardiovascular, respiratory, and musculoskeletal systems. In response to cardiorespiratory exercise, the cardiovascular system increases oxygen delivery to the skeletal muscle by increasing **cardiac output** as well as redistributing blood flow from non-essential organs. Furthermore, the skeletal muscle tissue extracts more oxygen from the blood to support the metabolic activities needed to fuel skeletal muscle activity.

During **steady-state exercise** at low intensities, **pulmonary ventilation** increases due to an increase in breathing frequency and tidal volume. In contrast, hyperventilation (over-breathing) occurs during maximal exercise intensities to buffer the acidic carbon dioxide that accumulates in the blood during anaerobic exercise. Common values for selected cardiorespiratory parameters at resting, submaximal, and maximal exercise are presented in Table 1.3.

Cardiac output

The product of an individual's heart rate (the number of times the heart contracts per minute) and stroke volume (the volume of blood ejected from the heart per minute).

Steady-state exercise

Exercise performed at an intensity whereby the body's physiological systems are maintained at a relatively constant value.

Table 1.3 Typical values for selected cardiorespiratory parameters during rest, submaximal, and maximal exercise for a healthy adult male

Physiological parameter	Rest	Submaximal exercise	Maximal exercise
Cardiac output	5 L/min	10–15 L/min	20–45 L/min
Stroke volume	50–80 mL/beat	110–130 mL/beat	110–130 mL/beat
Heart rate	50–70 beats/min	70–180 beats/min	180–220 beats/min
Skeletal muscle blood flow	15–20%	80–90%	80–90%
Systolic blood pressure	100–120 mmHg	120–180 mmHg	180–200 mmHg
Minute ventilation	5–6 L/min	35–150 L/min	150–200 L/min
Breath frequency	10–15 breaths/min	15–35 breaths/min	35–50 breaths/min
Tidal volume	0.5 L/min	0.5–3.0 L/min	3.0–5.0 L/min

Pulmonary ventilation

The product of an individual's breathing frequency (the number of breaths per minute) and tidal volume (the volume of air inhaled per minute).

Metabolism

Chemical processes that occur within a living organism to maintain life.

Metabolic acidosis

A decrease in blood pH below the body's normal pH of ~7.37–7.42.

Buffer

A chemical system within the body that aims to counteract a change in the blood pH, defined by the blood [H+].

Buffers and maintaining acid–base balance

The body must regulate acid–base balance during acute exercise to delay the onset of fatigue. **Metabolic acidosis** during exercise can impair energy substrate **metabolism** and skeletal muscle contraction decreasing the desired power output. Under physiological conditions, lactic acid produced immediately dissociates into lactate ($C_3H_5O_3^-$) and hydrogen ions (H^+) in solution. Hydrogen ions dissolved in a solution are acidic, and therefore decrease the blood pH. The pH scale, a measure of the relative acidity of a solution, ranges from 0 (extremely strong acid, such as hydrochloric acid) to 14 (extremely strong base, such as sodium hydroxide), with a pH of 7 indicating a neutral solution (such as water). Since many of the body's systems operate within an optimal pH range, the body counteracts increases in blood acidity during exercise by neutralising the rise in [H^+] using a combination of chemical (bicarbonate and phosphate), physiological (protein), and respiratory **buffers** to maintain blood pH within physiologic limits (pH = ~7.37–7.42).

The main method of controlling acid–base balance during acute exercise is by hydrogen carbonate ions (HCO_3^-) in the blood acting as a **proton** acceptor to neutralise H^+, forming carbonic acid ($H_2CO_3^-$), which dissociates into water (H_2O) and CO_2 in the blood via the reversible chemical reaction below. The excess CO_2 that accumulates in the blood is then expired (breathed out). As CO_2 accumulates in the blood and the blood pH decreases (i.e., becomes more acidic), the respiratory frequency increases, in turn increasing the blood pH by expelling excess CO_2.

$$H^+ + HCO_3^- \leftrightarrow H_2CO_3 \leftrightarrow H_2O + CO_2$$

Blood pH is also maintained by the buffering effects of proteins in the blood and surrounding cells, which also act as proton acceptors for H^+. Finally, phosphate ions (PO_4^-) act as proton acceptors in a similar way to HCO_3^-. In this way, some nutritional supplements act as buffers to improve anaerobic performance (see Chapter 12 for more details).

Proton

A subatomic particle with a positive electric charge.

Acute responses to musculoskeletal exercise

The musculoskeletal system also undergoes several different physiological responses during acute exercise to allow it to produce mechanical work. Such responses to acute exercise include an increase in **motor unit** and muscle fibre recruitment, muscle temperature, and muscle enzyme activity.

Motor unit

A motor neuron (nerve cell) and the skeletal muscle fibres that it innervates (services).

Acute cardiorespiratory and/or resistance exercise requires repeated skeletal muscle action to complete the desired physical task. Skeletal muscle actions rely on the actions of smaller fibres (called myofilaments) consisting of myosin (a thick myofilament) and actin (a thin myofilament). Myosin and actin slide past each other during skeletal muscle actions; hence, the process underlying skeletal muscle action is known as the sliding filament theory (Figure 1.3).

The body has two main skeletal muscle fibre types, slow- (type I) and fast-twitch (type IIa and IIx) fibres, and while some muscles contain predominantly slow- or fast-twitch fibres, most muscles contain a mixture of both fibre types. Slow-twitch fibres are highly fatigue resistant, but they have low force-generation characteristics, whereas fast-twitch fibres have high force-generation characteristics, but fatigue more quickly. The endowment of muscle fibre types within a skeletal muscle is mostly genetically determined; non-athletes may have a balanced distribution of slow-twitch (~45–55%) compared to fast-twitch fibres (~45–55%), endurance athletes possess a high percentage of slow-twitch (~70–85%) compared to fast-twitch fibres (~30–15%), and track sprinters possess a high percentage of fast-twitch (25–30%) compared to slow-twitch fibres (70–75%). In addition to exercise training, several factors such as sex, hormone concentrations, and ageing can cause some shifts in the fibre type distribution within muscles.

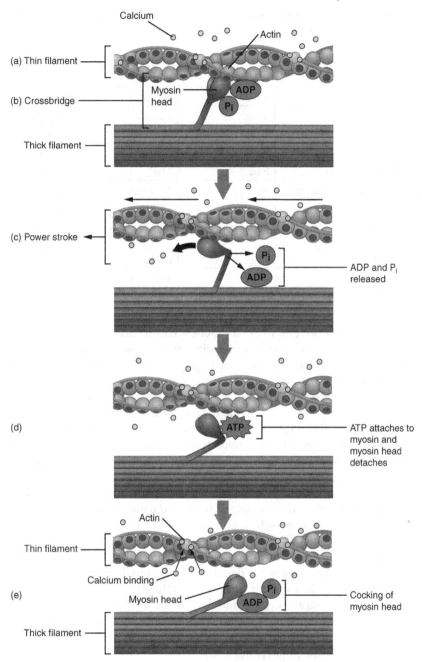

Figure 1.3 Skeletal Muscle Contraction (a) The active site on actin is exposed as calcium binds to troponin. (b) The myosin head is attracted to actin, and myosin binds actin at its actin-binding site, forming the cross-bridge. (c) During the power stroke, the phosphate generated in the previous contraction cycle is released. This results in the myosin head pivoting toward the center of the sarcomere, after which the attached ADP and phosphate group are released. (d) A new molecule of ATP attaches to the myosin head, causing the cross-bridge to detach. (e) The myosin head hydrolyzes ATP to ADP and phosphate, which returns the myosin to the cocked position.

Source: OpenStax https://cnx.org/contents/FPtK1zmh@8.25:fEI3C8Ot@10/Preface. Image converted to greyscale.

Table 1.4 A comparison of the physiological, neurological, and biomechanical properties of different skeletal muscle fibre types

Characteristic	Type I	Type IIa	Type IIx
Colour	Red	Red	White
Fibre size	Small	Medium	Large
Motor neuron size	Small	Large	Very large
Twitch velocity	Slow	Medium	Fast
Force production	Low	Medium	High
Phosphate resynthesis rate	Fast	Medium	Slow
Oxidative enzyme concentration	High	Medium	Low
Glycolytic enzyme concentration	Low	Medium	High
Major metabolic fuel source	Triacylglycerols	Phosphocreatine/ glycogen	Phosphocreatine/ glycogen
Mitochondrial density	High	High	Low
Capillary density	High	Medium	Low
Myoglobin content	High	Medium	Low

The different muscle fibre types play a practical role during exercise. When the external resistance is low, such as during low-intensity cardiorespiratory or resistance exercise, the body recruits predominantly slow-twitch (type I) skeletal muscle fibres, which are highly fatigue-resistant but have low force-generation characteristics. In contrast, high external loads, such as those encountered during maximal strength training, activate fast-twitch (type II) skeletal muscle fibres, which are more susceptible to fatigue but can generate higher forces (see Table 1.4 for a comparison between the physiological characteristics of the different skeletal muscle fibre types). Collectively, slow- and fast-twitch skeletal muscle fibres produce the movements required during an acute exercise bout.

Acute exercise may involve three different types of skeletal muscle actions: concentric, eccentric, and isometric. Concentric muscle actions involve the shortening of skeletal muscle fibres and occur when the contractile force of the muscle is greater than the resistance force, whereas eccentric muscle actions involve the lengthening of skeletal muscle fibres and occur when the contractile force is less than the resistive force. The skeletal muscle length remains constant during an isometric muscle action, which occurs when the contractile and resistive forces are equal. Exercises involving more eccentric muscle actions, such as walking downhill or plyometric training (e.g., bounding and hopping exercises) often result in more skeletal muscle damage 48–72 hours after exercise than exercise that involves predominantly concentric muscle actions (such as bicycling).

Prescribing physical activity and exercise

Due to the strong association between physical activity and health outcomes such as chronic disease and obesity, the World Health Organization has developed age-specific guidelines for physical activity[8] (Table 1.5). These guidelines are intended to help facilitate positive health outcomes for people of all ages.

Whether you are undertaking exercise for general health or to improve your competitive performance, when exercise sessions are repeated over multiple weeks and months chronic adaptations to exercise begin to occur. These chronic adaptations occur as a result of the specific loading and progression of exercise sessions and can be specific

Table 1.5 World Health Organization's physical activity guidelines

Group	Guideline
Children & Adolescents (5–17 years)	At least an average of 60 minutes of moderate-to-vigorous, mostly physical activity across the week On at least 3 days per week, vigorous-intensity aerobic activities as well as those that strengthen muscle and bone
Adults(18–64 years)	150–300 minutes of moderate physical activity or 75–150 minutes of vigorous physical activity per week At least 2–3 days per week of muscle-strength activities at moderate or greater intensity that involve all major muscle groups
Older Adults (65 years and older)	At least 150–300 minutes of moderate physical activity per week or at least 75–150 minutes of vigorous-intensity aerobic physical activity At least 2 days per week of muscle-strengthening activities at a moderate or greater intensity that involves all major muscle groups

Source: World Health Organisation Guidelines on Physical Activity and Sedentary Behaviour.[8]

Table 1.6 Example application of the FITT principle for targeted physiological adaptation

	Cardiovascular endurance	Muscular endurance	Muscular strength
Frequency (How often the exercise is performed)	3–5 times per week	3–5 times per week	3 times per week
Intensity (How hard the exercise is)	60–90% max heart rate	12+ repetitions, 2–4 sets	3–7 repetitions, 3–5 sets
Time (The duration of each individual exercise session)	>30 min	30–60 min	15–60 min
Type (The kind of activity completed)	Running Swimming Bicycling Walking	Free weights Circuit training Bodyweight exercises	Free weights Resistance machines

aerobic, anaerobic, or strength adaptations, depending on the goals of the individual. One of the simplest and most common methods to monitor and progress a training program is by using the FITT (frequency, intensity, time, and type) Principle. An example of how you may target different exercise goals using the FITT Principle is provided in Table 1.6. By changing one or more of the elements within the FITT Principle, one can continue to overload the body to promote adaptations.

Progressive overload

The continued incremental increase in training demand (duration or intensity) required to elicit an adaptive response.

It is important to adjust training loads as an individual progresses through an exercise program to ensure adequate training stress is applied; this is termed **progressive overload**. Following an initial exercise stimulus, the body is transiently fatigued due to acute changes, and subsequently recovers and adapts to that initial stimulus. This results in the body having a new baseline level of performance, which therefore requires a greater exercise stimulus to promote the next adaptation. If exercise is not followed by sufficient rest, it may result in the individual becoming over-trained. Conversely, if too much time follows between exercise bouts, the adaptations return to the initial baseline levels without further adaptation occurring. In this sense, the **periodisation** of training becomes important to ensure a sufficient balance between exercise stimulus and recovery.

Periodisation

The timing of exercise bouts to ensure sufficient exercise stimulus and recovery is provided to elicit the greatest response and adaptation.

Oxidation

Part of a chemical reaction that results in the loss of electrons. During fat oxidation, triglycerides are broken down into three fatty acid chains and glycerol.

Chronic adaptations to exercise

Adaptations that occur as a response to exercise are specific to the training stimulus applied and include changes to the cardiovascular, metabolic, respiratory, and muscular systems. Regular aerobic exercise, for example, enhances the ability of the body to use fat as fuel during exercise through increased transport of free fatty acids, fat **oxidation** and mitochondrial biogenesis (increase in the number and mass of mitochondria), and elicits the development of type I muscle fibres. These adaptations lead to an improved capacity to complete longer duration or higher intensity exercise while remaining within an aerobic state.

Exercise and prolonged training also stimulate the release of several hormones, including testosterone and growth hormone, which promote an **anabolic** effect on the body. These hormones increase protein synthesis and cell growth, leading to an increase in lean muscle mass and decreased fat mass. This chronic adaptation of an individual's body composition, which increases the amount of active tissue in the body, also leads to an increased metabolic rate for the individual. Growth hormone similarly stimulates cartilage formation and skeletal growth, encouraging bone formation. The mechanical loading of exercise, such as during foot strike while running, also elicits the remodelling of bone to adapt to the load under which it is placed; this is known as **Wolff's Law**. As is the case with all chronic adaptations to training, when the exercise stimulus is removed these adaptations revert to baseline levels.

Anabolic

An anabolic effect refers to the 'building up' and repair of tissues through increased protein synthesis and cell growth. It is the opposite of 'catabolism', which refers to the breakdown of molecules.

Wolff's Law

Bone in a healthy person will adapt to the loads under which it is placed. In this sense, an exercise stimulus results in bone remodelling that makes the bone stronger to resist that sort of loading.

Along with the more commonly discussed changes to our cardiovascular, metabolic, and muscular systems, exercise also affects our immune system. Following acute exercise, white blood cell numbers and activity decrease due to circulating hormones (catecholamines, growth hormone, cortisol, testosterone) and local inflammation. This acute-phase response can last from two to 72 hours post-exercise. The extent of these changes is influenced by the intensity and duration of exercise, with longer duration and higher intensity exercise eliciting a greater immunosuppressive response. As such, during the acute post-exercise phase individuals have a greater susceptibility to illness. However, when looking at chronic exercise involvement, there appears to be a J-shaped relationship between exercise and immune function. While sedentary behaviour or excessive exercise can result in immune dysfunction and a greater risk of illness, moderate amounts of regular exercise exert a protective effect on the immune system. Nutrition is also thought to play a role in maintaining immune function, through the adequate intake of specific micronutrients (e.g., iron, zinc, and vitamins A, E, and B_{12}) and sufficient carbohydrate availability during exercise bouts to help limit the rise in the stress hormone cortisol.

Recovering from exercise

Sufficient recovery is required following each bout of exercise (short-term recovery) and within each training block (long-term recovery) for the body to adequately adapt to the exercise stimulus. It is during this recovery period that the body replenishes energy stores and repairs damaged tissue to allow the body to develop and adapt in response to the stimulus. The simplest ways to recover from exercise are to have a rest day from training and to get good-quality sleep. Other common recovery methods include cold or contrast water immersion, compression garments, foam rolling, and massage. Nutrition plays a big part in the recovery process through the sufficient intake and timing of key macro- and micronutrients. The nutritional requirements during the recovery phase are dependent on the demands of the activity and so will vary between endurance and power-based sports. As an example, nutritional recovery strategies for endurance sports, such as a marathon, will focus on rehydration and the replenishment of carbohydrates, whereas power-based sports such as weightlifting will have a greater focus on increasing protein-building amino acids to assist in muscle repair and growth. More can be found about these requirements in Chapters 17 and 18.

Summary

This chapter has described the importance of physical activity for human health, the differences between physical activity, exercise, and sport, and physiological adaptations to sport and exercise. It has outlined the physiological responses to acute exercise, how exercise is measured and monitored, and the principles of exercise prescription to establish positive chronic adaptations in response to training. This chapter has high-lighted the importance of recovery to further promote these positive adaptations and avoid the risk of overtraining, injury, or illness and outlined how recovery can come in the form of appropriate prescription of rest, specific recovery interventions, and recovery nutrition strategies.

Chapter highlights

- Physical activity is vital for health and wellbeing, and daily physical activity levels can be maximised through participation in intentional exercise and recreational or com-petitive sports.
- The purpose of exercise is to improve or maintain:
  - aerobic and anaerobic capacity;
  - muscular endurance, strength, and power;
  - body composition;
  - flexibility;
  - balance.
- Exercise prescription involves the manipulation of frequency, intensity, time, and type of exercise.
- Metabolic equivalents (METs) are used to describe the amount of work performed during exercise based on the amount of oxygen consumed relative to rest. The energy expended can be expressed using kilojoules (kJ) or kilocalories (kcal).
- The intensity of exercise can be estimated using heart rate or rating of perceived exer-tion (RPE).
- The body responds to cardiorespiratory exercise by increasing the blood flow to the muscle, increasing the volume of air inhaled, and increasing the amount of oxygen delivered from the blood to the working muscles.
- The body responds to musculoskeletal exercise by increasing the temperature and enzyme activity within the muscle, and by recruiting more muscle fibres.
- Chronic adaptations that occur as a response to exercise are specific to the training stimulus applied and include changes to the cardiovascular, metabolic, respiratory, and muscular systems.
- Rest is important to avoid overtraining, promote recovery, and minimise the risk of injury and illness.
- Immune function is affected by exercise volume and intensity, with moderate amounts of exercise having a protective effect on the immune system.

References

1. Global Association of International Sports Federations. Definition of sport. SportAccord; 2012. Available from: https://web.archive.org/web/20121205004927/http://www.sportaccord.com/en/members/definition-of-sport
2. Eady J. *Practical sports development*. London: Pearson Professional Education; 1993.
3. Gellish RL, Goslin BR, Olson, RE. Longitudinal modelling of the relationship between age and maximal heart rate. *Med Sci Sports Exerc*. 2007;39(5):822–829.
4. Karvonen MJ. The effects of training on heart rate: A longitudinal study. *Ann Med Exp Biol Fenn*. 1957;35(3):307–315.

5. Borg GA. Psychophysical bases of perceived exertion. *Med Sci Sports Exerc.* 1982;14(5):377–381.
6. Foster C, Florhaug, JA, Franklin J. A new approach to monitoring exercise training. *J Strength Cond Res.* 2001;15(1):109–115.
7. American College of Sports Medicine. *ACSM's guidelines for exercise testing and prescription.* 11th ed. Philadelphia: Lippincott Williams & Wilkins; 2022.
8. World Health Organization. *WHO guidelines on physical activity and sedentary behaviour.* Geneva: World Health Organization; 2020. Available from: https://www.who.int/publications/i/item/9789240015128

2 Energy for sport and exercise

Matthew Cooke and Sam SX Wu

The human body requires a constant supply of energy to fuel working organs, including the brain, heart, lungs and muscles. The major energy currency within the human body is an energy-rich molecule known as adenosine triphosphate, or ATP. This chapter will explore how ATP is produced and the factors that impact how much is needed. Methods used to estimate energy expenditure and calculate individual energy requirements will be described. Finally, the chapter will conclude with a focus on recovery from sport and exercise.

Learning outcomes

This chapter will:

- define and describe the association between 'energy', 'power' and 'work' and explain their relationship with exercise intensity and duration of exercise and sporting events;
- compare and contrast the relative contributions of energy systems in relation to exercise intensity, duration and modality;
- discuss methods used to assess energy expenditure and determine the daily energy requirements of an individual;
- explain the interplay between energy systems that allows physical exercise to occur, as well as those systems' contribution to recovery.

At rest, the demand for ATP is low; however, sport and exercise can increase this demand as much as a thousandfold, requiring a coordinated metabolic response by the energy systems to replenish ATP levels. The contribution of each energy system is determined by the interaction between the intensity and the duration of exercise and is regulated by metabolic processes and the **central nervous system.**

Central nervous system

Consists of the brain and the spinal cord, and is responsible for receiving, processing, and responding to sensory information.

DOI: 10.4324/9781003321286-3

Table 2.1 Adaptations from aerobic and anaerobic resistance training

Aerobic training	Anaerobic resistance training
Increases in:	Increases in:
• Aerobic power output	• Anaerobic power output
• Muscular endurance at prolonged submaximal intensities	• Muscular endurance at high power outputs
• Capillary density	• Strength production
• Mitochondrial density and size	• Muscle fibre size
• Proportion of Type I muscle fibres	• Proportion of Type II muscle fibres
• Aerobic enzymes	• Anaerobic substrates

The relationship between energy, work and power

Energy exists in many different forms. Although there are many specific types of energy, the two major forms are kinetic energy and potential energy. Kinetic energy is the energy in moving objects or mass, such as mechanical energy and electrical energy. Potential energy is any form of energy that has stored potential and can be put to future use such as nuclear energy and chemical energy (ATP). With exercise, energy is the capacity to do work and is calculated as follows:

$$\text{Work done}\left(\text{Newton}\cdot\text{metres}\left[\text{N}\cdot\text{m}\right]\text{ or Joules}\left[\text{J}\right]\right) = \text{Force}\left(\text{N}\right) \times \text{Distance}\left(\text{m}\right)$$

Work done, measured in **Newton metres** or **Joules** is calculated as force multiplied by distance. For example, the greater the force required to move an object, or the further the distance of the object to be moved, the greater the work done. Power, also known as work rate, is the amount of work done over time:

$$\text{Power}\left(\text{Watts}\left[\text{W}\right]\right) = \text{Work done}\left(\text{J}\right) \div \text{Time}\left(\text{s}\right)$$

Therefore, the faster the rate at which work is completed, the higher the power output. With sufficient training, athletes can develop physiological adaptations that allow them to perform a larger amount of work in a short period of time, thus generating higher power outputs (see Table 2.1). Power output is often used in sports such as cycling and rowing to quantify training loads or as a measure of exercise performance. It is not uncommon for professional riders in the Tour de France to produce more than 1600 watts in the final sprint and reach 75 km/h after two weeks of gruelling cycling over the French Alps and having just completed 200 kilometres immediately prior to the sprint!

Energy in the human body

Chemical energy is a form of potential energy that is stored in the bonds of atoms and molecules. Within the body, the major energy currency is the ATP molecule, which comprises three components: An adenine ring (as part of adenosine), ribose sugar and three phosphate groups (triphosphate) (Figure 2.1).

Carbohydrates, protein, fats and alcohol (discussed in more detail in Chapter 4) are sources of energy in the diet. Under normal circumstances, more than 95 per cent of this food energy is digested and absorbed from the gastrointestinal tract, providing the body with its chemical energy needs (see Chapter 3 for more detail on digestion and absorption).

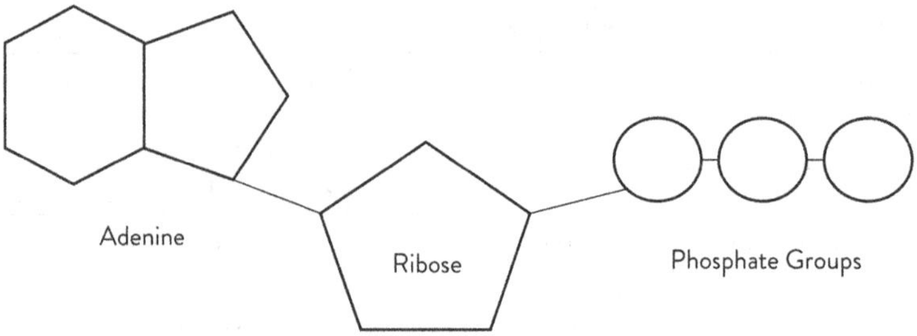

Figure 2.1 An ATP molecule.

In the presence of water, ATP can be broken down to form adenosine diphosphate (ADP). This process is known as **hydrolysis**. Living cells contain ten times more ATP than ADP. When ATP is hydrolysed to ADP, a large amount of energy is released. The release of this free energy from the high-energy bonds is used to drive energy-requiring reactions such as protein synthesis.

Hydrolysis

The breakdown of a compound by chemical reaction with water.

Catabolic reactions

Biochemical reactions that result in the breakdown of large molecules and give off energy in the form of ATP.

Anabolic reactions

Small molecules join to form a larger molecule in the presence of energy (ATP).

Reactions within a cell can be classed as either catabolic or anabolic. **Catabolic reactions** involve breaking molecules down into their smaller components; energy is released as a by-product of these reactions. **Anabolic reactions** involve combining simple molecules to form complex molecules, and energy in the form of ATP is required to support these reactions. Energy-yielding reactions (catabolic) within a cell are typically coupled to energy-requiring reactions (anabolic). The high-energy bonds of ATP thus play a central role in cell metabolism by serving as a usable storage form of free energy.

Production of energy: The role of metabolic pathways

Given the importance of energy, especially chemical energy in the form of ATP, it is not surprising that the human body has a number of important metabolic pathways to ensure its ATP levels remain relatively constant. A metabolic pathway is a linked series of **enzyme**-mediated biochemical reactions occurring within a cell.

Enzymes

Proteins that start or speed up a chemical reaction while undergoing no permanent change to their structure. Enzymes perform this function by lowering the minimum energy required (activation energy) to start a chemical reaction. Enzymes are involved in most biochemical reactions; without them, most organisms could not survive.

Cytoplasm

The semifluid substance contained within a cell.

The three main metabolic pathways for ATP resynthesis (Figure 2.2) are: (a) the phosphagen system (ATP-PCr, alactacid), (b) anaerobic glycolysis (lactic acid) and (c) oxidative phosphorylation (mitochondrial ATP production). Both the phosphagen system and glycolysis pathway occur in the **cytoplasm** (cytosol) of the cell. Oxidative phosphorylation occurs within the mitochondria. Mitochondria are known as the powerhouses of the cell. They are organelles that act like a digestive system to take in nutrients, break them down and create energy-rich molecules for the cell.

The phosphagen system

The phosphagen system is the quickest way to resynthesise ATP, and comprises three reactions (Table 2.2). Phosphocreatine (PCr) donates a phosphate to ADP to produce ATP. Despite its ability to rapidly resynthesise ATP, the total capacity of this high-energy

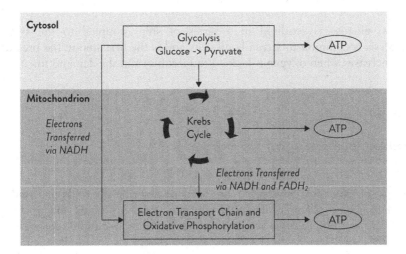

Figure 2.2 Metabolic pathways involved in ATP resynthesis.

Table 2.2 Three reactions of the phosphagen system

Reactants	Products	Enzymes Used
ATP + Water (H_2O)	ADP + Pi + Energy	ATPase
PCr + ADP	ATP + Cr	Creatine kinase
ADP+ADP	ATP + AMP	Adenylate kinase

Note: ATP: Adenosine triphosphate; ADP: Adenosine diphosphate: AMP: Adenosine monophosphate; Pi: Inorganic phosphate; PCr: Phosphocreatine; Cr: Creatine.

phosphate system to sustain maximal muscle contraction is about 4 seconds, assuming complete depletion of PCr and ATP. With this in mind, **creatine supplementation** has been investigated over the past few decades as a way to enhance exercise performance. Creatine supplementation can increase total creatine, specifically, PCr levels stored in the muscle, and thus enhance the rephosphorylation of ADP to ATP. Numerous studies have shown the benefits of creatine supplementation on exercise performance, especially that involving short-burst, high-intensity power-type movements, such as power lifting.[1] Creatine supplementation is discussed in more detail in Chapter 12.

Creatine supplementation

Supplementation with synthetic creatine can augment the level of creatine in the body and lead to enhanced performance of power activities.

Glycolysis

A major source of cellular energy comes from the breakdown of carbohydrates, particularly glucose. The complete oxidative breakdown of glucose to carbon dioxide (CO_2) and water (H_2O) is written as follows:

$$C_6H_{12} + 6O_2 \rightarrow 6CO_2 + 6H_2O$$

Within cells, glucose is oxidised in a series of steps coupled to the synthesis of ATP. **Glycolysis** is common to virtually all cells and is the first step in the breakdown of glucose. It increases when oxygen is lacking (anaerobic) and the demand for ATP is high.

Glycolysis

The breakdown of glucose to form two molecules of ATP.

The terms 'aerobic' and 'anaerobic' are used to describe the different conditions by which oxidation of food molecules especially glucose, fatty acids and proteins occur (known as respiration). Aerobic respiration occurs when adequate oxygen is present,

Box 2.1   Did you know? Aerobic vs anaerobic glycolysis

Before the 1980s, scholars and researchers referred to the complete oxidation of carbohydrates as 'aerobic glycolysis', as opposed to 'anaerobic glycolysis', which is often referred to now when pyruvate is converted to lactate (a temporary product formed when pyruvate combines with a hydrogen ion, H^+). The difference in terminology was based on the assumption that the extent of cell oxygenation was the primary determining factor for the complete oxidation of pyruvate via mitochondrial respiration or the production of lactate. This is inconsistent with the biochemistry of glycolysis. It is now understood that if the intensity of the exercise is high enough, lactate is produced regardless of normal oxygenation, or even hyper-oxygenation such as with the breathing of pure oxygen. Terms—'lactic glycolysis' versus 'alactacid glycolysis' for intense and steady-state exercise conditions, respectively—have been proposed as being more biochemically representative.[2]

anaerobic respiration occurs when a lack of oxygen is present and the demand for ATP is high. See Box 2.1 for more information.

Anaerobic glycolysis involves a series of ten steps (see Figure 2.2) that utilise glucose, either circulating in the blood or from the stored form of glycogen, to produce two ATP molecules, pyruvate and reduced coenzyme NADH. Glycolysis also produces **lactic acid**, predominantly during exercise performed at high intensities (see Chapter 1 for more information about lactic acid and buffering). Although the production of lactic acid will contribute to the local fatigue of the muscle, it is the only metabolic pathway that can keep up with the high demand for ATP resynthesis and, thus, allow the muscle to continue contracting at high intensities. The total capacity of anaerobic glycolysis to sustain maximal contractions is approximately 30 seconds.

When adequate oxygen is present (aerobic), pyruvate (the end-product of glycolysis) undergoes decarboxylation (a chemical reaction that removes a carboxyl group and releases CO_2) in the presence of **coenzyme** A (CoA) to produce acetyl CoA.

Acetyl CoA then enters the **Krebs cycle** (also known as the citric acid cycle or TCA cycle), which is the central pathway in oxidative metabolism and the first stage in cellular respiration (Figure 2.2).

Lactic acid

A by-product of anaerobic glycolysis that contributes to fatigue of the muscle.

Coenzyme

A substance that works with an enzyme to initiate or assist the function of the enzyme. It may be considered a helper molecule for a biochemical reaction.

Krebs cycle

A series of biochemical reactions that generate energy from the breakdown of pyruvate (the end-product of glycolysis).

Cellular Respiration

The Krebs cycle, in conjunction with oxidative phosphorylation, provides the vast majority (more than 95 per cent) of energy used by aerobic cells in humans. The Krebs cycle is a series of eight reactions that break down pyruvate to produce reduced coenzymes $NADH^+ + H^+$ and $FADH_2$, carbon dioxide and guanosine triphosphate (GTP), a high-energy molecule (Figure 2.2).

Electron transport chain

Electrons are passed through a series of proteins and molecules in the mitochondria to generate large amounts of ATP.

Cellular respiration

A series of metabolic reactions within the cell that generate energy (ATP) from nutrients.

Electron

Negatively charged subatomic particles.

Oxidative phosphorylation

The **electron transport chain** (ETC) is the next step in the breakdown of glucose and the final step in **cellular respiration**. Requiring oxygen to function, reduced coenzymes from the Krebs cycle and glycolysis are re-oxidised with their **electrons** transferred through the ETC to produce large amounts of ATP (Figure 2.2). Mitochondrial oxidative phosphorylation is the only source of ATP production that has the capacity to support prolonged exercise.

The total yield from the complete oxidation of a glucose molecule is 38 molecules of ATP. This comes from:

- a net gain of two ATP molecules from glycolysis;
- an additional two molecules from the conversion of pyruvate to acetyl CoA and subsequent metabolism via the Krebs (citric acid) cycle;
- the assumption that the oxidation of the reduced coenzymes, $NADH+ + H+$ and $FADH_2$, will produce three and two molecules of ATP, respectively.

Both glycolysis and the Krebs cycle give rise to ten molecules of NADH$^+$ + H$^+$ and two molecules of FADH$_2$ combined. In the case where two molecules of NADH$^+$ + H$^+$ produced by glycolysis are unable to enter mitochondria directly from the cytosol, the total yield is 36. The pathways involved in glucose degradation also play a central role in the breakdown of other organic molecules (discussed further in Chapter 4), such as nucleotides, amino acids and fatty acids, to form ATP.

Interaction among metabolic energy systems: Influence of sport and exercise

The interaction and relative contribution of the three energy systems during different exercise intensities and sporting activities have been of considerable interest to exercise scientists and biochemists. The first attempts to understand these interactions appeared in the literature in the 1960s and 1970s, using incremental exercise and periods of maximal exhaustive exercise. Although energy systems respond differently in relation to the diverse energy demands placed on them during daily and sporting activities, we now know that virtually all physical activities derive some energy from each of the three energy-supplying processes. With this in mind, the energy system most suited (dependent on the energy demands of the exercise) will contribute sequentially, but in an overlapping fashion, to provide energy (see Table 2.3 for examples of which energy system is best suited for various sporting activities).

Table 2.3 Energy systems used to support select sporting activities

Phosphagen (ATP-PCr, alactacid) system	*Anaerobic glycolysis (lactic acid) system*	*Oxidative phosphorylation (mitochondrial ATP production)*
Sprinting—performance is determined predominantly by the capacity of the ATP-PCr system because of the short distance covered. However, events longer than 100 m would require greater input from anaerobic glycolysis.	Swimming—performance is determined predominantly by the capacity of the ATP-PCr and glycolytic system because of the short distance covered. However, events such as the 1500 m would require input from oxidative phosphorylation.	Marathon running—although all energy systems would be activated, performance is determined predominantly by the capacity of oxidative phosphorylation, with input from anaerobic glycolysis during periods of sprinting.
Golf—given the explosive nature of the sport (i.e., club swing), performance is determined predominantly by the capacity of the ATP-PCr system.	Fencing—performance is determined predominantly by the capacity of the ATP-PCr and glycolytic system because of the numerous short, powerful bursts that last around 5–10 seconds.	Basketball—basketball games typically last about 50 minutes, which means performance is determined predominantly by the capacity of oxidative phosphorylation. However, the game also requires short bursts of explosive power and thus would need input from the ATP-PCr and glycolytic systems.

Compare the demands of a 100-metre sprint to a 42.2-kilometre marathon. The sprint is fast, with minimal oxygen breathed in during its 10-second duration, making the event almost exclusively anaerobic.[3] The marathon, on the other hand, is primarily an aerobic event completed in two to two-and-a-half hours at 80–85 per cent of an elite athlete's maximal capacity.[3] Despite the different demands of each event, all systems are activated at the start of exercise to maintain ATP levels and ensure adequate supply for maximal power output and intensity. The anaerobic (non-mitochondrial) systems, which are capable of supporting extremely high muscle force application and power outputs such as those during a 100-metre sprint, would be the predominant energy system used at these times. During a marathon race, the anaerobic system, which is limited in its capacity, is unable to meet the energy demands required by extended periods of intense exercise. The aerobic energy system (oxidative metabolism) is the only system that can resynthesise ATP at a rate that can maintain the required power and work output needed during the race. The aerobic system also plays a significant role in performance during high-intensity exercise, with a maximal exercise effort of 75 seconds deriving approximately equal energy from the aerobic and anaerobic energy systems.[2]

Quantifying energy expenditure: Applications in sport and exercise

Regardless of which energy system predominates during exercise, all energy systems contribute to the supply of energy and thus have important implications for performance and recovery. Measurement of an athlete's energy expenditure helps determine the daily energy requirements for the athlete's training and competition, to inform dietary requirements to help them achieve body composition and performance goals. For example, a power lifter training to increase muscle mass would aim to consume more energy than is expended to increase his body mass. Alternatively, a boxer attempting to lose weight would aim to consume less energy than he expends. Of course, the composition of the diet can also impact performance and body composition, as will be discussed in detail in other chapters.

So, how is energy expenditure measured? The rate of energy metabolism is directly proportional to the amount of heat the whole body produces. As such, the rate of metabolism can be quantified by measuring heat produced by the body. This direct measurement method is known as **direct calorimetry**. This relationship is represented in Figure 2.3.

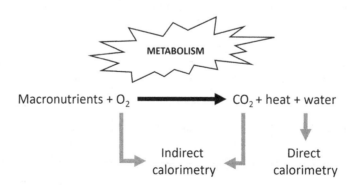

Figure 2.3 Aerobic metabolism pathway for macronutrients.

Direct calorimetry

A direct measure of heat transfer to determine energy expenditure.

Direct calorimetry requires a person to be placed in an insulated chamber, which allows all heat production within the chamber to be measured. Although this method is highly accurate, building a calorimeter is expensive and requires a lot of space in a laboratory. Furthermore, heat that is produced by the exercise equipment when in use may complicate measurements. Therefore, a cheaper and smaller—but still accurate—method known as **indirect calorimetry** is more widely used for measuring energy expenditure. The most common approach to measuring oxygen consumption is open-circuit spirometry. This involves collecting all exhaled gases into a mixing chamber, which is then processed and analysed by a metabolic cart (Figure 2.4). The metabolic cart analyses oxygen (O_2) consumed and carbon dioxide (CO_2) produced to calculate metabolic rate. Metabolic rate can be determined during rest (resting metabolic rate, RMR) or during submaximal or maximal intensity exercise. The maximal amount of oxygen that can be used by the body during high-intensity exercise is termed maximal aerobic capacity (VO_2max), and is commonly used as an indicator of cardiorespiratory fitness (see Chapter 1 for more information about VO_2max and cardiorespiratory fitness).

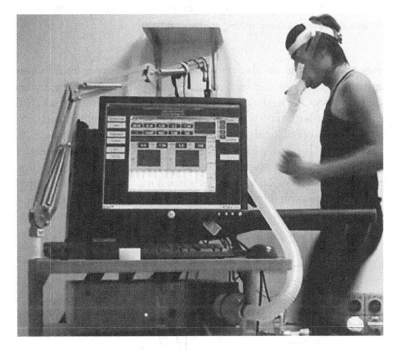

Figure 2.4 Indirect calorimetry using a mouthpiece connected to a metabolic cart.
Photo courtesy of Sam Wu

Indirect calorimetry

A method of estimating energy expenditure by measuring oxygen consumption and carbohydrate production.

CO_2 produced and O_2 consumed can also be expressed as a ratio (CO_2/O_2) to obtain a number that is normally between 0.7 and 1.0. This number is known as the **respiratory exchange ratio** (RER) and represents the composition of the mixture of lipids (fats) and carbohydrates oxidised through metabolism during submaximal exercise.[4] These estimations are based on knowledge of the exact amount of energy produced when metabolising carbohydrates, lipids and proteins with oxygen. Different types of macronutrients produce slightly different amounts of energy per litre of O_2 consumed (Table 2.4). However, as protein normally contributes negligible energy to exercise during aerobic exercise of less than two hours, a release of 4.82 kcal/L O_2 has been observed when burning a mixed macronutrient combination.[5] For ease of calculation, 5 kcal of energy per litre of O_2 is generally used to calculate energy expenditure during aerobic physical activity. Therefore, a person utilising 3 L/min of oxygen during a run would be expending approximately 15 kcal of energy each minute.

Respiratory exchange ratio

The ratio of carbon dioxide produced to oxygen consumed; used to indicate the relative contribution of substrates oxidised during submaximal exercise.

Ideally, tests to determine aerobic capacity and energy expenditure should be conducted in a controlled environment such as a laboratory to ensure accuracy and precision of results. Equipment specific to the athlete's sport, such as treadmills, bicycle ergometers, rowing machines and cross-country skis, is commonly used to maximise the relevance of results to the field. However, field tests are sometimes more appropriate, feasible and cheaper to conduct. Such tests, which are **maximally exhaustive** in nature, include the multistage shuttle run test (also known as the beep test), the yo-yo endurance test or the 2.4-kilometre run test (see Box 2.2). At times when a maximal test is not appropriate due to the possible risks of maximal exhaustion, a health or fitness professional may choose to administer a submaximal test. A submaximal test requires a lower intensity of exercise

Table 2.4 Energy produced per litre of O_2 when metabolising different macronutrients

Macronutrient	kcal/LO_2
Carbohydrate	5.05
Fat	4.69
Protein	4.49

Note: 1 kcal = 4.186 kj.
Source: Anonymous.[6]

and therefore is associated with a lower medical risk. Physiological data acquired during a submaximal test (commonly heart rate, blood pressure and ratings of perceived exertion) are then used to calculate and estimate the individual's maximal capacity.

Maximally exhaustive

Exercise that requires the participant to work at their maximal capacity until exhaustion.

Recovery from sport and exercise

During exercise, oxygen consumption increases to meet demands based on exercise intensity. Upon cessation of exercise, the increased oxygen consumption does not immediately return to pre-exercise levels but gradually returns to baseline. This recovery period is known as **excess post-exercise oxygen consumption** (EPOC). Previously termed oxygen debt, it was hypothesised that the increased oxygen uptake post-exercise was to repay the oxygen deficit created at the beginning of exercise when energy production was not sufficient to meet a sudden increase in energy demands.

Excess post-exercise oxygen consumption

An increased rate of oxygen consumption following high-intensity activity.

Box 2.2   Maximal tests of aerobic capacity and energy expenditure

The **multistage shuttle run** test, or beep test, requires participants to run repeats of 20 metres at increasing speeds every minute.

The **yo-yo endurance test** is a variation of the multistage shuttle run test with a higher initial running speed and different increments in speed.

The **2.4-kilometre run test, or Cooper 1.5-mile test**, involves running 2.4 kilometres on a hard, flat surface in the shortest time possible. VO_2max is calculated as (483/time in minutes) + 3.5.

Box 2.3   Estimating daily energy requirements

The daily energy expenditure for healthy adults can be calculated using a variety of equations and two commonly used examples are presented below. They are suitable for use with adults 19–78 years of age, but it is important to keep in mind that factors such as climate, body composition and surface area of the body can also influence resting energy expenditure.

Mifflin-St Jeor[7]

$$\text{For females : resting energy expenditure}\left(\frac{\text{kcal}}{\text{day}}\right) = 9.99 \times \left(\text{weight in kg}\right)$$
$$+ 6.25 \times \left(\text{height in cm}\right) - 4.92 \times \text{age in years} - 161$$

$$\text{For males : resting energy expenditure}\left(\frac{\text{kcal}}{\text{day}}\right) = 9.99 \times \left(\text{weight in kg}\right)$$
$$+ 6.25 \times \left(\text{height in cm}\right) - 4.92 \times \text{age in years} + 5$$

Harris Benedict[8]

$$\text{For females : resting energy expenditure}\left(\frac{\text{kcal}}{\text{day}}\right) = 447.593$$
$$+ \left(9.247 \times \text{weight in kg}\right) + \left(3.098 \times \text{height in cm}\right) - \left(4.330 \times \text{age in years}\right)$$

$$\text{For males : resting energy expenditure}\left(\frac{\text{kcal}}{\text{day}}\right) = 88.362$$
$$+ \left(13.397 \times \text{weight in kg}\right) + \left(4.799 \times \text{height in cm}\right) - \left(5.677 \times \text{age in years}\right)$$

Resting energy expenditure calculated from the above equations can be multiplied by a factor according to the individual's physical activity level (PAL) for an estimated total daily energy expenditure. These factors are defined as:

1.0–1.39:	Sedentary, activities of daily living, sitting in office
1.4–1.59:	Activities of daily living plus 30–60 minutes of light-intensity activity (e.g., walking)
1.6–1.89:	Activities of daily living plus standing, carrying light loads, 60 minutes of walking
1.9–2.5:	Activities of daily living plus strenuous work or highly active/athletic lifestyle.[9]

It is important to acknowledge that there is no clear classification for athletes of various fitness levels and training intensities. Therefore, using indirect or direct calorimetry should be encouraged for an accurate measurement of total daily energy expenditure.

The energy required for EPOC is supplied primarily by oxidative pathways and is required to return the body to its resting, dynamically balanced level of metabolism (**homeostasis**). EPOC can be divided into two portions: a rapid component and a slow component. The metabolic processes that contribute to the rapid component of EPOC include increased body temperature, circulation, ventilation, replenishment of O_2 in blood and muscle, resynthesis of ATP and PCr, and **lactate shuttling**. The underlying mechanisms of the slow component of EPOC are much less understood. Apart from a sustained elevation of circulation, ventilation and body temperature, the slow component has been attributed to the storage of fatty acids as **triglycerides**, and a shift of substrate use from carbohydrates to lipids. The duration of EPOC depends on various factors, the most important being exercise intensity and duration. Short-duration and low-intensity exercise has been shown to produce short-lasting EPOCs, while high-intensity exercise clearly elicits a more substantial and prolonged EPOC lasting several hours.[9] Several hormones released during physical activity also contribute to EPOC and would gradually return to baseline levels.[10]

Homeostasis

Processes used by living organisms to maintain steady conditions needed for survival.

Lactate shuttling

Lactate produced at sites of high glycolysis can be shuttled (moved) to other muscles where it can be used as an energy source.

Triglycerides

The main type of fat in human bodies and diets. They are made up of a glycerol backbone with three fatty acids attached.

Summary

This chapter has described how energy systems provide the human body with a continual supply of chemical energy in the form of ATP. Exercise increases the demands for this energy, but it is the intensity and duration of the exercise that ultimately determines the use of ATP and the fuel sources required for its resynthesis. Energy systems (phosphagen system, anaerobic glycolysis, and oxidative phosphorylation) alone or in combination contribute to the resynthesis of ATP during and following exercise and thus have important implications for performance and recovery. Finally, measurement of an individual's energy expenditure via direct or indirect methods helps determine their daily energy requirements for body composition, training and competition goals, and informs exercise programming for optimal performance.

Chapter highlights

- The two major forms of energy are kinetic energy and potential energy. Energy is the capacity to perform work and power is the rate of work completed.
- Chemical energy within the bonds of a fuel source can be extracted via a series of complex reactions specific to one of three energy systems: the phosphagen system

(ATP-PCr, alactacid), anaerobic glycolysis (lactic acid) and oxidative phosphorylation (mitochondrial ATP production).

- The phosphagen system is the quickest of the energy systems, with the capacity to resynthesise ATP for up to 6–10 seconds. It is predominantly used during very short, explosive movements.
- Anaerobic glycolysis is the second fastest, with the capacity to resynthesise ATP for up to 30–60 seconds. It is predominantly used in short-duration, high-intensity 'speed' events such as the 400-metre track sprint.
- The aerobic energy system has the slowest rate of ATP resynthesis. Its advantage over the anaerobic energy systems is that it has a much larger capacity and is able to supply energy for hours rather than seconds.
- All activities require an energy contribution from at least two energy systems. Under maximal-effort conditions, all three systems are activated at the beginning of exercise, but one energy system will predominate.
- Metabolic rate and energy expenditure can be assessed by determining heat production from the body or by measuring an individual's oxygen consumption and carbon dioxide production for a given period.
- EPOC is necessary to return the body to a dynamically balanced resting state and is influenced mainly by exercise intensity and duration.

References

1. Cooper R, Naclerio F, Allgrove J. Creatine supplementation with specific view to exercise/sports performance: An update. *J Int Soc Sports Nutr.* 2012;9(1):33.
2. Baker JS, McCormick MC, Robergs RA. Interaction among skeletal muscle metabolic energy systems during intense exercise. *J Nutr Metab.* 2010;2010:905612.
3. Newsholme EA, Leech AR, Duester G. *Keep on running: The science of training and performance.* Chichester, UK: John Wiley & Sons; 1994.
4. Peronnet F, Massicotte D. Table of nonprotein respiratory quotient: An update. *Can J Sport Science.* 1991;16(1):23–29.
5. Lemon P, Nagle F. Effects of exercise on protein and amino acid metabolism. *Med Sci Sports Exerc.* 1981;13(3):141–149.
6. Anonymous. Method of calculating the energy metabolism. *Acta Pædiatrica.* 1952;41:67–76.
7. Mifflin MD, St Jeor ST, Hill LA. A new predictive equation for resting energy expenditure in healthy individuals. *Am J Clin Nutr.* 1990;51(2):241–247.
8. Roza AM, Shizgal HM. The Harris Benedict equation reevaluated: resting energy requirements and the body cell mass. *Am J Clin Nutr.* 1984;40(1):168–182.
9. Kerksick CM, Kulovitz M. Requirements of energy, carbohydrates, proteins and fats for athletes. In: Bagchi D, Nair S, Sen CK, editors. *Nutrition and enhanced sports performance.* Amsterdam: Elsevier; 2014, pp. 355–356.
10. Borsheim E, Bahr R. Effect of exercise intensity, duration and mode on post-exercise oxygen consumption. *Sports Med.* 2003;33(14):1037–1060.

3   Digestion and absorption

Annie-Claude M Lassemillante and Sam SX Wu

The present understanding of digestion began in 1822 when William Beaumont studied how food was digested by inserting and removing food from the stomach of Alexis St Martin, who had a hole in his stomach as a result of a shooting accident. This chapter will describe the various processes involved in digestion and explore current knowledge on the impact of exercise on digestion and absorption and emerging evidence on training the gut.

Learning outcomes

This chapter will:

- describe the role of the digestive tract, including accessory organs such as the liver, pancreas and gall bladder, in the digestion and absorption of nutrients;
- identify and explain the role of key digestive enzymes and secretions in the digestion of nutrients;
- explain how normal digestion and absorption processes are impacted by exercise.

Digestion

Digestion is the process by which the body breaks down food into nutrients, which are essential for normal bodily functions. Digestion begins at the mouth, where food enters the body, and ends at the anus, where waste and undigested products leave the body.

During digestion, food is broken down mechanically and chemically. Mechanical processing involves breaking food into smaller pieces and mixing it with digestive secretions. Such breakdown includes chewing, opening and closure of **sphincters**, churning action of the stomach, **peristalsis** and **segmentation**. Chemical digestion involves the breakdown of **macromolecules** by enzymes to form smaller molecules such as glucose, amino acids and fatty acids. These smaller molecules are then absorbed through the gastrointestinal lining and transported to the liver to be metabolised and redistributed to other parts of the body (see Figure 3.1 for anatomy of the digestive tract).

Sphincters

Muscular rings that open or close to control the passage of food along the digestive tract.

DOI: 10.4324/9781003321286-4

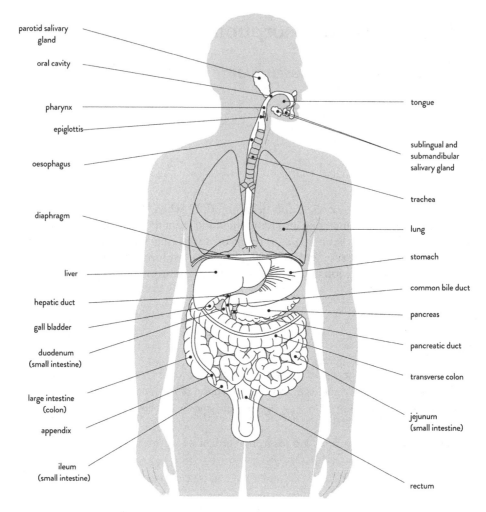

Figure 3.1 Components of the digestive tract and accessory organs.
Source: Hodgson, pp. 312–27.[1]

Peristalsis

The wave-like contractions of the longitudinal muscles of the digestive tract that propel food forward.

Segmentation

The contraction of the circular muscles of the digestive tract that leads to the mixing and breaking up of food.

Macromolecules

Proteins (polypeptides), digestible carbohydrates and fats (triglycerides) digested by humans.

Bolus

A portion, with respect to food, that is swallowed at one time.

Salivary amylase (or α amylase)

An enzyme in the saliva that breaks down amylose, a type of carbohydrate.

Lingual lipase

An enzyme secreted by the tongue that breaks down triglycerides, a type of fat.

Trachea

The tube leading to the lungs, more commonly known as the windpipe.

Mouth: The starting point of digestion

While digestion begins in the mouth, food is primarily broken down mechanically at this stage, with some chemical digestion of carbohydrates and fats (used mostly by infants as they suck on foods such as biscuits and rusks).

Chewing is the first stage of digestion, where the teeth and strong muscles of the jaw break food down into smaller pieces, thus increasing the surface area of the food exposed to digestive secretions. The tongue moves food around the mouth, mixing it with saliva that moistens and coats the food for easy movement down the oesophagus upon swallowing. The chewed food mixed with saliva is called the **bolus**.

Saliva is produced by the salivary glands and contains mucus, salts, water and digestive enzymes, namely salivary amylase (or α amylase) and lingual lipase. **Salivary amylase** begins the breakdown of specific bonds in starch molecules to produce maltose; however, this is only a small part of carbohydrate digestion. **Lingual lipase** begins the digestion of fats and is present in higher concentrations in the saliva of babies; its activity reduces with age due to reduced reliance on milk (and its fat content) for energy production and other physiological functions.

Oesophagus: Connecting the mouth to the stomach

The oesophagus connects the mouth to the stomach, with sphincters at both ends. Upon swallowing, the oesophageal sphincter opens, allowing the bolus of food to travel along the oesophagus. Peristalsis is responsible for the movement of food along this tube, allowing the bolus to reach the stomach even if the person swallowing is upside down. The respiratory tract and digestive tract share the pharynx (between mouth and oesophagus); a small flap, called the epiglottis, closes during swallowing to prevent food from entering the **trachea**.

At the stomach end of the oesophagus, the gastro-oesophageal sphincter opens for the bolus of food to enter the stomach. This sphincter also prevents the contents of the stomach from travelling up the oesophagus, hence protecting the oesophagus from the strong digestive secretions (hydrochloric acid) of the stomach. Gastro-oesophageal reflux disorder (GORD) is a condition in which this sphincter does not close properly for various reasons (for example, infection, long-term induced vomiting, pressure) resulting in a burning sensation caused by hydrochloric acid irritating the oesophageal lining.

Chyme

The mass of partially digested food that leaves the stomach and enters the duodenum.

Emulsification of fat

Involves the formation of smaller fat droplets suspended in the aqueous digestive juices. This process increases the surface area of fat for more efficient digestion.

Intrinsic factor

A glycoprotein produced in the gastric pits that binds with vitamin B12 to help in the absorption of vitamin B12.

Pepsinogen

Part of the zymogen enzyme family. These enzymes digest proteins and polypeptides (smaller proteins) in the body and are secreted in an inactive form to protect the digestive and accessory organ tissues themselves from being broken down. The enzymes can be activated by hydrochloric acid and other activated zymogens. The 'inactive' feature of these enzymes is very important to protect digestive and accessory organ tissues themselves from being broken down, as they are all made up of proteins.

Stomach: Where hydrochloric acid plays an important role

When the stomach is empty, it shrivels and forms internal folds, called rugae. This anatomical feature allows the stomach to increase its capacity from 50 millilitres to about 1.5 litres to accommodate food and/or beverages and gastric juices. The smooth muscles of the stomach (diagonal, circular and longitudinal) contract and relax in many directions. This creates a churning action to mix the food with gastric juices to form **chyme**. This mixing is very important for breaking chewed food into smaller pieces, for **emulsification of fat** and for increased contact of digestive enzymes with their target macromolecules.

In the gastric glands (also called gastric pits due to their appearance), specialised cells secrete the gastric juices needed for digestion in the stomach. Hydrochloric acid and **intrinsic factor** are produced at the bottom of the gastric pits. Cells in the middle section of the gastric pits secrete the proteolytic enzyme **pepsinogen**. Towards the entrance of the gastric pits, alkaline mucus is secreted, which protects the stomach lining from the strong hydrochloric acid. The presence of partially digested proteins in the stomach triggers the release of the hormone gastrin, which in turn triggers the gastric juices.

Hydrochloric acid is responsible for the acidic environment (pH 2) in the stomach and is important for:

- neutralisation of slightly alkaline salivary amylase, hence stopping starch digestion;
- **denaturation** of proteins;
- activation of inactive enzymes, notably activation of pepsinogen to pepsin;
- releasing vitamin B12 bound to proteins in food;
- killing harmful bacteria that can cause infection or food poisoning.

In food, vitamin B12 is bound to a protein; hence, it is not available for absorption. During digestion, hydrochloric acid denatures the protein-bound form of vitamin B12, thereby releasing it. The free vitamin B12 then binds with the intrinsic factor for transport to the small intestine, where it will be absorbed. The digestion of macronutrients from the mouth to the small intestine is outlined in Table 3.1.

Denaturation

The change that occurs in a protein's shape and structure and resulting in loss of function. This denaturation may occur due to external stressors such as chemicals, temperature, digestion or other factors.

Small intestine: The longest part of the digestive tract

Basic anatomy and physiology of the duodenum, jejunum, ileum and accessory organs

The small intestine is a long tube (4.5–7.5 metres) that comprises the duodenum, jejunum and ileum. The duodenum is a short section (30 centimetres) at the start of the small intestine, while the jejunum and ileum are the longer middle and end sections of the small intestine respectively. The pyloric sphincter controls the entry of chyme to the duodenum

Table 3.1 Action of digestive enzymes and their target nutrients

Region of digestive tract	Substrate	Enzyme	Secreted by	End-product
Mouth	Starch	Salivary amylase (α amylase)	Salivary glands	Shorter polysaccharide chains and dextrins
	Fat	Lingual lipase (minor contribution to fat digestion in adults)	Salivary glands	Diglycerides and fatty acids
Stomach	Protein	Pepsinogen *Activated to pepsin by HCl*	Parietal cells of stomach	Polypeptides
Small intestine	Starch	Pancreatic amylase	Pancreas	Maltose
	Sucrose	Sucrase	Small intestine	Glucose and fructose
	Maltose	Maltase	Small intestine	Glucose
	Lactose	Lactase	Small intestine	Glucose and galactose
	Fat	Pancreatic lipase	Pancreas	Fatty acids and glycerol
	Polypeptides	Trypsinogen *Activated to trypsin by enteropeptidases*	Pancreas	Tripeptides, Dipeptides and amino acids
	Polypeptides	Chymotrypsinogen *Activated to chymotrypsin by trypsin*	Pancreas	Tripeptides, dipeptides and amino acids
	Polypeptides	Procarboxipeptidases *Activated to carboxypeptidases by trypsin*	Small intestine	Tripeptides, dipeptides and amino acids
	Tripeptides	Intestinal tripeptidases	Small intestine	Dipeptides
	Dipeptides	Intestinal dipeptidases	Small intestine	Amino acids

and prevents intestinal contents from travelling to the stomach. The ileocecal valve allows entry of intestinal contents into the colon.

Enterocytes

Cells lining the intestines that are highly specialised for digestion and absorption.

Brush border

The microvilli-covered surface of the epithelial cells in the surface of the small intestine.

The small intestine coils around the peritoneal space, forming circular folds, and the intestinal lumen is covered with finger-like projections called villi (see Figure 3.2). Each individual villus is also covered with microscopic hair-like projections called microvilli,

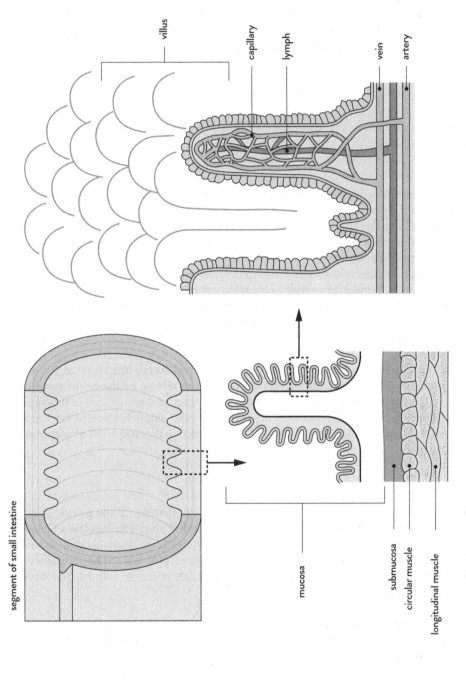

Figure 3.2 The intestinal folds and villi: important anatomical features that increase the surface area of the small intestine.

Source: Hodgson, pp. 312–27.[1]

which extend from the plasma membrane of the **enterocytes**. The folds, villi and micro-villi are responsible for the large surface area of the intestine; if these were all flattened, the small intestine would cover the surface of a tennis court. The **brush border** gets its name from the collection of villi, which look like the bristles on a brush. Many enzymes are secreted in the brush border and this is where macromolecules are broken down. Like the stomach, the brush border is covered by a protective layer of mucus with an additional layer of actin filaments, called the **glycocalyx**.

Glycocalyx

A protective mucus on the epithelial cells that is weakly acidic and consists of mucopolysaccharides.

While some enzymes are secreted in the brush border, other enzymes and digestive juices are secreted by accessory organs and are transported to the small intestine. The pancreas and gall bladder are accessory organs to the digestive tract that are responsible for secretion and storage of digestive juices needed in the duodenum. See Table 3.1 for enzymes and their respective macronutrients and end-products of digestion.

The pancreas produces and secretes many enzymes used for the digestion of all three macromolecules (see Table 3.1) as well as bicarbonate for acid neutralisation. Secretin is a hormone released in the blood when the cells lining the wall of the duodenum detect the presence of chyme. This leads to the release of pancreatic juices in this region of the small intestine, to production of bile by the liver, and to inhibition of hydrochloric acid production in the stomach.

The gall bladder is a small pouch that concentrates and stores bile secreted from the liver. The presence of fat in the duodenum stimulates the release of the hormone cholecystokinin (CCK), which signals the gall bladder to contract and release bile in this region of the small intestine. Bile acids and salts are needed for the emulsification of fat and the formation of small fat droplets, which are key to the effective digestion and absorption of this macronutrient.

Movement of chyme along the small intestine

Upon leaving the stomach, the acidic chyme enters the duodenum via the pyloric sphincter. Upon sensing the acid, the sphincter closes until the pH rises and it relaxes again to allow the chyme to enter the duodenum. Here the pancreatic juices neutralise stomach acid and the digestion of macronutrients continues (see Table 3.2). The frequency of opening of the pyloric sphincter is governed by stomach content, volume and chyme consistency. For example:

- gastric emptying is slower after a high-fat meal (hence high-fat chyme);
- gastric emptying is faster after a large meal. The stretching and expansion of the stomach drives the opening frequency of this sphincter;
- liquids pass through the small opening of the pyloric sphincter more easily than solid chyme.

Table 3.2 Hormonal control of digestion—selected hormones

Hormone	Secreted by	Triggered by	Response
Gastrin	Stomach	Presence of food in the stomach	Stimulates release of hydrochloric acid and pepsinogen. Increases gastric and intestinal movement of chyme.
Secretin	Small intestine	Presence of acidic chyme in the duodenum	Stimulates secretion of pancreatic enzymes in the duodenum. Reduces intestinal movement of chyme.
Cholecystokinin (CCK)	Small intestine	Presence of fats and/ or amino acids in the duodenum	Stimulates contraction of gall bladder to release bile into the duodenum. Secretion of pancreatic enzymes and juices into the duodenum.

Peristalsis propels the chyme along the small intestine, while the bi-directional flow of segmentation allows for mixing of chyme with pancreatic juices and bile for further emulsification of fat and mixing with other digestive secretions. By the time chyme reaches the **ileocecal valve**, digestion of nutrients is complete and most nutrients have been absorbed; only water and unabsorbed contents (such as fibre) remain. The latter serve as food for the gut bacteria residing in the small intestine and colon.

Ileocecal valve

The sphincter that separates the small and large intestine.

Colon (large intestine)

The colon is larger in diameter than the small intestine and comprises five regions: the cecum and the ascending, transverse, descending and sigmoid colon. The small intestine is connected to the colon at the cecum; at the other end of the colon are the rectum, an internal anal sphincter and an external anal sphincter, which control defecation. The colon serves to absorb water and some minerals from intestinal content, to sustain fermentation of intestinal content by gut bacteria and to form stools. **Transit time** in the colon can range from 12 to 70 hours, during which colon content changes from liquefied form to semi-solid form due to absorption of water and digestive secretions. The colon is coated with mucus for protection and as a lubricant, and bicarbonate is also secreted to neutralise acids produced by bacteria.

Transit time

Duration of content movement through the colon. This can be affected by factors such as illness, infection and type and intensity of exercise. When transit time is accelerated there is not enough time for water and other macro- and micronutrients to be absorbed, resulting in their loss in stools.

Stools are generally composed of undigested food, some undigested nutrients, some water, sloughed intestinal cells, bacteria and indigestible fibre. When stools reach the rectum, defecation is stimulated and expulsion from the body is governed by strong muscle contractions in the sigmoid colon and rectum. The internal anal sphincter relaxes automatically, while the external anal sphincter is under voluntary control; therefore, a person can decide when to defecate.

Absorption

The majority of nutrients are absorbed into the enterocytes of the duodenum, jejunum and/or ileum and transported to other parts of the body via the network of blood and lymphatic vessels in each villus (Figure 3.2). The nutrients move from the intestinal lumen into the enterocytes via different mechanisms:

- passive diffusion is when small molecules, such as water and small lipids, are freely absorbed into the enterocytes across the concentration gradient;
- facilitated diffusion occurs when a specific carrier is needed to transport nutrients (for example, water-soluble vitamins) through the enterocyte cell membrane;
- active transport uses energy to transport some nutrients, against the concentration gradient, from one side of the enterocyte cell membrane to the other. Amino acids are absorbed through active transport, as is glucose, which is absorbed via the transporter sodium-glucose linked transporter 1 (SGLT-1).

Once the water-soluble nutrients and small lipids are absorbed through the enterocytes, they enter the bloodstream and are transported to the liver for further metabolism and distribution to other parts of the body. Larger lipids and fat-soluble vitamins are not water-soluble, and hence cannot be transported easily in blood. Instead, they are first absorbed into the enterocytes, where they are packaged with some proteins to form chylomicrons. These are then released into the lymphatic vessels for transport around the body.

Summary

This chapter has described and explained the processes of digestion and absorption along the digestive tract. The digestive tract includes the mouth, oesophagus, stomach, small intestine, large intestine and accessory organs, including the pancreas and gall bladder. Food is propelled along the digestive tract by peristalsis and enzymes are responsible for the breakdown of macromolecules into simple molecules. Most of the nutrients are absorbed in the small intestines and water and some minerals are absorbed in the colon. Many hormones regulate digestion, which can also be impacted by exercise duration and intensity.

Chapter highlights

- Digestion is the process by which the body breaks down the food consumed into nutrients which are essential for normal bodily functions.
- Digestion includes mechanical breakdown of food and mixing (chewing, opening and closing of sphincters, churning action of the stomach, peristalsis and segmentation) and chemical breakdown of nutrients.

- Saliva lubricates and protects the mouth, moistens food and contains salivary amylase and lingual lipase. Salivary amylase secreted by salivary glands starts the digestion of starch.
- The oesophagus is the tube connecting the mouth to the stomach. The gastro-oesophageal sphincter prevents reflux of stomach content hence protecting the oesophagus against the strong stomach gastric juices.
- In the stomach, specialised cells in the gastric glands secrete the gastric juices needed for digestion. Secretion of these gastric juices is stimulated by the presence of the hormone gastrin.
- Hydrochloric acid is important for the neutralisation of salivary amylase, hence stopping starch digestion; denaturation of proteins; activation of inactive enzymes, notably activation of pepsinogen to pepsin; releasing vitamin B12 bound to proteins in food; and killing harmful bacteria that can cause infection or food poisoning.
- Small intestines comprise the duodenum, jejunum and ileum. The anatomical features of small intestines include circular folds, lining covered by finger-like projections called villi and each villus is covered by hair-like projections called micro-villi.
- Enzymes secreted by accessory organs, such as the pancreas, or brush border responsible for the chemical breakdown of nutrients in the small intestines.
- In the colon, water and some minerals are absorbed from intestinal content to form stools.

References

1. Hodgson JM. Digestion of food. In: ML Wahlqvist, editor. *Food and Nutrition: Food and Health Systems in Australia and New Zealand*. 3rd ed. Abingdon Oxon, UK: Routledge; 2011.

4   Macronutrients

Evangeline Mantzioris

The macronutrients—protein, fat, and carbohydrate—are essential nutrients that supply energy and are required in relatively large quantities for the body. They are also functional building blocks and have a diverse range of uses in the body, including growth and repair, precursors for hormones and components of the immune system. Alcohol is not considered a macronutrient, as despite providing energy, it is not essential as it is not required by the body per se and has toxic properties. Interestingly, all these macronutrients are composed of the same elements: carbon (C), oxygen (O), nitrogen (N), and hydrogen (H).

Learning outcomes

This chapter will:

- describe the chemical and biological properties of the macronutrients;
- outline the physiological and biochemical uses of macronutrients in the body;
- describe the health effects of under- and overconsumption of the macronutrients;
- explain the synthesis and metabolism of the macronutrients;
- outline the recommended intakes and dietary sources of the macronutrients.

Dietary energy, measured in kilojoules (calories; see Box 4.1) is the fuel essential for maintaining bodily functions and supporting physical activity. It originates from macronutrients—carbohydrates, proteins, and fats—metabolised during digestion.

Box 4.1   Calculating energy from macronutrients in food

To calculate the energy present in foods, you need to multiply the total amount of each of the macronutrients contained in the food (in grams) by the Atwater factors for protein, fat, and carbohydrate. The Atwater factors provide the available energy for each of the macronutrients regardless of the food from which they are derived.

DOI: 10.4324/9781003321286-5

Atwater Factors

- Protein: 17 kJ/g (4 kcal/g)
- Fat: 37 kJ/g (9 kcal/g)
- Carbohydrate: 17 kJ/g (4 kcal/g)

For example, a food label might indicate that there is:

- Protein: 9.6 g
- Fat (total): 3.2 g
- Carbohydrate: 43.0 g

In this case, the energy in kilojoules that is provided by each nutrient is as follows:

- Protein: 9.6 × 17 = 163.2 kJ (9.6 × 4 = 38.4 kcal)
- Fat: 3.2 × 37 = 118.4 kJ (3.2 × 9 = 28.2 kcal)
- Carbohydrate: 43 × 17 = 731 kJ (43 × 4 = 172 kcal)
- Total energy: 163.2 + 118.4 + 731 = 1012.6 kJ (38.4 + 28.2 + 172 = 238.6 kcal)

Protein

Proteins are essential nutrients, which provide 17 kJ/g (4 kcal/g) of energy and are made up of single units known as amino acids. Amino acids are the building blocks of the human body and are used to synthesise cells, muscles, organs, hormones, and immune factors, as well as acting as buffers to regulate the acidity or basicity of the body.

Chemical structure

Proteins are composed of amino acid chains, linked together by peptide bonds (chemical bonds between amino acids). Proteins vary according to the number and sequence of amino acids, the folding of the protein and the interaction with other chemical groups in the protein to induce chemical change. All of this leads to unique individual proteins, reflecting the variety of roles they play in your body.

All amino acids have the same basic chemical structure: a central carbon to which is attached a hydrogen group (H), an amino group (NH_2), a carboxylic acid group (COOH) and a side chain group. It is the side chain group that makes each of the amino acids different (see Figure 4.1). There are 20 different amino acids; nine are essential and the remaining 11 are non-essential.

Essential amino acids

There are nine amino acids that the human body requires but is unable to **synthesise**, and which therefore must be obtained from the diet. As such, they are termed essential (or indispensable). These are histidine, isoleucine, leucine, lysine, methionine, phenylalanine, threonine, tryptophan, and valine. The depletion of essential amino acids in the protein

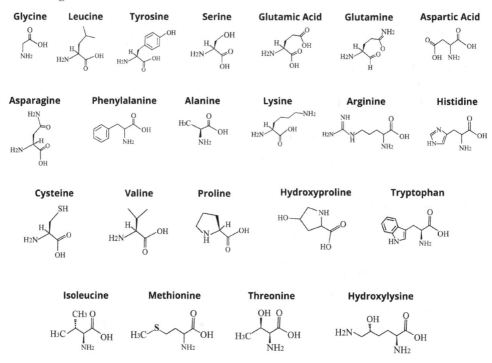

Figure 4.1 Chemical structure of amino acids.

pool in the body will begin to limit the production of proteins essential for growth (including muscles), repair, cell functioning and development.

Synthesise

To form a substance by combining elements.

Non-essential amino acids

There are 11 non-essential (or dispensable) amino acids that the body can synthesise, but that can also be provided by diet. In some conditions, a non-essential amino acid may become essential; in such cases, the amino acid is referred to as conditionally essential (or conditionally indispensable). Tyrosine is a conditionally essential amino acid, as the body uses tryptophan to make tyrosine: if tryptophan is limited it is then unable to synthesise tyrosine.

Protein foods are often categorised in reference to their quality, both in terms of the mix and amount of amino acids that they contain. Complete protein sources often refer to animal-derived proteins that contain, in the required proportions, all the essential amino acids. Plant proteins are termed incomplete, as they are missing one or more of the essential amino acids or have levels of an essential amino acid too low to meet requirements. Complementary proteins refer to the combination of two plant proteins to provide all the essential amino acids—for example, combining beans (lacking methionine) with grains (lacking lysine and threonine).

Uses in the body

Proteins have wide and varied roles in the human body: they are involved in the growth, repair and replacement of all cells (including blood, muscles, skeletal system, tissues, and organs), and are involved in regulating the homeostatic control and defence of the body.[3]

One of the main functional roles of proteins in the body is as enzymes, which accelerate chemical reactions in the body. Enzymes are synthesised from amino acids as well as other dietary components (for example, zinc and selenium). They are used by every organ and cell to assist in the repair and growth of the body. Enzymes also contribute to the synthesis of proteins involved in the homeostatic control of the body, immune function, fluid balance regulation, transportation of nutrients and other molecules, and detoxification of the body. In addition to protein's critical role in the growth and regulation of the body, protein can also be used as a source of energy if carbohydrate and fat intake is low (for instance, during times of starvation). If needed, muscle will be broken down to provide further energy if dietary intake of protein is also limited. Protein may also be metabolised for energy when energy demands are sustained over a long period of time in performance, such as in ultra-endurance events lasting 3–4 hours or more.

Box 4.2 Nutrient requirements

Nutrient requirements are a set of recommended intakes for macro- and micro-nutrients that best support healthy people to maintain good health. Nutrient requirements are set by regions or countries by analysing and synthesising the data from many thousands of peer-reviewed journal articles (the evidence base). The following table shows the names of the different categories that are used to express requirements around the world.

Country & Co-ordinating Body	Umbrella Term for Nutrient Reference Values	Average requirements—The average daily intake that meets the requirements of half of the healthy individuals	Recommended Intakes—The average daily intake that is sufficient to meet the nutrient requirements of nearly all healthy individuals	Acceptable Intake—The average daily intake, assumed for a group of apparently healthy people when there is insufficient evidence	Upper Intake Level—Maximum average daily nutrient intake level unlikely to cause adverse health effects to almost all individuals
Australia National Health & Medical Research Committee https://www.eatforhealth.gov.au/nutrient-reference-values	Nutrient Reference Values	Estimated Average Requirements (EAR)	Recommended Dietary Intake (RDI)	Acceptable Intake (AI)	Upper Level (UL)

European Union European Food Safety Authority https://www.efsa.europa.eu/en/topics/topic/dietary-reference-values	Dietary Reference Values	Average requirement (AR)	Population Reference Intake (PRI)	Adequate Intake (AI)	Tolerable Upper Intake Level (UL)
Ireland Food Safety Authority of Ireland https://www.lenus.ie/bitstream/handle/10147/44808/6367.pdf?sequence=1&isAllowed=y	Recommended Dietary Allowances for Ireland	Average Requirement (AR)	Population Reference Intake (PRI)	-	-
Japan Ministry of Health, Labour and Welfare https://www.mhlw.go.jp/content/10900000/000862500.pdf	Dietary Reference Intakes	Estimated Average Requirement (EAR)	Recommended Dietary Allowance (RDA)	Adequate intake (AI)	Tolerable upper intake level (UL)
UK Scientific Advisory Committee on Nutrition https://www.gov.uk/government/publications/sacn-dietary-reference-values-for-energy	Dietary Reference Values	Estimated Average Requirements (EAR)	Recommended Dietary Allowance (RDA)	Adequate Intake (AI)	Total Upper Intake Level (UL)
US + Canada The National Academies of Sciences, Engineering and Medicine https://ods.od.nih.gov/HealthInformation/nutrient recommendations.aspx	Dietary Reference Intakes	Estimated Average Requirement (EAR)	Recommended Dietary Allowance (RDA)	Adequate Intake (AI)	Tolerable Upper Intake Level (UL)

Recommended intakes for non-athletes

Protein in the body is continuously broken down and resynthesised. This process is known as protein turnover, with small amounts of protein lost in the stools. Dietary protein is required daily due to its ubiquitous role and limited storage in the body. In Australia, it is recommended that protein intake provides about 10–15% of the daily energy requirement. For the average adult who needs approximately 8700 kJ (2000 kcal) per day, this equates to about 50–75 g of protein per day. The NRV (Australia & New Zealand) recommendations for protein are based on a g/kg of body weight for each gender and age group (see Box 4.2 for an overview of international nutrient intake recommendations). The daily RDI for women aged 19–70 years is 0.75 g/kg and over 70 years is 0.94 g/kg of body weight. The RDI for men aged 19–70 years is 0.84 g/kg and for over 70 years is 1.07 g/kg of body weight. WHO has developed requirements for protein as well—it is set for over 18-year-olds as 0.83g/kg per day. However, this is assuming a protein digestibility-corrected amino acid value of 1.0, that is, the protein intake contains more than 100% of the requirements of all the essential amino acids. Requirements for athletes may differ, depending on their age and sport played, as discussed in Chapter 10.

Dietary sources

While animal products that are rich in protein are greatly valued for their high-quality protein, which provide a complete set of the essential amino acids in the proportions required, plant proteins provide a major source of protein for many millions of people around the world. Animal sources of protein also provide valuable additional nutrients that have limited presence in other foods, such as iron and zinc (present in meat), and calcium and vitamin B12 (present in dairy). Plant sources of protein (wheat, rice, pasta, legumes, nuts, and seeds) also provide carbohydrates, B-group vitamins, and fibre. This makes food sources of protein, compared to protein supplements, valuable for athletes and non-athletes to ensure they are getting a balanced diet with other macronutrients and micronutrients of importance in health, exercise, and performance.

Health effects of protein

Protein is important for the body's maintenance and health, and most Western populations consume adequate intakes for this. However, in developing countries the health problems associated with protein deficiencies are devastating, and it is the leading cause of death among children in these places.

In most cases, protein deficiency occurs in combination with an energy deficiency and is referred to as protein-energy malnutrition (PEM). Primary PEM occurs as the direct result of diets that lack both protein and energy. Secondary PEM arises as a complication of chronic illness, such as acquired immune deficiency syndrome (AIDS), tuberculosis, and cancer, due to increased nutritional requirements, limited oral intake, or malabsorption of nutrients. Acute PEM refers to a short period of food deprivation, as in the case of children who are often the appropriate height for their age but are underweight. Chronic PEM refers to long-term food deprivation that affects growth and weight and is characterised by small-for-age children.

In developed regions, protein deficiency is more likely to arise due to chronic illness or poverty and, as such, it is unlikely an athlete will have a compromised protein intake—unless it reflects a philosophical or religious reason that limits their intake of animal products. Chapter 6 will discuss planning diets for people who choose to follow a vegetarian diet.

Lipids

Lipids (or fats) are a large and diverse group of naturally occurring molecules, both in the diet and in the human body. They include fats, waxes, sterols, fat-soluble vitamins, monoglycerides, diglycerides, triglycerides, phospholipids, and esters. Dietary fats provide a concentrated form of energy (37 kJ/g, 9 kcal/g) and are also a vehicle in the diet for supplying fat-soluble vitamins (vitamins A, D, E, and K) and essential fatty acids (alpha-linolenic acid and linoleic acid). Importantly, and often under-considered, dietary fat provides important **organoleptic** properties to food that contains fats and to meals to which fats have been added. Lipids play critical roles in the body, including storing energy, cell signalling, and as the major structural component of cell membranes. While the intake of certain dietary fats (saturated and trans fats) is associated with the development of chronic disease, dietary fats are an essential part of the diet, providing essential fatty acids, vitamins, and other phytonutrients.

Organoleptic

The aspect of substances, in this case food and drink, that an individual experiences via the senses of taste, texture, smell, and touch.

Chemical structure

All lipids are compounds that are composed of carbon, hydrogen, and oxygen and are insoluble in water, but the different types of lipids that exist are structurally very diverse. There are four main categories: fatty acids, triglycerides, sterols, and phospholipids (see Figure 4.2).

Fatty acids

Fatty acids are composed of a chain of carbon (C) atoms, attached by single bonds. Each C atom can have up to four H atoms attached. The carbon chain has a carboxyl group at one end and a methyl group at the other end. Fatty acids can be classified according to the number of C atoms in the chain. Short-chain fatty acids have 2–6 C atoms, medium-chain fatty acids 6–12 C atoms, long-chain 14–20 C atoms and, finally, very long-chain fatty acids more than 20 C atoms. Fatty acids are, however, more often classified according to the number of double bonds present between the C atoms—the more double bonds in the chain, the more unsaturated the fatty acid.

Saturated fatty acids

Fatty acid chains that contain no double bonds between the C atoms are referred to as saturated fatty acids. They are mostly found in animal food products, such as meat, cheese, and butter, but are also present in some plant products, such as coconut and palm

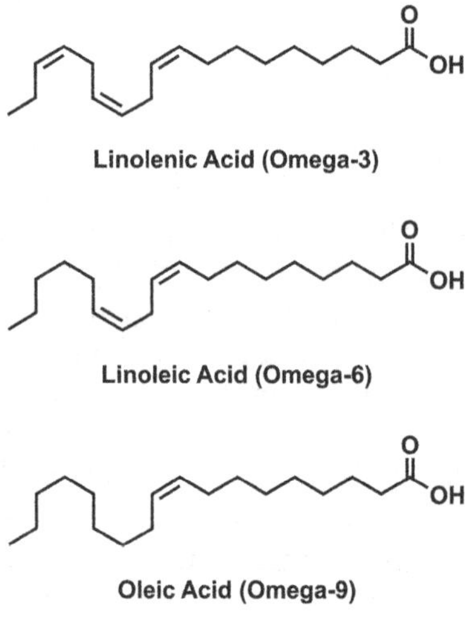

Linolenic Acid (Omega-3)

Linoleic Acid (Omega-6)

Oleic Acid (Omega-9)

Figure 4.2 Structural relationship of some fatty acids.

oils. Saturated fats are associated with an increased risk of cardiovascular disease; however, emerging research is beginning to show that their effect may not be as great as once thought.[3] The research and scientific debate in this area is continuing and as new high-quality evidence emerges this may lead to changes in dietary advice.

Monounsaturated fatty acids

Monounsaturated fatty acids contain one double bond in the C chain and are found in foods such as olives and olive oil, avocadoes, and some types of nuts. Monounsaturated fats (from olive oil) are one of the main components of the Mediterranean diet, which has been shown in both **epidemiological studies** and **intervention studies** to reduce risk and provide benefits in cardiovascular disease. It is important to note that the other components of the Mediterranean diet (vegetables, fruit, and grains) also play a role in good health.

Epidemiological studies

Studies that analyse the distribution (who, when, and where) and determinants of health and disease in a defined population by observation. Epidemiological studies include ecological, case-control, cross-sectional, and retrospective or prospective longitudinal cohort study designs.

Intervention studies

Studies in which researchers make changes to observe the effect on health outcomes; in nutrition and sport, this will include changes to diet and activity.

Polyunsaturated fatty acids

Polyunsaturated fatty acids (PUFAs) contain two or more double bonds in the C chain. PUFAs are further subdivided according to the position of the first double bond in the chain. When the double bond occurs on the third C atom from the methyl end, they are referred to as n-3 (or omega-3) fatty acids. If the first double bond occurs on the sixth C atom from the methyl end, they are referred to as n-6 (or omega-6) fatty acids. The parent fatty acids of the n-3 and n-6, alpha-linolenic and linoleic acid, respectively, are the essential fatty acids. They are known as essential, as the human body is unable to synthesise them, and, as such, must be obtained from the diet.

N-6 POLYUNSATURATED FATTY ACIDS

Linoleic acid (LA) is the parent fatty acid of the n-6 PUFA and, as it is essential, needs to be obtained from the diet. LA is found as a concentrated source in vegetable oils like safflower and sunflower oils, and salad dressings made from these oils. It is also present in some nuts and seeds. LA is important, as it can be metabolised through a series of reactions to form the longer-chain fatty acid, arachidonic acid (AA). AA can also be found in the diet (in meat). AA is the direct precursor of a diverse group of hormone-like substances known as eicosanoids, which play a critical role in the inflammatory process and in thrombosis (clot formation).

N-3 POLYUNSATURATED FATTY ACIDS

Alpha-linolenic acid (ALA) is the parent fatty acid of the n-3 PUFA, and like LA, it needs to be obtained from the diet. ALA is found in concentrated sources in flaxseed (linseed) oil, and in smaller amounts in canola oil. Walnuts, chia seeds, and green leafy vegetables also contain small amounts of ALA. ALA is metabolised through the same chain of reactions that converts LA to AA, to form the longer-chain fatty acids, eicosapentaenoic acid (EPA) and docosahexaenoic acid (DHA). EPA and DHA are found in fish, fish oil, and breast milk. Like AA, EPA is important, as it is the direct precursor of a diverse group of hormone-like substances known as eicosanoids; however, eicosanoids derived from EPA are anti-inflammatory and anti-thrombotic, compared to those derived from AA.

This biochemical difference between the two classes of fatty acids and their eicosanoids has been used therapeutically in the management of inflammatory diseases such as rheumatoid arthritis and psoriasis. DHA is found in concentrated amounts in the cellular phospholipids of the brain and neural tissue of humans and, as such, its role in foetal and early-life nutrition is critical.

TRANS FATTY ACIDS

Trans fatty acids (TFAs) are a chemical variation of unsaturated fats. In the **cis form** (the regular form), the C atoms that have double bonds and the H atoms are on the same side. In the **trans form**, the H-atoms are on opposite sides of the double-bonded C atoms, so that they look and act more like saturated fats.

Cis form

In a molecule, the C atoms that have double bonds and the H atoms are on the same side.

Trans form

In a molecule, the C atoms that have double bonds and the H atoms are on opposite sides.

TFAs naturally occur in dairy products and beef. In the food industry, manufacturers can produce TFAs by mixing H atoms with the unsaturated fatty acids, using a mixture of heat and pressure. This results in liquid oils being transformed into a solid state, making them very useful for producing certain foods, such as spreads and vegetable shortening for baking. However, these TFAs have been shown to be worse for cardiovascular disease compared to the equivalent amounts of saturated fat. The WHO has recommended that no more than 1% of dietary energy be derived from TFAs. In many countries, including Australia, Denmark, and the United States, there has been a reduction in TFA use in the food supply, either through voluntary initiatives or legislation.

TRIGLYCERIDES

Triglycerides are the main constituents of body fat (adipose tissue) in animals, including humans. They are made up of a glycerol backbone with three fatty acids attached. All triglycerides are composed of different types of fatty acids, from short-chain to long-chain. Triglycerides are also the main type of fat consumed in food, from both vegetable and animal sources.

STEROLS

Sterols are complex lipid molecules, having four interconnected carbon rings with a hydrocarbon side chain. The most familiar type of sterol is cholesterol, which is a critical component of cell membranes and a precursor to vitamin D, the sex hormones (oestrogen and testosterone) and the adrenal hormones (cortisol, cortisone, and aldosterone).

Cholesterol can be synthesised in the body and hence is not essential in the diet. Dietary cholesterol is only found in animal products. Cholesterol in the body can be classified as either high-density **lipoprotein** cholesterol (HDL-C) or low-density lipoprotein cholesterol (LDL-C) depending on whether it is part of a low-density lipoprotein (LDL) or high-density lipoprotein (HDL) molecule. LDL-C is referred to as 'bad' cholesterol, as LDL takes cholesterol to the blood vessels where it can form into atherosclerotic plaques, which can lead to blockages and myocardial infarction (heart attack). HDL-C is referred to as 'good' cholesterol, as HDL takes cholesterol away from the blood vessels to the liver, hence reducing the risk of a myocardial infarction.

Lipoprotein

A cluster of lipids attached to proteins that act as transport vehicles for the lipids in the blood. They are divided according to their density.

Plants synthesise many types of sterols, as well as stanols, which are structurally similar to sterols. Sterols and stanols are poorly absorbed by the body and reduce the absorption of cholesterol from the gastrointestinal (GI) system, which can have beneficial effects for cholesterol reduction. The food industry has added plant sterols to some types of margarines, milks, yoghurts, and cereals, which can lead to a reduction in cholesterol levels if at least 2–3 g/day of plant sterols or stanols are consumed.

PHOSPHOLIPIDS

Phospholipids have a unique chemical structure; they are soluble in both water and fat. They are similar to triglycerides, in that they have a glycerol backbone, but have only two fatty acids attached to the glycerol—the third position is taken up by a phosphate and a 'head-group'. It is the combination of the head-group, phosphate group and glycerol backbone that makes phospholipids soluble in water, while the fatty acids (the tail group) make them soluble in fats. This feature gives them a critical role, both in the body and in the food industry. Despite their importance, phospholipids make up only a small portion of the diet (<5%) and are not essential, as they can be synthesised by the body.

Phospholipids can freely move around the body, which enables them to transport other fats such as vitamins and hormones. They are also a critical component of the cellular membranes, where they form a phospholipid bilayer. The phospholipids assemble into two layers, with the hydrophilic (water-loving) ends on opposite sides, and the hydrophobic (water-fearing) ends facing each other on the inside. This arrangement allows for the transport of substances through the cellular membrane. Interestingly, the fatty acids attached to the phospholipids in the cellular membrane will reflect the dietary intake of fatty acids.

In the food industry, phospholipids (such as lecithin) allow foods to be emulsified, as in the production of salad dressings, mayonnaise, ice cream, and chocolate. Lecithin is found in eggs, liver, soybeans, wheat germ, and peanuts.

Recommended intakes for the general population

The Nutrient Reference Values from the NMHRC have no set RDI, EAR, or AI for total fat intake. However, there are recommendations for the intake of the essential fatty acids.[3]

Australian, US, UK, and EU dietary recommendations suggest limiting total fat to 20–35% of total energy intake. The WHO recommends that total fat intake should be less than 30%, saturated fats less than 10%, and trans-fats less than 1% of total energy intake. The WHO recommends an omega-6 fatty acid intake of 2.5–9% of energy and an omega-3 fatty acid intake of 0.5–2% of energy. This highlights the importance of reducing the intake of foods containing saturated fats and replacing them with oils and foods containing monounsaturated (olive, canola oil, avocado, almonds) or polyunsaturated fats (nuts, fish, polyunsaturated vegetable oils).

Carbohydrates

Carbohydrates, like fats and proteins, are molecules composed of C, H, and O atoms. They are ubiquitous in the diet—present in breads, cereals, grains, legumes, rice, pasta, vegetables, and fruit, although dairy is the only animal source of carbohydrates. Carbohydrates deliver the key source of fuel (energy) for the muscles and body, providing 17 kJ/g (4 kcal/g). Glucose, which is a monosaccharide (simple) sugar, is the exclusive source of energy for red blood cells and provides a significant portion of the energy that is required for the brain. Excess glucose in the blood is converted to the storage form of glucose, glycogen. The average person stores about 5000 kilojoules worth of glucose in the form of glycogen, which can be easily converted to glucose again to be used by the body when blood glucose levels begin to drop.

Carbohydrates have numerous biological functions in the body. Aside from their important role in providing energy, they also have a structural role. Ribose, which is a component of coenzymes and the backbone of RNA, is a five-C atom monosaccharide, and the closely related deoxyribose is a component of DNA. Carbohydrates also play key roles in the immune system and in blood clotting.

Chemical forms of carbohydrate

There are a wide variety of carbohydrates in the diet. They include simple carbohydrates (the sugars) and complex carbohydrates (the starches and fibre). Regardless of the length or complexity of the carbohydrate, they are all composed of sugar units (see Figure 4.3).

Monosaccharides

Monosaccharides are composed of a single unit of sugar and are the most basic units of carbohydrates. There are three monosaccharides or 'sugars': glucose, fructose, and galactose. The monosaccharides all have the same number of C, H, and O atoms but differ in their chemical structure. Monosaccharides are the building blocks of disaccharides and polysaccharides.

GLUCOSE

Glucose ($C_6H_{12}O_6$) serves as the essential energy source for the body; when people talk about blood sugar levels, they are referring to glucose in the blood. Most of the polysaccharides in the diet are composed of chains of glucose, with starch being the most common polysaccharide.

FRUCTOSE

The slightly different chemical structure of fructose results in it being the sweetest-tasting monosaccharide. Fructose occurs naturally in some fruits and honey. Fructose may be added to some foods, such as soft drinks, ready-to-eat breakfast cereals and desserts, and biscuit and cake mixes, through the use of high-fructose corn syrup.

GALACTOSE

Galactose is found in dairy products and sugar beets and is the least sweet-tasting monosaccharide.

Disaccharides

Disaccharides are composed of two glucose units and can be formed as pairs of any of the three monosaccharides. There are three disaccharides, and each contains glucose as one of the monosaccharide components. Sucrose, which is a common table sugar refined from cane sugar, is made up of glucose and fructose. Lactose is found in milk and is composed of galactose and glucose. Maltose, also known as malt sugar, is the disaccharide that is produced when amylase, an enzyme, breaks down starch.

Lactose intolerance

A condition that leads to the inability to digest lactose which results in bloating, abdominal discomfort, gas, or diarrhoea.

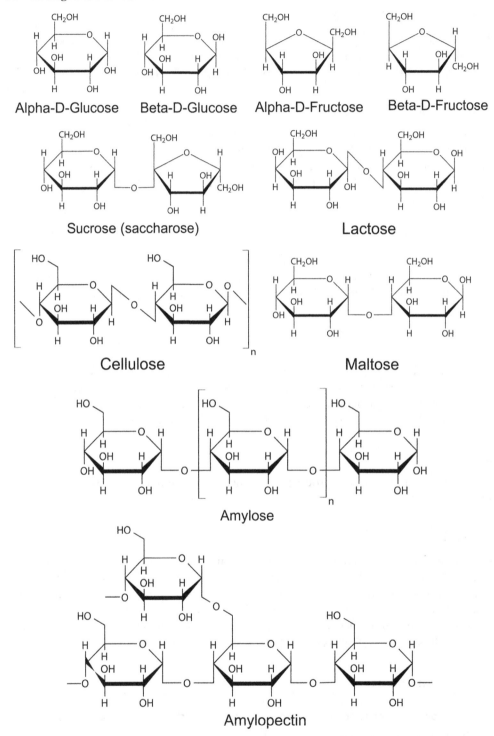

Figure 4.3 Chemical structure of carbohydrates

Lactose intolerance is common, with only about 30% of adults worldwide being able to digest lactose. Intestinal cells produce an enzyme called lactase, which breaks lactose down into galactose and glucose. When lactase activity is low in people, the lactose remains undigested in the intestinal tract and leads to a high concentration of contents in the intestine, which in turn draws fluid into the intestinal lumen and, in combination with the proliferation of bacteria that digest the lactose, leads to painful bloating, wind, or diarrhoea.

NON-NUTRITIVE SWEETENERS

Non-nutritive sweeteners are chemicals, found naturally that are extracted from plants (Stevia) or synthesised industrially (aspartame, saccharin), or are **sugar alcohols**, that have a sweet taste with either no kilojoules or reduced kilojoules compared to sugar. This allows the food industry to replace sugars with artificial sweeteners without adding kilojoules to the product. It was assumed that this would lead to significant weight loss in the community due to the decreased consumption of kilojoules, but research shows a lack of the predicted effect. Whether this is due to people increasing their consumption of other foods or the artificial sweeteners affecting metabolism in other ways is still being debated among researchers.[4] In 2023 the WHO, following an extensive systematic review, advised that "non-sugar sweeteners should not be used as a means of achieving weight control or reducing the risk of noncommunicable diseases" such as diabetes and heart disease.[7]

> **Sugar alcohols**
>
> Carbohydrates that have been chemically altered. They provide fewer kilojoules as they are not well absorbed and may have a laxative effect. They include sorbitol, mannitol, and xylitol. While they have fewer kilojoules they can still lead to elevation in blood glucose levels and, hence, can have an impact on blood glucose control in people with diabetes; as such they need to be considered in the diet.

Complex carbohydrates

Complex carbohydrates include oligosaccharides, which contain between three and nine monosaccharide units, and polysaccharides, which contain ten or more monosaccharide units.

Oligosaccharides

Oligosaccharides are found in a variety of foods. Starch, which is found in a wide variety of foods, such as wheat, maize potato, and rice, contains the α-glucan oligosaccharide maltodextrin. Maltodextrin is used in the food industry as a sweetener, fat substitute, and to modify the texture of food through its thickening properties.

The oligosaccharides that are not α-glucans include raffinose, stachyose, verbascose, inulin, and fructan, and are found in legumes, artichokes, wheat, and rye, and in the onion, leek, and garlic family. The fructans (including inulin) have unique properties in the GI system and are referred to as prebiotics. Prebiotics remain undigested in the GI system and promote the growth of select bacteria that improve human health. Consumption of these foods leads to alteration in the flora of the gut, with a domination of *bifidobacteria* and *lactobacillus*, and the production of short-chain fatty acids (SCFAs). SCFAs, also referred to as volatile fatty acids (VFAs), are important for colonic health as they are the primary energy source for colon cells and have anti-carcinogenic and anti-inflammatory properties.

Prebiotics

Food components that are not digested in the gastrointestinal system but are used by the bacteria in the colon to promote their growth.

Polysaccharides

GLYCOGEN

Glycogen is found in limited amounts in food, with a small amount found in meat. However, it is its role in the body that is critically important and of interest to nutritionists, including sports nutrition professionals. Glycogen is a secondary form of energy storage (~5000 kJ (1200 kcal/g) in the average person). When blood glucose levels increase following a meal, insulin is released, which stimulates the uptake of glucose into cells and storage as glycogen. Conversely, when blood glucose levels decrease due to a lack of dietary intake of carbohydrates or depletion of blood glucose levels from exercise, the pancreas releases glucagon, which stimulates the liver and muscles to release and break down glycogen and release glucose (known as glycogenolysis). Glucose can also be derived through gluconeogenesis, which is a metabolic pathway that leads to glucose formation from substrates such as lactate, glycerol, and glucogenic amino acids.

Glycogen is a highly branched structure, containing up to 30,000 glucose units that surround a protein core. Glycogen in the muscle, liver, and fat cells is stored in a hydrated form with three or four parts of water per part of glycogen. This explains the dramatic weight loss that is seen with low-carbohydrate diets. In this scenario, as blood glucose levels decrease, glycogen is converted back to glucose to supply the brain and muscles with fuel, which also releases the water, hence contributing to the weight loss observed.

STARCH

Starch is the form in which plants store glucose to use for energy. Some common starches include amylopectin and amylose. Both contain hundreds to thousands of glucose units linked together, as is the case with glycogen. Starch is found in many different foods including wheat, rice, lentils, maize, beans, and tuber vegetables.

Resistant starch is one type of starch that resists digestion in the small intestine and is fermented in the large intestine by bacteria into short-chain fatty acids. These SCFAs are important as they protect the bowel against cancer and are also absorbed into the bloodstream and may be involved in lowering blood cholesterol. Resistant starch is found in unripe bananas, potatoes, and lentils. Additionally, resistant starch can be added to 'high-fibre' breads and cereals. It is also considered to be a form of insoluble fibre, which is discussed below.

Fibre

While there are many definitions of fibre, most simply, dietary fibre is a carbohydrate that is not digested by the body. Fibre is the parts of the edible portions of plants that are not digested or absorbed in the small intestine, that go on to be partially or completely fermented in the large intestine and that promote beneficial physiological effects. These beneficial effects include laxation of bowel movements, reduced blood cholesterol and beneficial modulation of blood glucose levels. Dietary fibre can include polysaccharides, oligosaccharides and lignin. The recommended intake for dietary fibre ranges from 25 to 35 g/day. As there is a variety of types of fibre in food, researchers and nutritionists classify them into two different groups according to their physiological actions in the body.

Soluble fibre

Soluble fibre dissolves in water to form gels. The process of dissolving into a gel slows down digestion. Soluble fibres are found in oat bran, barley, nuts, seeds, legumes, and in some fruits and vegetables. Soluble fibre is commonly linked with reducing the incidence of cardiovascular disease and protecting against diabetes, by reducing blood cholesterol levels and lowering blood glucose levels.

Insoluble fibre

Conversely, insoluble fibre does not dissolve in water and is found in wheat bran, some vegetables and wholegrains. Insoluble fibre absorbs water and expands, adding bulk to stools and speeding its transit through the intestines, thereby promoting bowel movements and ameliorating constipation.

Glycaemic response, index, and load

Glycaemic response

The glycaemic response is defined by the length of time it takes for glucose to be absorbed from foods that have been consumed, regardless of whether the foods contain disaccharides or polysaccharides. A low glycaemic response indicates that the glucose is slowly absorbed over a longer period of time, resulting in a steady and modest rise in blood glucose levels after consumption of the food. A high glycaemic response indicates that the glucose is absorbed more quickly and that there is a sharp immediate rise in blood glucose levels. Other factors in food that will affect the glycaemic response, through their ability to delay or enhance the absorption of glucose, include:

- fat content (delays gastric emptying);
- acid content (delays gastric emptying);
- protein content (delays gastric emptying);
- amount and types of fibre (soluble fibre has a lower glycaemic index than that of insoluble fibre);
- type of starch (depending on the structure of the molecule, which affects the rate of enzyme digestion);

- level of processing (wholegrain bread has a lower glycaemic index than that of whole-meal bread);
- sugar type (fructose and lactose have lower glycaemic index tha n that of glucose).

Glycaemic index

The glycaemic index is a system that ranks foods according to their potential to increase blood glucose levels, relative to the reference food of white bread (which is given a glycaemic index rank of 100). Foods are considered high glycaemic index if they rank above 70, and low glycaemic index if they rank below 55. The glycaemic index of foods is also affected by the level of fat, protein, and fibre in them and, in drinks, the amount of carbonation. As such, it is important to appreciate that the glycaemic index does not always correlate with the overall healthiness of foods, as it does not consider the level of other micronutrients, sugar, and saturated fat. For example, some cola-based soft drinks and sweetened chocolate hazelnut spread have a lower glycaemic index than that of pumpkin, white rice, and couscous.

Glycaemic load

Glycaemic load is a measure that takes into account the amount of carbohydrates in the portion of food consumed, together with the glycaemic index of the food. A large intake of a food with a low glycaemic index could result in a high glycaemic response, compared to consuming a small portion of a high glycaemic index food, which will cause a smaller glycaemic response.

$$\text{Glycaemic load} = \frac{(\text{Glycaemic index} \times \text{amount of available carbohydrate})}{100}$$

As foods are rarely consumed in isolation or in set quantities, the use of the glycaemic load will describe the glycaemic response more accurately. While general health recommendations for the population focus on the selection of foods with a lower glycaemic index to promote satiety and confer health benefits, for the athlete, knowledge of the glycaemic index of foods is also important for implementing nutrition plans to optimise performance. Meals before exercise focus on consuming low glycaemic index foods to enable a sustained release of glucose in the blood. However, during and after exercise, high glycaemic index foods are preferred to promote a quicker glycaemic response, allowing the absorbed glucose to be utilised for performance and to replace lost glucose, respectively.

Satiety

The feeling of fullness and satisfaction after consuming food which inhibits the need to eat.

Recommended intakes of carbohydrates

In Australia, the percentage of energy derived from carbohydrates (CHO) is recommended in the range of 45–65% of total energy, which is the same recommendation in

America and Europe, while the UK recommends 50% of energy intake. For an average person consuming 8700 kJ/day (2000 kcal/day), this equates to 230–330 grams of CHO per day. The recommendation is that carbohydrates should predominantly be derived from wholegrain, low-energy dense sources and/or from low glycaemic index foods. This recommendation is not, however, used to determine the requirement for fuelling exercise and performance for athletes, which will be discussed in Chapter 10.

In 2015, the WHO recommended that free sugar intake should be less than 10% of total energy intake and that further health benefits could be attained with a reduction to less than 5% of dietary energy for adults and children.[6] For adults, this equates to about 20–25 g/day for the average person. Free sugars refer to the monosaccharides and disaccharides added to foods and drinks by the food industry, as well as those incorporated in food preparation at home. It is important to note that this does not include foods that naturally contain these sugars, such as milk, fruit, and some vegetables.

Sugars have been enjoyed in the diet for many centuries, as they provide sweetness and palatability (taste) to many foods; however, in recent years the intake of free or added sugars has increased significantly, leading to excessive intake and undesirable health outcomes. The impact of **hyperglycaemia** on cells and tissues in the body is also cause for concern. It is often difficult for the consumer to ascertain which foods contain sugars, as they assume various names on food labels, including brown sugar, raw sugar, corn sweeteners, corn syrup, dextrose, glucose, maltose, molasses, honey, or high-fructose corn syrup. An indirect impact of eating large amounts of added sugars is that they may replace other nutrient-rich foods and result in nutrient deficiencies. Foods such as lollies, cakes, biscuits, doughnuts, muffins and chocolate, and drinks such as sports drinks, soft drinks, and fruit drinks, all have high amounts of added sugar with few other nutrients in them, so they are referred to as **nutrient-poor**. Of particular concern for the athlete is the quantity of sports drinks they may consume to enhance exercise performance, in terms of both general and dental health. Even, if they are 'rinsing and spitting', the sugar will stay in contact with their teeth for a period of time and can have a direct impact on the development of dental cavities.

Hyperglycaemia

Elevated blood glucose levels.

Nutrient-poor

A food or meal that has a low content of nutrients relative to energy content.

Alcohol

Although consumed by some in the diet, alcohol is defined as a drug since it affects brain function. While alcohol can have some potential health benefits at low to moderate intakes, the harmful effects of alcohol, including accidental deaths, violence, and motor vehicle accidents, generally outweigh any benefit. WHO reports that alcohol is involved with the death of 3 million people annually, and responsible for 5.1% of the global burden of disease. Therefore, any potential health benefit of alcohol must be considered against the risk it poses to individuals and society. It is included in this chapter as it is a macronutrient, providing energy to the body (29 kJ/g or 7 kcal/g); however, it is not necessary to include it when planning diets and nutritional intakes for people, including athletes, due to the negative health and performance effects (discussed below).

Chemistry of alcohol

From the chemist's perspective, alcohol refers to compounds containing a hydroxyl group (–OH), which include methanol, ethanol, isopropyl alcohol, glycerol, butanol, and pentanol. However, for most people, the term 'alcohol' is used to describe alcoholic beverages containing ethanol.

Alcohol (ethanol or ethyl alcohol) is a two-carbon compound, with five hydrogen and one hydroxyl group attached (C_2H_5OH). Alcohol is normally consumed in alcoholic beverages, and the addition of any added sugars and fats along with the percentage of alcohol must therefore be considered when determining the kilojoules consumed. A standard drink—regardless of the concentration of ethanol it contains—is defined as containing 10 grams of alcohol.

Metabolism of alcohol

Ethanol is readily absorbed in the jejunum and is one of the few substances that is absorbed from the stomach. It is distributed evenly throughout the body fluids, as it moves across cellular membranes, including the blood–brain barrier, breast, and placenta. As such, blood and all organ systems (including the brain, breast milk, and the foetus) reach a peak concentration of alcohol very quickly after consumption. Most alcohol is metabolised in the liver, although a small percentage is metabolised as it passes through the stomach wall, which is known as first-pass metabolism. A small amount of alcohol is passed through the urine and some is excreted in the breath, which is why breath testing can be used to detect blood alcohol levels.

Alcohol can be metabolised via three pathways.[8] The major pathway is through alcohol dehydrogenase in the liver. Ethanol is converted to acetaldehyde, followed by the conversion of acetaldehyde to acetic acid by aldehyde dehydrogenase. The lack of this enzyme in some people leads to alcohol flush reaction (Asian flush), which is characterised by facial flushing, light-headedness, palpitations, and nausea.

The second pathway for ethanol metabolism occurs in the smooth endoplasmic reticulum (ER) system and is referred to as the microsomal ethanol-oxidising system (MEOS) with cytochrome P450. The microsomes are induced in the ER after chronic alcohol consumption and, like alcohol dehydrogenase, ethanol is converted to acetaldehyde.

The third pathway for the metabolism of ethanol to acetaldehyde is through an enzyme called catalase; however, this is a very minor pathway, unless alcohol is consumed in a fasted state.

Health effects of alcohol

Ethanol is a depressant of the brain and nerve tissues (central nervous system) and affects several neurochemical processes, leading to an increased risk of suffering mental health problems, including alcohol dependence, depression, and anxiety. Alcohol also impacts on other physiological processes in the body. Alcohol increases the risk of developing several chronic diseases (high blood pressure, cardiovascular disease, and liver disease) as well as certain cancers (mouth, throat, oesophageal, liver, colorectal, and breast). Importantly, if consumed as part of after-game celebrations, alcohol can limit athletes' ability to adhere to nutrition recovery plans (see Chapter 11).

Alcohol recommendations

Since alcohol does not provide any essential nutrients, and because it is also a drug, it is not listed in the nutrient reference recommendations. In Australia, the NHMRC has provided guidelines for consumption, which balance the health risks with any benefits. Healthy adults should drink no more than 10 standard drinks a week, and no more than four standard drinks on any one day to reduce the risk of harm from alcohol. The less you drink, the lower the risk of harm. Children and people under 18 years of age should not drink alcohol to reduce the risk of harm from alcohol. For women who are pregnant or planning a pregnancy or breastfeeding, they should not drink alcohol to prevent harm from alcohol to their unborn child or baby.

In 2022, the American Cancer Society listed acetaldehyde (a metabolite of alcohol consumption) as a known cancer-causing agent and the World Cancer Fund recommended there was no safe level of intake.[1, 5] In 2022, Canada's guidance on alcohol and health recommends drinking two standard drinks or less per week so that you are likely to avoid alcohol-related consequences for yourself and others.[2]

Summary

This chapter has explained how the macronutrients, protein, fat, and carbohydrate, play a key role in nutrition. They are metabolised to provide energy for the body and act as building blocks for cells, tissues, and organs, and/or are precursors to essential hormones, immune mediators, and enzymes. Alcohol, which provides energy, is not strictly considered a macronutrient as it also has drug-like properties in the body and can negatively affect health as well as sporting performance. While this chapter provides the background on macronutrients, it is important to remember that people eat food, not nutrients; the application of this nutritional information to food is presented in Chapter 6.

Chapter highlights

- Protein, fat, and carbohydrate are referred to as macronutrients, which provide energy.
  - Protein 17 kJ/g (4 kcal/g)
  - Carbohydrate 17 kJ/g (4 kcal/g)
  - Fat 37 kJ/g (9 kcal/g)
- Both protein and fat contain essential elements required to sustain life: the essential amino acids and essential fatty acids, respectively, as well as other essential vitamins.
- Amino acids are the building blocks of muscles, organs, hormones, enzymes, and inflammatory mediators.
- Lipids (fats, triglycerides, and cholesterol) are also the precursors to sex hormones and Vitamin D. Fatty acids form an integral part of the cellular phospholipid bilayer in cells.

- Carbohydrates are an important source of glucose for exercise and performance but also supply essential B-group vitamins and fibre.
- While alcohol provides energy, it is not recommended due to its deleterious health effects and impact on training and performance for athletes.
- For athletes, these requirements need to be modified according to the athlete's training and competition schedule.

References

1. American Society. *Known and probable carcinogens.* https://www.cancer.org/healthy/cancer-causes/general-info/known-and-probable-human-carcinogens.html
2. Canadian Centre on Substance Abuse. *Canada's guidance on alcohol and health.* https://ccsa.ca/canadas-guidance-alcohol-and-health
3. Dehghan M, Mente A, Zhang X. Associations of fats and carbohydrate intake with cardiovascular disease and mortality in 18 countries from five continents (PURE): A prospective cohort study. *Lancet.* 2017;390(10107):20150–20162.
4. Fowler SP, Williams K, Resendez RG. Fueling the obesity epidemic? Artificially sweetened beverage use and long-term weight gain. *Obesity.* 2008;16(8):1894–1900.
5. World Cancer Research Fund International. *Alcoholic drinks and cancer risk.* https://www.wcrf.org/diet-activity-and-cancer/risk-factors/alcoholic-drinks-and-cancer-risk/
6. World Health Organization. *Guideline: Sugar intake for adults and children.* Geneva: World Health Organization; 2015.
7. World Health Organization. *Use of non-sugar sweeteners: WHO guideline.* Geneva: World Health Organization; 2023.
8. Zakhari S. Overview: How is alcohol metabolized in the body? *Alcohol Res Health.* 2006; 29(4):245–254.

5   Micronutrients and antioxidants

Gina Trakman

Micronutrients are substances that humans need in small quantities for normal physiological function. Micronutrients have roles in almost every human body system; they are required for energy metabolism, nervous system function, bone and teeth health, blood health, eye health, fluid balance, and as antioxidants. This chapter looks at the interactive roles (related to athletic training and performance) of micronutrients, athletes' micronutrient requirements, the effect of micronutrient deficiency on athletic performance and the relationship between oxidative stress, antioxidants/phytonutrients, and exercise.

Learning outcomes

This chapter will:

- describe the functions, that are relevant to health, athletic performance, and training, of B-group vitamins, vitamin D, calcium, sodium, potassium, chloride, iron, folate, magnesium, and zinc;
- identify common micronutrient deficiencies among athletes and outline the impact of micronutrient deficiencies on athletic performance;
- identify food sources of micronutrients of concern for athletes;
- explain the mechanisms that influence iron absorption in athletes;
- define and describe the implications of oxidative stress for athletic performance;
- identify common antioxidants and phytonutrients and discuss whether athletes should use antioxidant or phytonutrient supplements.

Micronutrients

Water soluble

Compounds that can be dissolved in water and are found in the aqueous parts of the body (or food). Water-soluble vitamins are not stored in the body; they are excreted in the urine.

It is important to consume micronutrients in the correct amount via the diet (Figure 5.1) because deficiencies and excesses in intake can negatively affect general health. There are

DOI: 10.4324/9781003321286-6

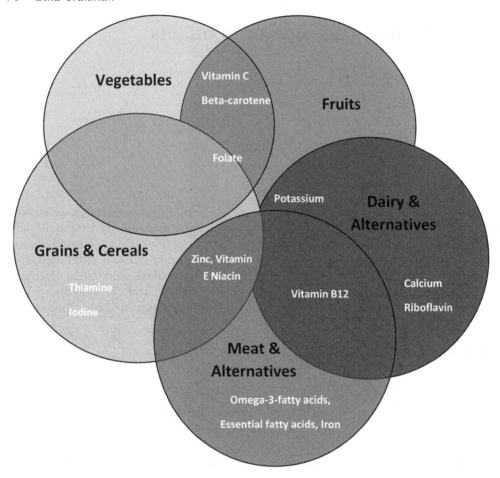

Figure 5.1 Food sources of micronutrients.

Source: Gina Trakman.

two types of micronutrients—vitamins and minerals. Vitamins are organic compounds—they are classed as **water-soluble** (B-group vitamins and vitamin C) or **fat-soluble** (A, D, E, K). Minerals are inorganic chemical elements (such as magnesium) or compounds of elements (such as sodium chloride). Minerals are grouped based on the quantities that they are required in by the body. The recommended intake for the macrominerals (calcium, chloride, magnesium, phosphorus, potassium, sodium, sulphur) exceeds 100 micrograms per day. Microminerals (copper, iron, zinc, molybdenum, manganese, selenium, fluoride) are needed in smaller amounts.

Fat soluble

Compounds that can be dissolved in lipids (fats or oils) and are found in the lipids of the body (or food). Fat-soluble vitamins are stored in the body.

Determining micronutrient requirements

Exercise can lead to increased micronutrient utilisation and degradation, as well as losses of minerals in sweat and urine. Athletes also often have high lean muscle mass and, therefore, may need extra micronutrients for muscle repair and maintenance.[1] However, there is insufficient evidence to set specific nutrient recommendations for active individuals and athletes' dietary intake is generally assessed against population-based guidelines, such as the Food and Agricultural Organization (FAO)/World Health Organization (WHO) vitamin and mineral requirements in human nutrition (international), the Dietary Reference Intakes (Canada and America), the European Food Safety Authority Dietary Reference Values, and the National Healthy and Medical Research Council (NHMRC) Nutrient Reference Values for Australia and New Zealand. The recommended intakes listed in these guidelines are usually set to cover the needs of the majority (98%) of the healthy population and, therefore, overestimate the needs of almost all healthy people, meaning general micronutrient recommendations may cover the potentially increased requirements of athletes. Further, athletes have high energy needs and can usually avoid nutrient deficiencies by eating balanced, nutritious diets that meet their increased energy needs. Circumstances in which athletes' needs may differ from the general population and where they are at risk of deficiency are discussed in more detail throughout this chapter.

B vitamins, iodine, chromium, and energy metabolism

Many of the B vitamins (thiamin, riboflavin, niacin, pantothenic acid, vitamin B_6, and biotin) are needed for energy production, protein and fatty acid synthesis, and carbohydrate metabolism. Several B-vitamins are cofactors in the Krebs cycle, a series of chemical reactions that results in the release of chemical energy (and carbon dioxide). The minerals iodine, chromium, and iron are also involved in energy metabolism. Iodine is a structural component of thyroid hormones, responsible for the regulation of growth, development, and metabolic rate, and chromium is required for insulin function and glucose metabolism.

During exercise, skeletal muscle's use of energy increases up to a hundredfold.[1] In fact, thiamin and riboflavin requirements are sometimes reported as 'micrograms per 100 kilocalories', because of their importance in energy production.[2] Since B vitamins are widely distributed throughout foods (Figure 5.1), most athletes can achieve adequate intakes provided they eat a balanced diet. However, deficiencies in riboflavin and vitamin B_6 have been reported in female athletes who are vegetarian or have eating disorders.

Mild riboflavin and vitamin B_6 deficiencies do not appear to lead to diminished aerobic capacity. Despite the lack of evidence for their efficacy, B vitamin supplements are often marketed to active individuals, with claims that they are required in 'times of physical stress' to support energy production and reduce fatigue. Supplementation is unlikely to be harmful because B vitamins are water-soluble and thus are excreted in urine. However, athletes should be aware that extreme intakes of vitamin B_6 via supplementation can lead to sensory neuropathy; niacin can reach toxic levels, causing itchy, red or warm skin, dizziness, leg cramps, muscle pain and insomnia; and excess folate supplementation can mask vitamin B_{12} deficiencies.

Calcium, Vitamin D, and bone health

Calcium is a structural component of bone. It combines with phosphorus to form hydroxyapatite, a hard, crystalline structure that gives bones their strength. Vitamin D increases the absorption of calcium and phosphorus from the gut. Magnesium and fluoride also play a role in mineralising bones. Finally, several proteins associated with bone turnover (for example, osteocalcin) require vitamin K for their synthesis. One of the best dietary sources of calcium is the dairy food group, such as milk, cheese, and yoghurt. Phosphorus is found in most foods that are high in protein. Small amounts of vitamin D are also found in dairy, eggs, mushrooms, and fortified margarine; however, to achieve adequate levels of vitamin D, appropriate exposure to sunlight is needed. Vitamin D exists on the skin as 7-dehydrocholesterol, which is activated upon exposure to ultraviolet B (UVB) rays. Sun exposure recommendations vary depending on the season, time of day, proximity to the equator, age, the amount of skin exposed and Fitzpatrick skin phototype.[3] To achieve adequate Vitamin D status, in winter, in areas such as the UK and Norway, as much as 40 minutes to 2 hours of sun exposure per day may be required,[4] while just 6 minutes per day would be sufficient for a light-skinned person during summer in the north-east of Australia.[5]

Regular exercise (especially resistance activity) increases bone density by stimulating bone-building mechanisms. However, overtraining is known to decrease the production of the sex hormone oestrogen, which plays a vital role in maintaining bone mass, especially in females. Low bone mass and density will increase the risk of stress fractures and thus can have a detrimental effect on an athlete's ability to perform. Female athletes with eating disorders are at particular risk of stress fractures because their calcium intake is likely to be low, and it is probable that they have menstrual dysfunction, which is associated with decreased oestrogen production.[6]

Calcium status is difficult to measure because the bone acts as a calcium reservoir and serum calcium levels are maintained within a relatively small window. So, it is important to ensure an adequate intake of calcium to supply the body's calcium needs and limit the loss of calcium from bones. Vitamin D status is measured based on circulating levels of 25-hydroxycholecalciferol (25(OH) D). Cut-off points for deficiency vary (see Table 5.1).

Vitamin D deficiency appears to be widespread among athletes and non-athletes, with 24%, 23%, 37%, and 40% of the populations in the US, Australia, Canada, and Europe, respectively, reported to have sub-optimal serum Vitamin D levels and >20% of the population in India, Tunisia, Pakistan, and Afghanistan reported to have a mild-to-moderate Vitamin D deficiency.[7] Data specifically related to athletes is limited. In general, the athletes at the greatest risk of vitamin D deficiency are those with dark skin, those who compete indoors, and those who live at high altitudes. All athletes with diagnosed deficiency should take a vitamin D supplement as prescribed by their doctor or dietitian.[8] It is also recommended that (pending nutritional assessment) athletes with disordered

Table 5.1 Vitamin D status based on serum 25(OH)D (nmol/L) levels

Reference	*Vitamin D Status: 25(OH) D levels (nmol/L)*
Sports medicine[8]	Sufficient: 100 Insufficient: 50–80 Marginal Deficiency: 25–50
General population[5]	Adequate: >50 Mild deficiency: 30–49 Moderate deficiency: 13–29 Severe deficiency: <13

eating and **amenorrhea** supplement their diet with 1500 micrograms of calcium and 400–800 International Units (IU) of vitamin D per day.

Amenorrhea

The absence or cessation of menstruation. Primary amenorrhea is defined as the failure to reach menarche, often characterised by a delay in the first menstrual period beyond 15 years of age. Secondary amenorrhea is defined as the absence of 3–6 consecutive menstrual periods.

Calcium and Vitamin D: Other roles

Calcium has additional roles in muscle contraction, nerve conduction and blood clotting. Emerging evidence indicates that vitamin D also has a role in muscle tissue function. The discovery of a vitamin D receptor in skeletal muscle provided a biologically plausible explanation for observations that athletic performance improves in the summer and with exposure to UVB radiation. More recent research has shown that vitamin D status is correlated with jumping height and velocity, muscle strength, and muscle power. However, at present, there is insufficient evidence to set an 'optimal' level for Serum 25(OH) D for athletes or to recommend vitamin D as an **ergogenic aid**.[8]

Ergogenic aid

Any substance or aid that improves physical performance.

Iron, Vitamin B$_{12}$, folate, and blood health

Iron is a structural component of **haemoglobin,** a protein in red blood cells that is responsible for the transport of oxygen to tissues. Iron is also a cofactor for enzymes that participate in the electron transport chain, a series of reactions that are needed for the synthesis of ATP, the body's energy carrier (see Chapter 2). Given its role in energy production and cell metabolism, it is clear that iron is an essential nutrient for athletes, especially endurance athletes. Iron losses of athletes can be more than 70% higher than those in the general population.[9] Requirements, however, are often not met. **Iron deficiency anaemia** (IDA) is the most common nutrient deficiency among the general population and athletes with around 15–35% of female athletes and 5–11% of male athletes having iron deficiency.[10] Athletes who are at particular risk of iron deficiency include:

- athletes consuming energy-restricted diets (low iron consumption);
- adolescent athletes (periods of rapid growth increase iron needs);
- vegetarian athletes (plant sources of iron are poorly absorbed);
- female athletes who are menstruating (iron is excreted through blood loss);
- athletes who undertake altitude training (increased production of red blood cells requires iron, along with other nutrients such as vitamin B$_{12}$ and folate);
- endurance athletes, especially runners (pounding the pavement destroys red blood cells, often described as 'foot strike **haemolysis**');

- athletes who are injured (iron is needed for wound healing);
- athletes who donate blood.

Iron losses in urine, sweat, and via gastrointestinal bleeding have also been suggested to contribute to IDA in athletes. In addition, there has been a growing interest in the influence of exercise on iron regulation via the hormone hepcidin (see Box 5.1).

Box 5.1   Exercise and hormonal regulation of iron[10, 11]

- Hepcidin is a protein made in the liver that regulates the release of iron from the intestines, special immune cells (erythrocyte-recycling macrophages), and liver cells into plasma. Hepcidin levels are lowest in the morning and increase throughout the day.
- When hepcidin levels are high, iron absorption and recycling are reduced, leading to lower plasma iron levels.
- Hepcidin levels are increased by inflammation. Accordingly, the exercise-initiated inflammatory response leads to high hepcidin levels. This effect is temporary and typically occurs in the three to six hours after exercise.
- Low-carbohydrate diets also increase inflammatory markers and therefore exacerbate exercise-induced increases in hepcidin, with some studies showing athletes on a low-carbohydrate high-fat diet have greater increases in hepcidin than those on a carbohydrate-rich diet.
- Post-exercise increases in hepcidin may be less in those with already low plasma iron levels, but the type and intensity of exercise are not likely to have an impact.
- The sex hormones oestrogen and testosterone can reduce hepcidin levels. Low energy availability can lead to reduced levels of sex hormones; therefore, athletes experiencing low energy availability may be at increased risk of iron deficiency for reasons not directly related to inadequate dietary intake.

Athletes will likely benefit from consuming iron-rich foods and oral iron supplements outside the window where iron absorption is compromised (i.e., three hours after exercise and in the evening).

Haemoglobin

The protein unit in the red blood cell that carries oxygen.

Iron deficiency anaemia

Depletion of iron levels in the blood that leads to low levels of haemoglobin and small pale red blood cells, which limits their capacity to carry oxygen.

Haemolysis

The rupture of red blood cells.

There are a range of biomarkers used to assess iron status, including total iron binding capacity (TIBC), serum ferritin (SF), transferrin saturation, haemoglobin (Hb), and mean cell volume (MCV). Iron depletion occurs in three stages, as depicted in Figure 5.2.

Iron is carried around the blood by a protein called **transferrin**; when blood iron stores are low, TIBC increases so that transferrin can bind to more of the available iron and, at the same time, SF levels drop. When transferrin saturation (serum iron/TIBC) is below 16%, the body experiences early functional iron deficiency. If iron deficiency progresses further, the body is unable to make haemoglobin and the MCV of red blood cells decreases, leading to iron deficiency anaemia (IDA).

Transferrin

An iron transport protein in the blood.

Work capacity

The total amount of work a person can sustain over a defined period of time.

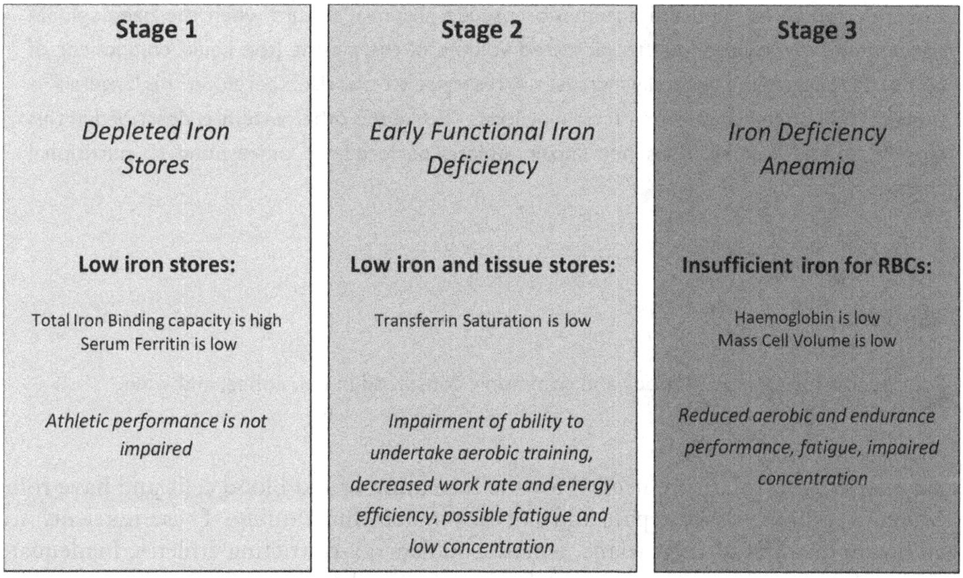

Stage 1	Stage 2	Stage 3
Depleted Iron Stores	*Early Functional Iron Deficiency*	*Iron Deficiency Aneamia*
Low iron stores:	**Low iron and tissue stores:**	**Insufficient iron for RBCs:**
Total Iron Binding capacity is high Serum Ferritin is low	Transferrin Saturation is low	Haemoglobin is low Mass Cell Volume is low
Athletic performance is not impaired	*Impairment of ability to undertake aerobic training, decreased work rate and energy efficiency, possible fatigue and low concentration*	*Reduced aerobic and endurance performance, fatigue, impaired concentration*

Figure 5.2 Stages of iron deficiency

The final 'stage' of iron deficiency, IDA, has detrimental effects on athletic performance, and aerobic performance in particular, and also impacts concentration and, therefore, the ability to make tactical decisions during play.[10] Correction of IDA with supplements increases **work capacity**, reduces heart rate, and decreases lactate concentrations.[10] While stage 1 and stage 2 iron deficiency have not consistently been shown to impact athletic performance, they can lead to lethargy and mood disturbance, which may impact an athlete's ability to train properly. Supplementation in individuals with early functional iron deficiency (stage 2) may improve performance, but research findings are mixed.[12] Reversing iron deficiency via oral iron supplementation can take up to three months and oral iron supplements are often poorly absorbed and cause gastrointestinal upset. Strategies to improve tolerance include trialling different forms of iron and using alternate-day iron supplementation protocols.[13] Transdermal iron patches have not been shown to improve iron status in athletes.[14] In some individuals, iron infusions, which rapidly correct haematological markers of iron status, may be preferred.

The ideal scenario is to prevent iron deficiency from developing. In this context, at-risk athletes should be regularly screened (via blood tests). Consideration must be given to factors that can influence ferritin, plasma iron, and Hb, such as exercise-induced inflammation, high blood volume due to training and heat adaptations, time of day, and hydration status (see **sports anaemia**). In addition to regular monitoring, athletes should focus on preventing the development of IDA by obtaining adequate iron from foods. Red meat, chicken, fish, and eggs are the best dietary sources of iron. Wholegrains, leafy greens, nuts, and seeds also provide some iron. These vegetarian sources should be combined with vitamin C to increase absorption. Consumption of **tannins** and calcium should be avoided when eating iron-rich foods because they inhibit iron absorption.

Sports anaemia

Also referred to as dilutional anaemia or pseudo-anaemia, occurs when the haemoglobin concentration is 'diluted' due to increased volume of the plasma (the liquid component of blood). Plasma volume generally increases in response to exercise; therefore, this 'anaemia' is transient and often fluctuates with training loads. Unlike the other anaemias described in this chapter, sports anaemia does not impair athletic performance or respond to nutritional changes.

Tannins

Polyphenols found in plant foods and commonly consumed in tea, coffee, and wine.

Vitamin B_{12} and folate are needed for the formation of red blood cells and have roles in protein synthesis, tissue repair and nervous system functioning. These nutrients are often low in the diets of vegetarians, females, and energy-restricting athletes. Inadequate intake of folate and vitamin B_{12} will lead to folate deficiency anaemia and vitamin B_{12} deficiency anaemia respectively. These anaemias are also associated with decreased endurance performance.[2] Folate is found in green leafy vegetables and wholegrains; vitamin B_{12} is found exclusively in animal foods—meat, chicken, fish, eggs, and dairy.

Zinc and magnesium

Zinc and magnesium are cofactors for several enzymes involved in energy metabolism. Zinc also has roles in growth, building, and repairing muscle tissue, and in immune status—all relevant functions for athletes. Magnesium is needed for immune function, protein synthesis and muscle contraction. Athletes may experience magnesium and zinc loss through sweat, urine, and faeces, but mineral losses are difficult to measure accurately. Endurance athletes have been found to have impaired zinc status in several studies.[2] Magnesium deficiencies have also been reported amongst athletes, although the magnesium status of athletes and non-athletes is similar, indicating that increased physical activity may not drive magnesium deficiency. Both zinc and magnesium deficiencies occur predominantly among vegetarian, female, and weight-class athletes. Zinc deficiency can impair athletic performance by reducing cardiorespiratory function, muscle strength, and endurance. Likewise, magnesium deficiency has been reported to increase oxygen requirements for performing submaximal activities.[15]

Magnesium supplementation to correct pre-existing deficiencies has been shown to improve performance. On the other hand, there is limited data to confirm the beneficial effect of zinc supplementation on performance. Zinc may have an indirect effect because it has been shown to enhance immune function and, therefore, could protect athletes' ability to train.[16] In general, however, single-dose zinc supplements are not recommended because they can interfere with the absorption of iron and calcium and lead to zinc **toxicity**.

Toxicity

Occurs when nutrients are consumed in very high amounts and cause health problems. For example, very high levels of vitamin A consumed by pregnant women have been linked to birth defects. Toxicity is most likely to occur with overconsumption of fat-soluble vitamins and some minerals.

Potassium, sodium, chloride, and fluid balance

Sodium is the main **cation** in extracellular fluid, potassium is the main cation in intracellular fluid, and chloride is the main **anion** in intracellular fluid. Together, these **electrolytes** maintain fluid balance. Sodium and phosphorus also act to ensure acid–base balance of body fluids and both sodium and potassium have additional roles in nerve-impulse transmission and muscle contraction. Athletes experience electrolyte losses through sweat and, therefore, have higher sodium and chloride needs than the general population.[15]

Cations

Positively charged ions, which means they have gained electrons.

Anions

Negatively charged ions, which means they have lost electrons.

Electrolytes

Salts that dissolve in water and disassociate into charged particles called ions.

Sodium and chloride are often found together in foods as sodium chloride (salt). Table salt, soy sauce, and other commercial sauces, processed foods, meat, milk, and bread are all sources of sodium chloride. The estimated global daily mean sodium intake is almost double the FAO/WHO recommendations of 2.0 g/day.[17] Therefore, many athletes would meet their increased salt needs incidentally. However, for athletes participating in endurance events, sports drinks containing electrolytes are frequently recommended. This is discussed in more detail in Chapter 11. Most athletes can meet their potassium needs through regular food intake by including potassium-rich foods such as fruit, vegetables, and dairy.

Antioxidants

Pathogenesis

The biological mechanism that leads to the development of diseases.

Antioxidants prevent **oxidative stress** and have been extensively studied for their potential ability to reduce the **pathogenesis** of many chronic diseases. Vitamin C (found in fruits and vegetables) and vitamin E (found in oils, nuts, seeds, and wheat germ) have antioxidant functions. Vitamin E is fat-soluble and, therefore, acts within cell membranes to prevent polyunsaturated fatty acids (PUFAs) and other phospholipids from being oxidised. After vitamin E has performed its antioxidant function, it will have an unpaired electron; Vitamin C regenerates vitamin E by donating an electron to (re) neutralise vitamin E.

Phytonutrients, found in plant foods, also have antioxidant functions. Common phytonutrients include:

- anthocyanins (found in tart cherries/Montmorency cherries);
- beta-carotene (found in orange and green fruits and vegetables);
- curcumin (found in turmeric);
- isoflavones (found in soy);
- lycopene (found in tomatoes);
- resveratrol (found in grapes and wine);
- quercetin (found in fruits and vegetables).

Antioxidants

Substances that decrease **free radical** damage by donating an electron to 'neutralise' free radicals.

Free radicals

Also referred to as reactive oxygen species, free radicals are highly reactive chemical species that can damage cellular components, resulting in cell injury or death. They are usually produced by oxidation and contain an unpaired electron.

Oxidative stress

Occurs when the body's production of free radicals occurs at a rate higher than the body's ability to neutralise them.

In addition to these food sources, the body has several **endogenous** antioxidant systems. The mineral selenium and the amino acids cysteine and taurine have roles in these systems, as donors for thiol-based antioxidants.

Endogenous

Substances that originate or derive from within the body, in this case from body stores.

Antioxidants and specific phytonutrient supplements are popular among athletes, but their use is controversial. The arguments and evidence for and against antioxidants and phytonutrient supplementation in athletes are outlined in Table 5.2.

In addition to being studied for their potential to reduce oxidative stress, the effect of antioxidant supplementation on performance and recovery has been assessed. There is limited evidence to support their use in these situations.

Although there are varying opinions on the utility of antioxidant supplements, diets rich in antioxidants and phytonutrients are encouraged by most experts because these compounds have a role in immune function and eye health and are associated with reduced incidence of several non-communicable diseases, including cancer and cardio-vascular disease. Antioxidants and phytonutrients commonly co-occur with each other and with micronutrients in minimally processed, whole plant foods, and choosing these foods over isolated antioxidant or phytonutrient supplements is likely to offer greater benefits in terms of improving athletic performance and recovery, disease prevention and general dietary adequacy.

Practical tips for increasing antioxidants and phytonutrients include:

- Aim to have two servings of fruit and five servings of vegetables daily. Add fruit to breakfast cereals and choose it as a snack. Add vegetables to main meals (grate into sauces, put on sandwiches) and snack on cherry tomatoes, carrots, celery, and cucumber;
- Choose whole grains over processed grains;
- Swap some meat/chicken/fish meals for tofu and legumes;
- Snack on nuts;
- Choose dark chocolate as a sweet treat.

Table 5.2 Arguments for and against antioxidant and phytonutrients supplementation

Expert Body	Argument		Evidence
The International Society of Sports Nutrition (ISSN)[15]	Yes	• Exercise increases oxygen consumption and has been shown to damage molecules in blood and skeletal muscle. • Athletes often have poor diets and consume inadequate amounts of antioxidant-rich foods.	"Vitamins C and E may decrease oxidative damage caused by vigorous training schedules and may also help support a healthy immune system"
The Australian Institute of Sport (AIS)[18]	Maybe	• The amount of free radicals produced increases with exercise intensity, duration of exercise, in hot environments, and at high altitudes. Overtraining can lead to chronic oxidative stress, which has been associated with chronic fatigue, team performance decrements, muscle atrophy, and illness	Polyphenols, Quercetin, Tart cherry juice, exotic berries, curcumin, and antioxidants vitamins E and C are listed as category B supplements, which indicates that they are "Deserving of further research and could be considered for provision to athletes under a research protocol or case-managed monitoring situation"
The American College of Sports Medicine (ACSM)[19]	No	• Regular physical activity up-regulates the body's endogenous antioxidant systems, and thus aids in fighting free radical damage. • There is insufficient evidence to support antioxidant supplementation for general health. • The presence of free radicals leads to the expression of skeletal muscle proteins that result in positive adaptations to training; high-dose supplementation can blunt these adaptations.	"…The current literature does not support antioxidant supplementation as means to prevent exercise-induced oxidative stress"
The International Olympic Committee (IOC)[8]	No		"…athletes should not use antioxidant supplements but should focus on consuming a well-balanced, energetically adequate diet that is rich in anti-oxidant containing foods"

Phytonutrients (also known as phytochemicals)

Naturally occurring chemicals that plants produce to protect themselves from damage by insects and microorganisms. Phytonutrients have purported beneficial effects on human health, including supporting immune function and reducing cancer risk.

Summary

This chapter has provided an overview of micronutrient requirements for athletes. Micronutrients and antioxidants are needed in small amounts for normal physiological functioning. They are distributed throughout the food supply and have roles relevant to athletic performance, including energy production, maintenance of bone health, control of fluid balance, muscle contraction, nerve impulse control, and balancing oxidative stress in the body (see Table 5.3). Although athletes have increased needs for certain micronutrients, athlete-specific, quantitative micronutrient recommendations do not exist, and recommendations for the general population are used to plan athletes' micronutrient intakes. Athletes with low energy intakes or other risk factors for nutrient deficiency should be monitored. Where nutrient deficiencies are confirmed, they should be addressed through changes to dietary intake and prudent use of dietary supplements supervised by a medical or nutrition professional. Correction of deficiency can improve performance, but micronutrient intakes above physiological requirements are unlikely to offer ergogenic benefits. Some experts argue that antioxidant supplements may enhance recovery from

Table 5.3 Summary of functional roles of micronutrients related to athletic performance

Function	*Micronutrient*
Energy, macronutrient metabolism, and macronutrient synthesis	Thiamin (B_1) Riboflavin (B_2) Niacin (B_3) Pantothenic acid (B_5) Biotin Pyridoxine (B_6) Iodine Chromium Iron Zinc Magnesium
Muscle contraction	Magnesium Sodium
Fluid balance	Sodium Potassium Chloride Phosphorus
Bone health	Vitamin D Vitamin K Calcium Phosphorus Magnesium
Blood health	Vitamin B_{12} Vitamin K Iron Folate
Immune function	Vitamin C Iron Zinc

exercise by reducing oxidative stress, but others caution that these should be avoided due to potential adverse effects on adaptations to training.

Chapter highlights

- There is insufficient evidence to set specific quantitative micronutrient recommendations for athletes which differ from the general recommendations.
- Athletes have increased needs for iron, sodium, and potassium and may also have increased B vitamin, magnesium, and zinc requirements, but this is yet to be demonstrated in research studies.
- Most athletes can meet their micronutrient needs by consuming a balanced diet that contains adequate energy.
- Certain athletes are at risk of nutrient deficiency. Common risk factors include being female, being vegetarian, participating in endurance activities, consuming an energy-restricted diet, and having disordered eating behaviours.
- The most common deficiency among athletes is iron deficiency; endurance athletes are at high risk of developing iron deficiency due to inadequate dietary intake, increased iron losses, and the impact of intense exercise on hepcidin, a hormonal regulator of iron levels.
- Low serum levels of magnesium, zinc, and vitamin D, and low intakes of riboflavin and vitamin B_6 are also reported among athletic populations.
- Deficiencies should be addressed by altering dietary intake. In most instances, micronutrient supplementation is also warranted and has been shown to improve performance. Supplementation should be based on blood test results and nutritional analysis and be supervised by qualified professionals.
- Micronutrient intakes (through food or supplements) above physiological requirements are very unlikely to have any ergogenic effects.
- Antioxidants, phytonutrient supplements (vitamins A, C, and E and selenium), and food polyphenols have received much attention for their potential ability to enhance recovery from exercise by reducing oxidative stress. At present, there is a lack of consensus on antioxidant supplementation.

References

1. Woolf K, Manore MM. B-vitamins and exercise: does exercise alter requirements? *Int J Sport Nutr Exerc Metab.* 2006;16(5):453–84.
2. Lukaski HC. Vitamin and mineral status: effects on physical performance. *Nutrition.* 2004;20(7–8):632–44.
3. Gilchrest BA. Sun exposure and vitamin D sufficiency. *Am J Clin Nutr.* 2008;88(2):570S–7S.
4. Kift R, Rhodes LE, Farrar MD, et al. Is sunlight exposure enough to avoid wintertime vitamin D deficiency in United Kingdom population groups? *Int J Env Res Public Health.* 2018;15(8): 1624.
5. Nowson CA, McGrath JJ, Ebeling PR, et al. Vitamin D and health in adults in Australia and New Zealand: a position statement. *Med J Aus.* 2012;196(11):686–7.
6. Sale C, Elliott-Sale KJ. Nutrition and athlete bone health. *Sports Med.* 2019;49(2):139–51.
7. Amrein K, Scherkl M, Hoffmann M, et al. Vitamin D deficiency 2.0: an update on the current status worldwide. *Eur J Clin Nutr.* 2020;74(11):1498–513.
8. Powers, S, Nelson WB, Larson-Meyer E. Antioxidant and Vitamin D supplements for athletes: sense or nonsense? *J Sports Sci.* 2011;29 Suppl 1:S47–55.

9. Hinton PS. Iron and the endurance athlete. *Appl Physiol Nutr Metab.* 2014;39(9):1012–8.

10. Sim M, Garvican-Lewis LA, Cox GR, et al. Iron considerations for the athlete: a narrative review. *Eur J Appl Physiol.* 2019;119(7):1463–78.

11. Ganz T. Hepcidin. *Rinsho Ketsueki.* 2016;57(10):1913–7.

12. Burden RJ, Morton K, Richards T, et al. Is iron treatment beneficial in, iron-deficient but non-anaemic (IDNA) endurance athletes? A systematic review and meta-analysis. *Br J Sports Med.* 2015;49(21):1389–97.

13. McCormick R, Dreyer A, Dawson B, et al. The effectiveness of daily and alternate day oral iron supplementation in athletes with suboptimal iron status (Part 2). *Int J Sport Nutr Exerc Metab.* 2020;30(3):191–6.

14. McCormick R, Dawson B, Sim M, et al. The effectiveness of transdermal iron patches in athletes with suboptimal iron status (Part 1). *Int J Sport Nutr Exerc Metab.* 2020;30(3):185–90.

15. Kerksick CM, Wilborn CD, Roberts MD, et al. ISSN exercise & sports nutrition review update: research & recommendations. *J Int Soc Sports Nutr.* 2018;15(1):38.

16. Kreider RB, Wilborn CD, Taylor L, et al. ISSN exercise & sport nutrition review: research & recommendations. *J Int Soc Sports Nutr.* 2010;7(1):7.

17. World Health Organization. *Guideline: sodium intake for adults and children.* World Health Organization; 2012.

18. Australian Institue of Sport. *AIS sports supplement framework.* Australian Government Australian Sports Commission; 2017.

19. Thomas DT, Erdman KA, Burke LM. Position of the Academy of Nutrition and Dietetics, Dietitians of Canada, and the American College of Sports Medicine: nutrition and athletic performance. *J Acad Nutr Diet.* 2016;116(3):501–28.

6 Translating nutrition
From Nutrients to Foods

Adrienne Forsyth

The preceding chapters provided an overview of the nutrients needed for good health and performance. However, planning a nutritious diet is a complex task because individuals consume nutrients as part of whole foods within the context of a diet influenced by a range of sociocultural, environmental, and individual factors. The factors that influence dietary intake will be discussed in later chapters. This chapter will explore how to meet nutrient requirements through food and identify appropriate food choices to meet the macro- and micronutrient requirements of athletes.

Learning outcomes

This chapter will:

- introduce the rationale for food-based dietary recommendations;
- explore how whole-food diets can be used to meet individual nutrient requirements;
- identify food sources of macro- and micronutrients required by athletes;
- present foods and food combinations to meet individual nutrient requirements.

Food is made up of more than nutrients

Chapters 4 and 5 described the role of a number of nutrients in health and performance. It is tempting to try to put together a magic bullet nutrient supplement to meet these needs. However, consuming nutrient requirements in the form of food provides more than consuming supplements alone.

Synergistic

The interaction of two or more substances, in this case nutrients, to produce a combined beneficial effect that is greater than the sum of its individual effects.

DOI: 10.4324/9781003321286-7

Ischaemic heart disease

Also called coronary artery disease, a group of diseases including angina, myocardial infarction, and sudden coronary death. The pathogenesis of this disease involves the restriction of blood flow in the coronary arteries that results in reduced blood flow, and hence oxygen supply, to the heart muscle.

There are many benefits of consuming nutrients as part of whole foods rather than from supplements. To begin with, some nutrients are absorbed better as part of whole foods. For example, the lactose in milk may assist with calcium absorption. Foods can also have a **synergistic** effect in promoting nutrient absorption and function. When plant sources of iron, such as beans, are consumed with a source of vitamin C, such as citrus fruit, the vitamin C assists with iron absorption and therefore increases iron availability in the body. Many nutrients are also more effective when consumed as part of a whole-food diet. Omega-3 fatty acids derived from eating fish are often found to be more effective in preventing conditions such as **ischaemic heart disease** than omega-3 supplements alone. Whole foods also often bundle nutrients in a convenient package. For example, dairy foods such as milk contain not only calcium but also magnesium and phosphorus, which work with calcium to help build and maintain strong bones. Alongside vitamins and minerals, foods provide a range of other compounds with beneficial actions, such as fibre and phytonutrients. Foods also often conveniently provide nutrients where they are needed. Whole grains are good sources of B vitamins, and B vitamins are needed to derive energy from the carbohydrates in whole grains. Vitamin E is found in plant oils and helps to prevent oxidisation of the oil and minimise damage from free radicals in our bodies. Whole foods also have the added benefit of providing pleasure, creating an opportunity for socialisation, and promoting rest and relaxation during eating. On the other hand, supplements can be expensive, run the risk of toxicity with overconsumption, and may contain unwanted compounds or contaminants, which is particularly problematic for many competitive athletes.

Having established the importance of consuming nutrients as part of a whole-food diet, this chapter will now discuss how foods consumed can meet individual nutrient requirements.

Dietary guidelines

Dietary guidelines are developed by leading health organisations, often national government departments, to help the population make food choices that will meet their dietary requirements and promote good health. Dietary guidelines are presented as a series of food and/or nutrient recommendations, often accompanied by a pictorial guide, that are easy to interpret and adopt with limited nutrition literacy. The guidelines are developed by expert panels based on the analysis of data from published research. As nutrition science continually evolves, so do dietary guidelines. They are reviewed and updated periodically to reflect advances in research, population dietary trends/preferences, changes in the food supply, and other national priorities. Newer guidelines are likely to reflect current literature and recommendations regarding trans fat, salt, sugar, non-nutritive sweeteners, and highly processed foods. Some, including the latest Brazilian and Canadian guidelines, include recommendations for how to eat such as cooking at home and eating with others. They may also incorporate recommendations that support planetary health as well as human health with sustainable dietary choices.

The World Health Organization publishes guidelines, including food and nutrition recommendations, based on high-level evidence that may be used to inform national dietary guidelines.[1] Their healthy diet recommendations for adults are presented in Table 6.1, and readers are encouraged to become familiar with the dietary guidelines in their own country which may be found here: https://www.fao.org/nutrition/education/food-based-dietary-guidelines. Local guidelines are important because they present food-based advice that is reflective of the foods available and commonly consumed in the local context. Sports nutrition professionals may also seek out dietary guidelines for countries where their athletes will be travelling as a starting point to identify food sources of key macronutrients in that region. However, it is important to remember that advice in these guidelines is intended for healthy individuals to maintain good health. Individuals with

Table 6.1 World Health Organization's healthy diet recommendations for adults[1]

Recommendation	Description/notes
Eat fruits, vegetables, legumes (e.g. lentils, beans), nuts, and whole grains (e.g. unprocessed maize, millet, oats, wheat, brown rice) every day.	The recommended daily intake for an adult includes 2 cups of fruit (4 servings), 2.5 cups of vegetables (5 servings), 180 g of grains, and 160 g of meat and beans. Red meat can be eaten 1–2 times per week, and poultry 2–3 times per week.
Eat at least 5 portions of fruit and vegetables a day (at least 400 g).	Potatoes, sweet potatoes, cassava, and other starchy roots are not classified as fruit or vegetables.
Limit total energy intake from free sugars to around 12 level teaspoons (which is equivalent to 50 g) but ideally less than 5% of total energy intake for additional health benefits.	Most free sugars are added to foods or drinks by the manufacturer, cook, or consumer, and can also be found in sugars naturally present in honey, syrups, fruit juices, and fruit juice concentrates.
Limit total energy intake from fats to less than 30%.	Unsaturated fats (e.g. found in fish, avocado, nuts, sunflower, canola, and olive oils) are preferable to saturated fats (e.g. found in fatty meat, butter, palm and coconut oil, cream, cheese, ghee, and lard). Industrially-produced trans fats (found in processed food, fast food, snack food, fried food, frozen pizza, pies, cookies, margarines, and spreads) are not part of a healthy diet.
Limit salt to less than 5 g per day (equivalent to approximately 1 teaspoon) and use iodized salt.	

medical conditions that require specialised medical nutrition therapy should seek advice from a qualified dietitian. Athletes with specific dietary requirements may use the dietary guidelines as a starting point and should seek individualised advice from a sports nutrition professional.

There is also increasing interest in ensuring dietary guidelines promote environmentally sustainable choices. Athletes wanting to make sustainable food choices are encouraged to limit food packaging and food waste, choose seasonal produce, and consider adopting a **flexitarian**, plant-based approach to meet but not exceed protein requirements.[2]

Flexitarian

A flexible alternative to a vegetarian diet. Flexitarian dietary patterns are predominantly plant-based, often include dairy products and eggs, and may occasionally or strategically incorporate other animal food sources such as meat, poultry, and fish.

Where dietary guidelines include food selection guides, i.e., a recommended number of servings from different food groups, it is important for athletes to understand that these have been designed to provide only enough energy to meet the needs of the smallest and least active person. Athletes often expend more energy and therefore have higher energy requirements, so they may need to consume more servings of each of the food groups to meet their energy and nutrient requirements. Personalised eating plans should be developed for individual athletes based on their size, sex, body composition, activity levels, individual preferences, and sport-specific requirements. For example, some athletes may prefer or require more carbohydrate-rich wholegrain foods, while others require or prefer more protein-rich options.

Dietary guidelines are useful tools to guide decision-making about food for the general public and are important for athletes to follow to maintain good health. However, athletes typically have performance, recovery, or body composition goals that are also important to consider when developing an eating plan. Elite athletes looking to gain a performance edge may benefit from an eating plan that considers the amount and timing of food sources of macronutrients and select micronutrients. Other chapters in this book will discuss the timing and amounts of macro- and micronutrients needed to achieve performance, recovery, and body composition goals. This chapter will provide practical recommendations for food sources of macronutrients and key micronutrients.

Food sources of macronutrients

Carbohydrates

The characteristics of carbohydrate-containing foods differ depending on the type of carbohydrate. Foods rich in mono- and disaccharides, often referred to as sugar/s, tend to be sweet.

Sugars can be naturally occurring in food or be added to foods in the form of sucrose, what we commonly refer to as "table sugar". Sugar-containing foods include:

- added sugars in confectionary (candies or lollies);
- naturally occurring sugars in fruit (in the form of fructose);
- naturally occurring sugars in milk (in the form of lactose);
- table sugar, honey, and maple syrup.

Foods rich in polysaccharides, often referred to as starchy foods, include:

- breads, rolls, wraps, bagels, muffins, and crumpets;
- breakfast cereals, oats, and porridge;
- rice, pasta, and noodles;
- potato, sweet potato, and corn.

Some carbohydrate foods provide more nutrition than others. In addition to naturally occurring sugar, fruit also contains fibre and vitamins and milk also contains protein and minerals. Confectionary and other highly processed foods with added sugars can provide enjoyment and increase the palatability of foods but are not health-promoting as they contain no or very little nutrition. Recommended sources of carbohydrates for good health are whole and minimally processed foods, preferably higher fibre options, such as wholegrain bread, brown rice, and potatoes in their skins. For athletes, the timing of fibre intake is important; high-fibre foods may be avoided in the hours leading up to an intense training session to avoid gastrointestinal (GI) discomfort. Some people also experience unpleasant symptoms, such as gas, bloating, constipation, and diarrhoea, after consuming some types of carbohydrates. Strategies for managing GI problems will be discussed in Chapter 15.

Protein

Protein is commonly consumed in animal foods. Meat, poultry, fish, eggs, and dairy products such as milk, cheese, and yoghurt are all sources of protein. However, individuals may limit their intake of animal sources of protein due to the cost, or their personal preference to avoid animal food sources for ethical, environmental, or religious reasons. Animal sources of protein may also contain high levels of saturated fats, but intake of these fats can be minimised by selecting lean cuts of meat, skinless poultry, fish, and reduced-fat dairy products. Nuts, seeds, and legumes such as beans, lentils, and chickpeas are good protein-containing food options for vegetarian athletes and those looking for lower-fat or less expensive sources of protein. It is important to keep in mind that vegetable sources of protein are considered incomplete (i.e., they do not contain all of the essential amino acids) or limiting (i.e., they contain very small amounts of the essential amino acids relative to requirements). So, vegetarians should aim to consume a variety of protein-containing foods to obtain all essential amino acids. See Table 6.2 for examples of complementary proteins.

These foods can be simply combined to make complete proteins—for example, peanut butter (legumes) on toast (grains), or beans (legumes) and rice (grains). An eating plan that regularly includes legumes, grains, nuts, and seeds is likely to contain all of the amino acids needed to make complete proteins. Athletes need to keep in mind that most

Table 6.2 Food sources of complementary proteins

Food	Limiting amino acid(s)	Complementary food
Legumes	Methionine	Grains, nuts and seeds
Nuts and seeds	Lysine	Legumes
Grains	Lysine, threonine	Legumes
Corn	Tryptophan, lysine	Legumes

Source: Adapted from American Society for Nutrition.[3]

Table 6.3 Plant-based sources of protein

Legumes	Nuts	Seeds	Grains
Lentils	Walnuts	Pumpkin seeds	Teff
Peas	Almonds	Sunflower seeds	Rice
Peanuts	Brazil nuts	Flaxseeds	Wheat
Beans	Cashews	Chia seeds	Quinoa
(kidney, pinto, black, chickpeas)	Pecans		Oats

plant-based sources of protein contain less protein than animal sources. For example, 100 g (3.5 ounces) of cooked legumes such as chickpeas or lentils contains approximately 7 g of protein, while 100 g (3.5 ounces) of lean beef or chicken contains approximately 30 g of protein. So, those following a **vegan dietary pattern** will need to carefully plan their intake to ensure they are able to consume sufficient protein. Examples of plant-based sources of protein are listed in Table 6.3. Animal proteins are also typically more readily digested than plant sources of protein. High biological value (HBV) protein foods are those that contain all essential amino acids and are readily digestible. Most meat, fish, poultry, eggs, and milk products are considered HBV protein foods.

Vegan dietary pattern

A plant-based dietary pattern that strictly avoids all foods derived from animals.

Leucine

An essential amino acid, which is required for muscle protein synthesis.

The amino acid **leucine** plays a role in stimulating muscle protein synthesis, making it an important part of the diet for athletes, especially masters athletes (Chapter 24) and those recovering from injury (Chapter 16). Whey protein, which makes up 20% of the protein in dairy foods, is a good source of leucine, so dairy foods and whey protein supplements are popular among athletes.

Table 6.4 Food sources of macronutrients

Carbohydrate sources	Protein sources	Fat sources
Bread	Milk	Avocado
Rice and other grains	Eggs	Nuts
Pasta	Beef	Fish
Corn	Chicken	Peanut butter
Oats and cereals	Fish	Olive oil
Sweet potato	Tofu	Canola oil
Fruit	Legumes	Seeds

Fats

To reduce their risk of developing chronic diseases, it is important for athletes to limit their intake of saturated fats and consume moderate amounts of unsaturated fats. Saturated fats are found predominantly in animal products; they are in the fat on red meat, in chicken skin, and in cream. Palm and coconut oils are also sources of saturated fat and are often found in commercially prepared baked goods and deep-fried foods. Where possible, these fats should be replaced with health-promoting mono- and polyunsaturated fats. Monounsaturated fats are found in olive oil and walnuts and are known to help reduce the risk of developing chronic diseases such as diabetes and cardiovascular disease. Omega-3 polyunsaturated fats are found predominantly in fish and help to reduce inflammation, which can support a number of healthy functions including joint health and circulation. For athletes with lower energy requirements, intake of fat may need to be minimised to limit total energy intake. Table 6.4 lists examples of food sources of macronutrients.

Food sources of micronutrients

Each eating occasion presents an opportunity for athletes to nourish their bodies. Athletes should choose nutrient-dense foods as often as possible to support their bodies' increased nutrient requirements. Athletes may have increased demands for calcium, iron, B vitamins and antioxidants, including vitamins C and E. With careful planning, these needs can be met with a whole-food diet. See Table 6.5 for examples of some food sources of these nutrients. It is important to note that the amount of a nutrient that can be absorbed and used by the body, a concept known as bioavailability, can vary. For example, Table 17.2 outlines components in food that affect the bioavailability of iron.

Some athletes may choose to take vitamin and mineral supplements in an effort to meet their nutrient needs. All athletes should be encouraged to consume a whole-food

Table 6.5 Food sources of select micronutrients

Foods rich in calcium	Foods rich in iron	Foods rich in vitamin C
Milk	Beef	Citrus fruit
Yoghurt	Lamb	Tomatoes
Cheese	Beans	Berries
Fortified plant-based milks (soy, rice, almond)	Fortified breads and cereals	Bell peppers (capsicum)

diet that aligns with dietary guidelines to meet their nutrient needs; however, should they have concerns about their dietary intake or specific health issues to address, vitamin and mineral supplements may be considered. The nutrient supplement should be selected through consultation with a doctor or sports nutrition professional.

It is important to understand that individual foods can be sources of many different nutrients. For example, milk contains protein, carbohydrate, and calcium as well as other vitamins and minerals. It is also important to consider that some foods that are good sources of some nutrients may also contain large amounts of trans or saturated fats, sugars, salt, and food additives. For example, commercial peanut butter is a source of protein but is commonly made with added fats, sugar, and salt.

Combining foods: Meals for athletes

Since foods are consumed as part of meals and in the context of a whole diet, it is important to consider how different foods may fit together to create a healthy eating pattern for athletes. Recreational athletes may focus on developing a healthy eating plan to promote good health, while highly competitive athletes may follow carefully designed eating plans to maximise performance and attain optimal body composition. There are a number of considerations when creating an eating plan with athletes:

- the amount and timing of carbohydrate and protein intake may be adjusted based on energy expenditure and sport-specific requirements (see Chapters 9 and 10 for more details);
- fat intake may be adjusted to support appropriate energy intake and body composition goals (see Chapters 13 and 20 for more details);
- fibre may be avoided prior to a training session/event to minimise GI disturbances (see Chapter 15 for more details);
- special dietary requirements and personal preferences as well as cultural, religious, and philosophical values should be considered as part of an individualised dietary plan to maximise satisfaction with and adherence to the diet;
- a variety of enjoyable flavours and textures may be used to encourage consumption;
- food safety should be considered, especially for athletes eating on the go or travelling in foreign countries (see Chapter 27 for more details);
- convenience is important for busy athletes juggling training, work, study, caring responsibilities, and/or other commitments;
- access to an appropriate selection of ready-to-eat meals, and support for meal planning and time management can assist athletes to eat well;
- cooking skills may need to be taught to support athletes to prepare their own healthy meals.

There is no one best meal plan for athletes. The points listed above can all be considered when developing a personalised eating plan that meets the needs and preferences of an individual athlete. It is important to remember to update eating plans as athletes move through different stages of training, competition, growth, and development. Dietary needs will be different at different life stages (child vs adolescent vs young adult vs older adult) and points in sporting seasons (pre-season vs competition season vs off-season), and approaches to eating may change with life events such as studying, working, and living with others. A flexible approach, that works with an athlete's current situation and is regularly adapted based on performance goals, health measures, and personal preferences is ideal. Some simple meal ideas that can be adjusted for macronutrient content and personal preferences are included in the accompanying box.

Box 6.1   Examples of modifiable meals for athletes

Sample meal 1: Beef and black bean burrito
   Possible modifications based on individual needs:

- add rice to increase carbohydrate
- increase the amount of meat and/or beans to increase protein
- add vegetables like tomato and bell peppers (capsicum) to increase micronutrients and aid the absorption of iron from beans
- omit beans to reduce the fibre content

Sample meal 2: Fish curry with rice
   Possible modifications based on individual needs:

- use cauliflower rice to reduce carbohydrates or add potato to increase carbohydrates
- add additional sources of protein (meat, poultry, tofu, legumes) to boost protein content
- add vegetables like carrots and broccoli to increase fibre and micronutrient content

---

Summary

This chapter has described how food contains more than just nutrients and how dietary guidelines can be used to plan a nutritious foundation diet. Athletes will benefit from learning more about food and nutrition so that they can participate in developing their own eating plans. Sports nutrition professionals should support athletes to develop individualised eating plans that align with their personal preferences, values, and circumstances, support their health and development, and achieve their performance-related goals.

Chapter highlights

- A whole-food diet provides more benefits than can be gained by consuming nutrients alone.
- Dietary guidelines are designed to help the general population maintain good health and can be the basis of a foundational dietary plan for athletes.
- Athletes often require more food to meet higher energy, macro-, and micronutrient requirements.
- Carbohydrate-rich foods can be selected to maximise performance and minimise GI discomfort.
- Protein can be obtained from a number of plant and animal sources to meet an athlete's protein requirements.

- Athletes can usually meet all of their vitamin and mineral requirements with a carefully planned whole-food diet.
- Athletes may benefit from additional individualised dietary advice from a sports nutrition professional.

References

1. World Health Organization. *Healthy diet*. Cairo: WHO Regional Office for the Eastern Mediterranean; 2019. https://apps.who.int/iris/bitstream/handle/10665/325828/EMROPUB_2019_en_23536.pdf
2. Meyer NL, Reguant-Closa A, Nemecek T. Sustainable diets for athletes. *Curr Nutr Rep*. 2020;9:147–62.
3. American Society for Nutrition. *Protein Complementation*; 2011. https://nutrition.org/protein-complementation/

7 Dietary intake and energy availability

Nikki A Jeacocke

Understanding the dietary intake of athletes is important to determine the adequacy of their diet to meet their nutritional needs as a human, as well as the additional requirements through their chosen sport/s' training and competition demands. There are a range of factors that impact and influence an athlete's food choices and subsequent dietary intake. Sports nutrition professionals working with athletes are experts in knowing 'what an athlete should' consume to meet their individual needs and will work with an athlete to identify 'what the athlete does' consume. Vital to this exploration is also understanding 'why' an athlete makes their specific food and fluid choices, and what key influences are at play. This chapter will explore a range of intrinsic and extrinsic factors that influence athlete food intake and will deep dive into the interplay disordered eating, eating disorders, low energy availability, and relative energy deficiency in sports (REDs) may have on an athlete.

Learning outcomes

This chapter will:

- identify the range of intrinsic and extrinsic factors that influence food choices in athletes;
- explain body image, disordered eating, and eating disorders and their impact on an athlete's relationship with food, exercise, and their body;
- explain low energy availability and relative energy deficient in sport, what they are, and why they are important for athlete health and performance;
- describe the relationship between disordered eating, an eating disorder, low energy availability, and REDs.

Factors influencing athlete food choice

Through training, athletes strive on a daily basis to enhance their physical capacity in order to optimise competition performance. Although sometimes appearing superhuman, athletes (just like all humans), require food and fluid to sustain life and maintain bodily functions. Dietary guidelines are evidence-based documents that provide the general population with advice on dietary patterns, food groups and foods that provide the required nutrients to promote overall health and prevent chronic disease.[1] Over 100 countries

DOI: 10.4324/9781003321286-8

worldwide have developed dietary guidelines that are adapted to suit their population in relation to eating habits, food availability and culinary culture.[1] Despite the existence of these guidelines, defining what individuals should eat, there are a range of factors that influence and impact the food choices made by an athlete.[2,3] These are grouped below according to intrinsic and extrinsic factors.

Extrinsic factors:

- food availability;
- food security;
- seasonality of fresh produce;
- financial capacity to purchase food;
- cost of food available for purchase;
- cultural factors that impact the ingredients that are readily available and the food items 'usually cooked' including customs and traditions;
- availability of cooking facilities and equipment;
- social constructs including work patterns, housemates, and dependents;
- environmental conditions including temperature (for example, a preference for hot food on a cold day and vice versa);
- sport-related requirements including competition and training demands;
- peer-related impacts including beliefs and intake of other athletes;
- culture of the sport;
- influential figures such as parents and coaches; and their knowledge and food beliefs;
- impact of marketing, media, and social media and the influence they have on food choices.

Intrinsic factors:

- hunger and appetite including the impact exercise can have on these;
- nutrition knowledge including for everyday life and sport;
- food values and beliefs and importance placed on nutrition for life and sport;
- taste and food preferences;
- food allergies and/or intolerances and gastrointestinal discomfort;
- religious beliefs;
- cooking skills of the individual;
- resting metabolic rate and body composition;
- drive to change or manipulate body composition and/or weight;
- medical and neurodevelopmental conditions, for example, diabetes mellitus, anxiety, depression, neurodivergence, an eating disorder, or irritable bowel syndrome;
- the individual's relationship with food, exercise and body;
- body image including thoughts, feelings, and perception of one's body and the behaviours the athlete engages in as a result of these.

A range of these factors may remain constant over time, whereas some are more fluid and their impact on an athlete's food choices may vary over short-, medium-, and long-term time points. When working with an athlete, understanding the complex interaction of extrinsic and intrinsic factors at play for the athlete is vital to ensure nutrition interventions are suited to meet the requirements of the individual. The identification of these factors and their impact helps to explain why the application of generic nutrition concepts is insufficient when working with all humans, including athletes, and therefore an individualised approach to nutrition assessment, intervention, and management is required.

Eating and relationships with food

Body image forms a critical component of an athlete's relationship with their body and subsequent food choices. Body image refers to the thoughts, feelings, and perceptions an individual has about their body; and the behaviours they engage in because of these. An individual who accepts, appreciates, and respects their body may be described as having a positive body image, whereas body dissatisfaction occurs when an individual has persistent negative thoughts and feelings about their body.[4] Positive body image is a protective factor and can make an individual less susceptible to developing an eating disorder, whereas body dissatisfaction places someone at higher risk for developing an eating disorder.[4]

All athletes sit on a spectrum of eating behaviour which ranges from optimised nutrition to disordered eating, through to an eating disorder (Figure 7.1).[5] Optimised nutrition is described as individualised nutrition practices that are safe, supported, purposeful, and individualised and best balance health and performance for the athlete.[5] Within this space an athlete would be considered to have a resilient body image; overall positive (but not always) thoughts and feelings around food, their body, and exercise patterns; as well as flexibility in their eating patterns and exercise behaviours. Whilst this is the 'optimal' space, for a variety of reasons, not all athletes consistently sit in this zone. There is a range of factors that may elicit an athlete to move along the spectrum of eating behaviour including but not limited to injury, illness, selection, deselection, retirement (whether forced or voluntary), dieting, changes to body weight and/or shape, manipulating body weight and or shape, start of preseason training, comments including unsolicited comments about body weight and/or shape, and making weight for competition.[5]

Disordered eating (DE) occurs as thoughts and feelings about one's body lead to changes in eating and exercise behaviour that are problematic but fail to meet diagnostic

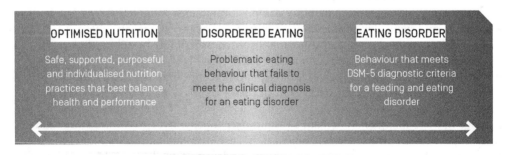

Figure 7.1 The spectrum of eating behaviour in the high-performance athlete.

Source: The Australian Institute of Sport (AIS) and National Eating Disorders Collaboration (NEDC) position statement on disordered eating in high-performance sport.[5]

criteria for an eating disorder, whether this be due to lesser frequency or lower level of severity of the behaviours.[5] Examples of DE include:

- increase in exercise outside of training sessions;
- reducing energy intake;
- restricting specific food groups or food types;
- rigidity around eating and/or exercise behaviours;
- bingeing and/or purging with less regularity;
- obsession with 'healthy' eating.

Eating Disorders (EDs) sit on the right of the spectrum of eating behaviour and involve specific criteria that meet the American Psychiatric Association's (2013) Diagnostic and Statistical Manual of Mental Disorders (5th Edition, DSM-5),[6] including problematic eating behaviours, distorted beliefs, preoccupation with food, eating, and body image. There are five eating disorders detailed in the DSM-5 including Avoidant Restrictive Food Intake Disorder (ARFID); Anorexia Nervosa (AN); Bulimia Nervosa (BN); Binge Eating Disorder (BED); and Other Specified Feeding and Eating Disorders (OSFED).[6] An ED is a serious, but treatable mental illness that can affect any athlete, in any sport, at any time, crossing boundaries of gender, age, body size, culture, socio-economic background, athletic calibre, and ability.[5]

Creating a safe sporting environment for all athletes is an important component of working to reduce movement across the spectrum with the aim of decreasing the rates of DE and EDs. This requires a whole of sport approach to first identify and then work to increase protective factors and reduce harmful factors.

Box 7.1 Case study: 24-year-old female track and field athlete

An athlete's ability to implement suggested nutrition strategies will provide further clues as to where they sit on the spectrum of eating behaviour. A 24-year-old track and field athlete reveals during her initial nutrition consultation she does not eat carbohydrates after 3 pm as she read in a magazine it causes weight gain. The sports nutrition professional explored this further and provided education on the need for carbohydrates to help meet the nutrition recovery requirements from her afternoon training session. The athlete and the sports nutrition professional brainstormed together practical examples of how she could add carbohydrates to dinner, considering the range of intrinsic and extrinsic factors discussed in the chapter above, for example, financial capacity, taste preferences, and cooking skills. At the follow-up consult, she had not added carbohydrate to her dinner. They explored together the potential reasons and the athlete confided she was 'so scared' she would gain weight and simply could not add the carbohydrate to dinner. She opened up about her body image concerns, fear of gaining weight, and limited carbohydrate-containing foods she considered 'safe' to eat. This information formed a critical piece of the puzzle to understanding the athlete as an individual, where she sat on the spectrum of eating behaviour and allowed the sports nutrition professional to plan the steps ahead.

Prevalence rates of disordered eating and eating disorders in athletes range from 0% to 19% in males and from 6% to 45% in females.[7] Within the literature, there tends to be a higher prevalence of DE and EDs in athletes compared to non-athletes.[5] Among athletes, there are higher-risk sports including aesthetically judged; gravitational; and weight class sports; although it is important to remember DE and EDs can occur in any athlete, in any sport, at any time.[5] More research is required to better understand the prevalence of DE and EDs within athletes.

Both DE and EDs are serious and can impact athlete health and performance. Whilst prevention is ideal, early identification and timely intervention are vital to reduce the impact on an athlete's health and performance.

Box 7.2   A note on weight

If asked to describe what an athlete with an eating disorder 'looks' like, many people might describe someone with low body weight and/or someone who has lost a significant and noticeable amount of weight. Weight loss is often thought of as a sign of an eating disorder; however, there are two key issues with this weight-centric approach to viewing, assessing, and identifying an eating disorder:

1. Someone may be suffering from an ED and not lose any weight, their weight may fluctuate, or they may sit at a 'normal' or 'higher' body weight. If relying on low body weight, or weight loss, to identify an ED, many EDs will go undiagnosed.
2. It can take a significant amount of time before weight loss is noticeable. Therefore, weight loss should not be relied upon as an early warning sign. It may be that disordered eating thoughts and behaviours are well entrenched before weight loss is apparent.

Energy availability

Energy availability and its associated terms are important concepts to understand when working with athletes. In the past, energy balance was considered a simple equation where energy balance was achieved when energy intake was equal to energy expenditure. To drive weight loss, it was thought that disrupting energy balance by either reducing energy intake, increasing energy expenditure, or a combination of both was required. Or, if weight gain was the aim, altering energy balance by increasing energy intake, decreasing energy expenditure, or a combination of both. Contemporary understanding of energy balance includes complex physiological interactions within the human body beyond the oversimplified energy balance described above. Key terms and concepts include:

- Energy intake (EI) = energy intake through food and fluid;
- Energy Availability (EA) = the energy available to support a human's body functions once the energy commitment to exercise has been taken from dietary intake;[5]
- Energy Availability (EA) = (Energy Intake (EI) – Exercise Energy Expenditure (EEE)) / Fat-Free Mass (FFM);[8]
- Adequate EA occurs when an athlete has enough energy available to cover the energy cost of exercise and for optimal bodily functions;

- Low Energy Availability (LEA) occurs when there is a mismatch between energy intake and exercise load leaving insufficient energy remaining for other bodily functions.[5] LEA can occur due to a reduction in EI, an increase in exercise energy expenditure, or a combination of these;[9]
- LEA can be classified as i) Adaptable LEA which involves exposure to LEA that is linked to mild, reversible, or benign effects, and signals an adaptive partitioning of energy and the plasticity of human physiology or ii) Problematic LEA, which involves exposure to LEA that is linked to greater and possibly ongoing disruption to various body systems. The impact of problematic LEA may vary depending on the body system and the individual, and also the duration, magnitude and frequency of the LEA.[10]

Relative energy deficiency in sports

The collective impact of problematic LEA on an athlete's health and performance is known as relative energy deficiency in sports or REDs. The literature and understanding of LEA and its impact on health and performance have grown over time. In 1997, the concept of the Female Athlete Triad was formalised by the American College of Sports Medicine.[11] The Female Athlete Triad described the interrelationship of eating disorders, amenorrhoea, and osteoporosis/bone injuries in female athletes.[11] The Female Athlete Triad was further refined in 2007 to highlight that each corner of the Triad involved a spectrum between health and disease.[12] The health end of the triad described optimal energy availability, eumenorrhea, and optimal bone health, whereas the disease end of the spectrum involved low energy availability with or without an eating disorder, functional hypothalamic amenorrhea, and osteoporosis.[12] In 2014, a broader concept was developed by an International Olympic Committee working group to expand the impact of LEA to include additional health and performance impacts and include male athletes as a population at risk.[9] This concept was coined relative energy deficiency in sport and has been updated in 2018 and again in 2023.[8,10] The 2023 consensus statement builds on the previous work, incorporating the >170 original research publications in relation to REDs that have been published since 2018. Key emerging areas of research have demonstrated the magnifying role of low carbohydrate availability on REDs independent of low energy, increased the evidence between the interaction of mental health and REDs, and the impact of LEA on males.[10] The updated statement also presents a summary of practical clinical guidelines for assessing LEA and provides guidelines for safe and effective body composition assessment to help prevent REDs.

According to Mountjoy et al.,[10] the updated definition of REDs is:

a syndrome of impaired physiological and/or psychological functioning experienced by female and male athletes that is caused by exposure to problematic (prolonged and/or severe) low energy availability. The detrimental outcomes include, but are not limited to, decreases in metabolic function, reproductive function, musculoskeletal health, immunity, glycogen synthesis, and cardiovascular and haematological health, which can all individually and synergistically lead to impaired well-being, increased injury risk, and decreased sports performance.

REDs can impact athletes' health and performance, as demonstrated via the REDs Conceptual Model (Health) and REDs Conceptual Model (Performance) summarised

REDs Health Impact

Low energy availability can lead to:
• Impaired Reproductive Health
• Impaired Bone Health
• Impaired Gastrointestinal Function
• Impaired Energy Metabolism/Regulation
• Impaired Haematological Function
• Urinary Incontinence
• Impaired Glucose and Lipid Metabolism
• Mental Health Issues
• Impaired Neurocognitive Function
• Sleep Disturbance
• Impaired Cardiovascular Function
• Reduced Skeletal Muscle Function
• Impaired Growth and Development
• Reduced Immunity

REDs Performance Impact

Low energy availability can lead to decreases in:
• Power Performance
• Athlete Availability
• Training Response
• Recovery
• Cognitive Performance/Skill
• Motivation
• Muscle Strength
• Endurance Performance

Figure 7.2 Summary of REDs Conceptual Model (Health) and REDs Conceptual Model (Performance).[10]

Source: Modelled from Mountjoy et al.[10]

in Figure 7.2. This figure highlights the central role LEA plays in the development of REDs and how problematic LEA is potentially associated with a range of health and performance impacts.

Relationship between DE/EDs and LEA/REDs

Low energy availability as the exposure variable and REDs as the outcome of problematic LEA; can occur in isolation or in combination with disordered eating or an eating disorder (Figure 7.3). Either may proceed the other, and the investigation of one necessitates the assessment of the other.[5]

Multidisciplinary Team Approach to DE/EDs and LEA/REDs

When working with athletes, Wells et al. highlight the importance of engaging in a multidisciplinary team approach in relation to prevention, early identification, and treatment of DE and EDs.[5] The authors coined the term Core Multidisciplinary Team (CMT) which includes the doctor, psychologist, and sports nutrition professional. Whilst all those working in sport have a role to play in the prevention and early identification of DE and EDs, the CMT have further responsibilities within management and treatment.[5] A multidisciplinary approach is also recommended when working with an athlete with LEA and associated REDs.[8, 10] A CMT may exist within a sporting organisation organically and it may be 'easier' to engage and work as a cohesive unit. For practitioners working in isolation, maybe through a smaller sporting organisation or as a practitioner within private practice, the creation of a CMT may be required. Whether it be an internal or external CMT, or a combination of these, communication is vital within and between the CMT, the athlete, coaches, and other performance support staff.

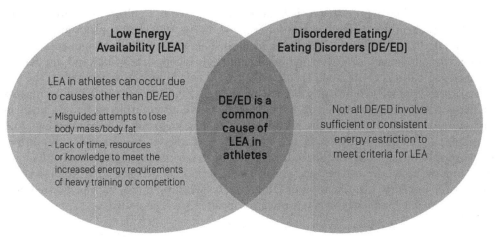

Figure 7.3 Eating disorders/disordered eating can occur in the absence or presence of low energy
   availability.

Source: The Australian Institute of Sport (AIS) and National Eating Disorders Collaboration (NEDC) position
statement on disordered eating in high-performance sport.[5]

Box 7.3   Case study: 17-year-old male basketball player

A 17-year-old male basketball player is referred to a sports nutrition professional for a nutrition assessment. He is fatigued and tired in training and is struggling with ongoing upper
respiratory tract infections and low iron levels.

   During his initial nutrition assessment, it is apparent he is still growing and finding it
hard to meet his energy requirements for sport and growth. He has poor nutrition
knowledge related to everyday life as a growing teenager, as well as the extra requirements for his busy training and competition schedule. The sports nutrition professional
establishes relatively early on in the consult that the athlete most likely has LEA and
needs to increase his energy intake to meet his energy requirements. Given his poor
nutrition knowledge, it would be easy to assume that with appropriate nutrition education for growth and sport, the LEA should be corrected, and this might be an 'easy fix'.

   However, the sports nutrition professional noticed some red flags as the consult progressed. He talked about his body, his drive to increase lean mass, his fear of gaining fat,
and some rigidity in thinking about food. The sports nutrition professional explored
these with the athlete further and realised the LEA was also accompanied by poor body
image and disordered eating behaviours. The sports nutrition professional discussed
their concerns with the athlete and his parent and suggested engaging a psychologist and
doctor for further assessment and management via a multi-disciplinary team.

   It would have been easy for the sports nutrition professional to focus on the lack of
knowledge of this athlete as the 'problem' and quickly jump into providing education as
the solution. Whilst increased knowledge would be beneficial, the lack of knowledge was
only part of a bigger picture for this athlete. He may have left the consult armed with
increased knowledge, but no capacity to put the knowledge into practice due to the
poor body image and disordered eating behaviours at play.

Within sporting organisations, it is important to create a culture and environment where the prevention, early identification, timely intervention, and appropriate management of DE, EDs, LEA, and REDs are prioritised. There are two key components of this: (1) policies, guidelines, and working documents that identify the issues and discuss the strategies to address them, and (2) education for all role holders that focuses on the key issues for each of these different stakeholders. Language is a key focus of the documents and education. How sports nutrition professionals talk about athletes' bodies, to them and about them, is important in creating safe sporting environments. How, when, and why sports nutrition professionals measure and assess athletes' weight and body composition should be carefully considered. All role holders within sport, from the athlete to their support network, coaches, and performance support staff, have a part to play in the prevention and early identification of DE and EDs. Working up to, but not beyond professional capacity is important to ensure appropriate care is provided.

Summary

This chapter has explored the intrinsic and extrinsic factors that influence dietary intake and relationship with food, disordered eating, eating disorders, low energy availability, and REDs. Athletes strive through their training to drive physiological changes to improve their performance in competition. Dietary intake can enhance these adaptations, with guidelines available covering what food, macro- micro-nutrients athletes should consume. Athletes are not robots who eat what they are told, rather complex individuals who have a range of intrinsic and extrinsic factors that will impact their dietary choices. An athlete's relationship with their body, food, and exercise all impact food choices. Within this body image, disordered eating and eating disorders are complex, often misunderstood, but important areas to understand. Low energy availability as the exposure variable and REDs as the outcome variable can significantly impact athlete health and performance. All those involved in sports should have a working knowledge of these areas and understand their specific professional roles and responsibilities when working with athletes.

Chapter highlights

- When working with athletes, it is important to gain an understanding of them as an individual to help identify the specific intrinsic and extrinsic factors that impact their food selection.
- Intrinsic and extrinsic factors influencing an athlete's food choices can remain static or change over time.
- Body image refers to the thoughts, feelings, and perceptions an athlete has about their body; and the behaviours they engage in because of these.
- Positive body image is a protective factor in developing disordered eating or an eating disorder.
- Body dissatisfaction can increase the risk for an athlete to develop an eating disorder.
- All athletes sit on the spectrum of eating behaviour, from optimised nutrition to disordered eating through to an eating disorder.
- Athletes can move up and down the spectrum of eating behaviour throughout their careers and into their lives after competitive sports.
- Optimised nutrition describes individualised nutrition practices that are safe, supported, purposeful, and individualised.

- Disordered eating occurs as thoughts and feelings about an athlete's body lead them to change their eating and exercise behaviour. Disordered eating behaviours can be the same as eating disorder behaviours but occur less frequently or with lower severity than occurs in eating disorders.
- Eating disorders are clinically diagnosed medical conditions requiring specific criteria to be met for diagnosis.
- Disordered eating and eating disorders can occur in any athlete, in any sport, at any time.
- REDs results from prolonged exposure to low energy availability.
- There is a wide range of impacts of LEA on athletes' health and performance.
- Disordered eating and eating disorders can occur in isolation or in combination with LEA and REDs, and vice versa. Assessment and identification of one necessitates the assessment of the other.
- A whole of sport approach to working with disordered eating, an eating disorder, LEA, and REDs is required.

References

1. Food and Agriculture Organisation of the United Nations. *Food-based dietary guidelines.* 2023. https://www.fao.org/nutrition/nutrition-education/food-dietary-guidelines/en/
2. Birkenhead K, Slater G. A review of factors influencing athletes' food choices. *Sports Med.* 2015;45:1511–22.
3. Thurecht R, Pelly F. Key factors influencing the food choices of athletes at two distinct major international competitions. *Nutrients.* 2020;12:924.
4. National Eating Disorders Collaboration. *Body Image Fact Sheet.* 2022. https://nedc.com.au/assets/Fact-Sheets/NEDC-Fact-Sheet-Body-Image.pdf
5. Wells KR, Jeacocke NA, Appaneal R, et al. The Australian Institute of Sport (AIS) and National Eating Disorders Collaboration (NEDC) position statement on disordered eating in high performance sport. *Br J Sports Med.* 2020;54:1247–58.
6. American Psychiatric Association. *Diagnostic and Statistical Manual of Mental Disorders (DSM-5).* 5th ed. American Psychiatric Pub; 2013.
7. Reardon CL, Hainline B, Aron CM, et al. Mental health in elite athletes: International Olympic Committee consensus statement. *Br J Sports Med.* 2019;53(11):667–99.
8. Mountjoy M, Sundgot-Borgen J, Burke L, et al. IOC consensus statement on relative energy deficiency in sport (RED-S): 2018 update. *Br J Sports Med.* 2018;52:687–97.
9. Mountjoy M, Sundgot-Borgen J, Burke L, et al. The IOC consensus statement: beyond the Female Athlete Triad—Relative Energy Deficiency in Sport (RED-S). *Br J Sports Med.* 2014;48:491–7.
10. Mountjoy M, Ackerman K, Bailey D, et al. The 2023 International Olympic Committee's (IOC) consensus statement on Relative Energy Deficiency in Sports (REDs). *Br J Sports Med.* 2023;57:1073–1097.
11. Ottis CL, Drinkwater B, Johnson M, et al. American College of Sports Medicine position stand: The female athlete triad. *Med Sci Sports Exerc.* 1997;29:i–ix.
12. Nattiv A, Loucks AB, Manore MM, et al. American College of Sports Medicine position stand. The female athlete triad. *Med Sci Sports Exerc.* 2007;39:1867–82.

8 Dietary assessment

Yasmine C Probst and Joel C Craddock

The preceding chapters have provided an overview of the nutrients needed for good health and performance. To understand the nutrients that come from the everyday diets of individuals or populations, it is necessary to collect information about what people eat. Dietitians and nutritionists use many different types of tools, referred to as dietary assessment methods, to collect this information. To translate the food information into nutrient outcomes, they also need to use tools called food composition databases. This chapter will explore some of the most common dietary assessment tools and address some considerations to be aware of when using food composition databases.

> **Learning outcomes**
>
> **This chapter will:**
>
> - describe common methods of dietary assessment, with a particular focus on their strengths and limitations;
> - outline how food information can be translated to nutrient outcomes;
> - discuss how dietary guidelines and nutrition policies can be used with dietary assessment information;
> - describe aspects of dietary assessment important in sports, including the timing of snacks or meals relative to training and competition.

What is dietary assessment?

Dietary assessment is the process of determining what a person or group of people are eating and drinking. This is fundamental to the skills of a sports nutrition professional but may also be important for other health and fitness professionals to gain an understanding of people's food habits. Dietary assessments can be obtained at the time foods and drinks are consumed, or they can be performed retrospectively, after foods and drinks have been eaten, often relying heavily on a person's memory. To help capture the required information, a range of assessment methods have been developed and refined over time, each with its own advantages and disadvantages. These factors are unique to the situation in which the assessment method is being used and the individual or group with whom it is being used. Capturing dietary information for a five-year-old child, for example, will have many different considerations compared to capturing dietary information from an

DOI: 10.4324/9781003321286-9

adult who lives alone and does all of their own cooking and shopping. Not only will the types of tools used need to be considered but the impact of other factors will also need to be thought through. These other factors include things such as bias and literacy, which will be addressed below in relation to each of the specific assessment methods. The assessment methods vary in terms of how they are undertaken but also in relation to the form in which the food information is collected. This form can be using pen and paper, or it can be in various digital formats including the use of smartphone apps. After the food information has been collected, careful consideration needs to be given to how the information will be used. Is nutrient information needed from the foods that were reportedly eaten or will these foods be related to dietary guideline recommendations? These two options will be discussed later in this chapter.

Dietary assessment methods

Estimated food record

A form of dietary assessment in which a person records all of the food and drink they have consumed over a specific period of time (commonly one, three, or seven days) by estimating the weight or serving size of the item.

The types of dietary assessment methods that are commonly used include those based on recall and memory, such as the 24-hour recall,[1, 2] the diet history interview,[3] and the food frequency questionnaire.[4, 5] Other assessments capturing intake at the time of consumption—namely, the food record or food diary—may also be used in isolation or in parallel with the other methods. These tools are categorised into whether they are capturing actual intake or usual intake information. The food record or food diary is the most suitable tool to capture actual food intake information. This assessment method requires a person to write down the names and brand names of all foods and beverages consumed by meal occasion and to quantify the amount consumed. The way in which this quantity is determined creates the differentiating factor between an **estimated food record** and a **weighed food record**. As the name suggests, an estimated food record only requires an estimate of the portion size in terms that the person recording the foods can relate to. A weighed food record, on the other hand, requires the person recording the foods to accurately measure and weigh all items to be consumed. This includes a breakdown of ingredients required for a food that is cooked as part of a recipe and requires the person to take the measuring equipment with them to all eating occasions and locations. As a result, although the accuracy of the weighed food items *should* be higher than an estimated record, often subconscious or conscious changes to the types of food eaten occur and the actual intake is distorted. To reduce the impact of this bias, digital food records have been developed whereby the user takes photographs of the food and beverage items being consumed before and after consumption. Using images to capture the food items also reduces the burden related to the number of days of recording. A requirement for more days often results in less detailed information being provided, which also substantially affects the accuracy. As a result, the common durations are 3–4-day estimated food records, which include at least one weekend day.

Weighed food record

A form of dietary assessment in which a person records, with weights and volumes, all of the food and drink they have consumed over a specific period of time.

A 24-hour dietary assessment follows a structured approach to dietary assessment by capturing information about foods and beverages consumed during the previous day or 24-hour period. Often administered by an interviewer in a conversational manner, this form of assessment alone cannot capture usual intake information about the diet unless it is repeated over a number of occasions. During a 24-hour recall, the interviewer follows a multiple-pass approach to guide the interviewee's recall of their food and beverage intakes. This approach begins with a free-flowing recall of all items in the order they were consumed. The process is conducted uninterrupted to allow the person to recall an unprompted food list. This list is then addressed from the beginning to obtain further detail about the food item types, accompanying foods and commonly forgotten items, as well as the portion size of each of the foods and beverages recalled. The recalls often follow a meal-based format in terms used by the person, although the eating occasion, timing and location may also be collected depending upon the requirements.

Like the 24-hour recall, the diet history interview is based on the memory of the person recalling their food and beverage consumption. The process is largely interviewer-led though addresses usual intake. This usual intake period generally covers a one-month period but can vary substantially, from one week up to one year. The diet history interview follows a similar format to the 24-hour recall; however, its open-ended nature lends itself to the recall of foods and beverages that are consumed less frequently, during different seasons, or at eating occasions such as birthdays. Guided by the interviewer, a diet history interview is a skill-based dietary assessment method traditionally undertaken by trained dietitians. Often followed up with a checklist of commonly forgotten foods, the diet history interview provides information about the foods eaten by a person, the frequency at which those foods are eaten and the portion size they are usually eaten. This portion size may be guided by household measures such as measuring cups and spoons, by pictorial portion guides or using food models. Both the diet history interview and the 24-hour recall have been digitised; the structure of the 24-hour recall lends itself particularly well to this format, with the prompts provided by an avatar on screen rather than in person by the interviewer. This format allows large numbers of people to recall their intakes without the need for additional resources.

Usual intake information may also be collected using a food frequency questionnaire. The questionnaire includes a list of food items suited to the purpose of the information being collected. For example, if the purpose is to determine calcium intake, then only calcium-containing foods need to be included. The food list may comprise single food items or it may group foods with similar characteristics. The person completing the questionnaire identifies how often the food is consumed based on the pre-determined frequency categories provided. Food frequency questionnaires may span wide time intervals, with some even referring to the previous year of intake. Food frequency questionnaires can be quantified or semi-quantified, meaning that they may also require information about the portion size most often consumed for each item in the food list. The portion sizes can refer to a standard size that may relate to dietary guidelines, or they may be displayed as images or different size options for each food choice. The inclusion of portion size information may result in improved response rates. Food frequency questionnaires are commonly self-administered, meaning they do not require an interviewer to ask the questions. This does, however, leave the tool open to interpretation by the person reporting their intake and may lead to missed sections or skipped food items that are seemingly not of relevance.

These dietary collection methods all provide options for detailed dietary assessments for an athlete but can be time-consuming and rely heavily on nutrition-trained experts to administer and analyse. Digital or online versions of these tools exist which can help to streamline the dietary assessment. For example, the Automated Self-Administered 24-Hour (ASA-24) dietary assessment tool is a self-administered web-based tool which can provide high-quality 24-hour diet recalls and/or single or multi-day food record assessments. Digital dietary assessment may provide advantages in data collection, allow for analysis in real time and also enhance participant compliance.

Translating dietary intakes to nutrient outcomes

The above section has outlined a number of methods that can be used to find out what food and beverages are being consumed by a person. These methods all result in information related to specific foods and beverages, which may not be practical if someone needs to determine how much protein or energy they are consuming. To translate the food and beverage information to nutrient information, tools referred to as **food composition databases** are used. These databases contain a list of foods available in the food supply and their nutrient information, including both macronutrients and micronutrients. Each country has its own unique food composition database, as many foods are affected by local processing, harvesting, soil conditions, UV exposure, food regulatory environments, and many other factors. There is specialised software available to make the use of food composition tables fast and efficient. Although the software is useful, it does require the user to have a basic understanding of which food composition database to choose. If many dietary assessments need to be translated, as is common in research, the person or people using the software also need to ensure they use it consistently and follow the same assumptions. It needs to be appreciated that not every food item found on the supermarket shelf will appear in a food composition database, but generic versions of most foods do exist and, therefore, careful choices for the correct food matches need to be made. Where no matching food information is available between survey and reference databases, food label information may be used, but this is considered lower quality data as it is often based on calculations and limited to the nutrients required to be listed under the various regulatory codes and policies.

Food composition databases

Databases that contain lists of key foods available in the food supply and their nutrient information including energy, macronutrients and micronutrients.

There are two main types of food composition databases used globally: a **survey database** and a **reference database**. The survey database contains a complete nutrient set for all the foods listed and is based on the food items reported in the country-specific national nutrition survey for which it was developed. Some of this nutrient information is calculated or borrowed from other overseas databases but a majority is based on the reference food composition database. The reference database contains fewer food items, although a higher proportion of the items have been analysed in the laboratory to identify the amounts of nutrients in the foods. As a result, some foods may not include the same number of nutrient values and the database may, therefore, be considered incomplete. Most countries have their own survey and reference databases to describe their local foods and relevant nutrient information. For instance, in Australia, the survey databases are referred to as AUSNUT (Australian Nutrient) databases and the reference database is the Australian Food Composition database. The most recent AUSNUT database contains over 5700 food and beverage items, while the most recent Australian Food Composition database contains slightly more than 2500 food and beverage items.[6,7] However, not all countries have a suitable reference database whilst others may be incomplete, outdated, or unreliable. Subsequently, the Food and Agriculture Organization of the United Nations created a global reference database to assist countries in obtaining high-quality food composition data which has been scrutinised for accuracy.[8]

Survey database

Databases that are specifically developed for the analysis of all foods reported in national nutrition surveys. For example, in Australia, AUSNUT 2011-13 was developed for the Australian Health Survey 2011–12.

Reference database

Databases developed from a wide range of foods that are primarily analysed in the laboratory. For example, in the United States, the USDA national nutrient database for standard reference is the reference database which forms part of the FoodData Central system.

Box 8.1   European food consumption surveys

Food consumption surveys across the European region use a range of dietary assessment methods from food records in Austria and Italy to 24-hour recalls in Belgium and Spain and 48-hour dietary recalls in Finland and Croatia. The surveys aim to capture representative food and beverage consumption for the given country with some targeting the whole population from children to adults and others targeting only sub-populations such as pregnant women in Latvia. The survey ranges in size from almost 300 child respondents in Cyprus to over 13,000 national respondents in Germany. A detailed summary of survey information can be found on the European Food Safety Authority website (EFSA), <https://www.efsa.europa.eu/en/microstrategy/food-consumption-survey>.

Using dietary guidelines and policies in practice

There are a number of ways to use information collected from a dietary assessment. The most common approach compares food consumed to national dietary guidelines. While each country has their own set of dietary guidelines specific to its population, cuisine, and food systems, they all aim to maximise intake from nutritious whole foods and limit consumption of foods that are highly processed and high in added sugars, salt, and saturated fats. This comparison can be made using data collected through any of the assessment methods described in this chapter, although care needs to be taken that any recommendations based on this comparison are relevant for the individual client. For this reason, readily available and consumer-friendly resources are used to guide discussions with clients around portion sizes and the balance and types of foods being consumed. Conversations based on dietary guidelines are generally considered to be within the scope of practice for trained nutrition, exercise, and fitness professionals. However, more specific and personalised dietary planning is the speciality of dietitians; hence, when working with athletes it is best to refer to a dietitian if not specifically trained as one.

Other useful tools that can be aligned with dietary assessment outcomes are nutrient reference values (see Chapter 4). Similar to dietary guidelines, these vary from country to country depending on the nutritional requirements and/or deficits within each country. After translating food and beverage information to nutrient intakes, the appropriate nutrient reference ranges can be used as a comparator to determine the adequacy of intake. A person consuming insufficient amounts of important nutrients may need to increase or balance the foods that they are eating. Given that insufficient intake of some nutrients can result in deficiency symptoms, while overconsumption can result in toxicity symptoms, adjustments based on nutrient concerns are best supported by a trained sports nutrition professional. The sports nutrition professional will be able to consider the medical, lifestyle, and exercise-related factors relevant to the individual and identify any possible medication interactions or underlying concerns as to why the nutrient levels are outside of the normal ranges. Diet quality tools may also be useful to evaluate an athlete's overall intake. An online tool designed specifically for athletes for this function is the Athlete Diet Index (ADI). The ADI assesses diet quality for athletes and considers the nutritional requirements, timing of intake, and evaluates dietary habits which can support regular training.[9]

It is important to note, however, that nutrient information taken directly from a dietary assessment and translated using a food composition database or other tool can be affected by advantages and disadvantages such as bias (see limitations in Table 8.1). For this reason, if a sports nutrition professional expresses concern they will likely suggest further medical intervention.

Applying dietary assessment to sports

Although dietary guidelines are developed for a country's general population, the messages are often applicable to many sporting practices as well. Athletes can follow dietary guidelines for a foundation diet of high quality which promotes general health and well-being. This is often overlooked by athletes as their focus may be on meeting certain nutrient targets for their sport (such as protein intake for strength-based sports) rather than their overarching intake.

It should be noted, however, that the level and types of training undertaken by athletes will likely require additional or modified guidance to optimise health and well-being.

Table 8.1 Summary of common dietary assessment methods

Assessment method	Recording type	Strengths	Limitations
Food record	• Prospective (recorded as they are consumed) • Self-administered	• Actual intake information • Using images reduces burden	• Increased days are affected by the burden • Social desirability bias creates changed intakes • Requires literate persons
24-hour recall	• Retrospective (reflects back on dietary intake) • Multiple pass method • Interviewer assisted	• Quick to administer • Repeated recalls can give usual intake information • Structured approach	• Affected by memory • Affected by social desirability bias
Diet history interview	• Retrospective • Interviewer prompted	• Usual intake information • Captures in-depth information	• Affected by memory • Affected by social desirability bias • Requires interviewer • Requires 30–60 minutes to complete
Food frequency questionnaire	• Retrospective • Self-administered • Can be interviewer-assisted	• Usual intake information • Can be completed over multiple attempts • Can be tailored to requirements, for example, nutrient type	• Length of food list affects accuracy • May not be quantified • Often overestimates intake

Athletes often engage in long or intensive training sessions and/or competitive events which require athletes to be at optimum performance for a sustained period. The timing of such events may last for a season or for shorter intermittent periods of time throughout the year. The idea of **nutrition periodisation** for these events should be considered and ideally discussed with a sports nutrition professional. This approach to nutrition and sport considers the physiological needs of the individual, the specific determinants of success for the sport being undertaken, the training and recovery plans in the long, medium, and short term and the associated nutrition interventions that are possible when considering the periodised training or planned event performance.[10]

A common tool used in practice, however, is app-based tracking using smartphone technology. This approach allows an athlete to monitor their food and beverage patterns in near real time. The high level of variability of apps, while expressed as a want by the athletes,[11] creates concern over the credibility of the tools in an unregulated space. Similarly, real-time monitoring of intake at the time of consumption using sensor-based technologies, similar to heart rate monitoring, is also emerging though in many instances cost prohibitive in relation to food consumption. The need for personalised technologies for athletes continues to expand but should be supported by a sports nutrition professional to avoid potential misinterpretation of information that is often country- and sporting-code-specific.

Nutrition periodisation

The strategic use of nutritional interventions during different phases of a training plan

Following a dietary assessment, many factors need to be addressed with the athlete. Are they in an off-season period? Are they training or are they competing? The type of sport being undertaken, whether it is primarily strength- or endurance-focused, and the athlete's age, health status, and sex should also be addressed. Many sports require careful timing of an athlete's fluid intake, snacks, and meals relative to their training schedule and intensity and their competitive games or events. The composition of these meals needs to be carefully managed. Too much or too little of key nutrients, such as protein, carbohydrate, and fat, which all provide energy to the body, can disrupt optimal performance and result in an athlete feeling lethargic or bloated or experiencing stomach cramps. Dietary planning needs to ensure that the athlete follows a generally healthy, balanced diet with personalised adjustments made to the above nutrients via key foods as needed.

For a dietary assessment of an athlete, a diet history interview will likely capture the most in-depth food and beverage information and also allow for a history of subjective factors—such as mood and perceived effects on performance—to be obtained. The interviewer has the ability to focus on key training and periods in the lead-up to an event while also considering other lifestyle-related factors that may impact the individual. Variations in dietary assessments due to the variable lifestyles of many athletes should also be taken into account. On some occasions, more detail may be required, and a food record or diary may be used as well. This provides accountability for the athlete if they have been asked to follow a very specific eating plan and also raises awareness of serving sizes in relation to recommended portion sizes. The food record can also capture the time of the meals and record the time of training to allow for meal plans to be tailored based on feedback from the athlete. A food diary should also endeavour to capture fluid intakes, even though beverages are often more intermittently consumed.

In the lead-up to an event, a 24-hour recall may also provide useful insights. Common recommendations for some sports, such as the timing and composition of pre-game meals and snacks, can be monitored with a quick recall. The recall can also capture information about food intake following an event and allow adjustments to be made to the food choices if needed to promote recovery. Sports nutrition professionals should be consulted to ensure any meal plans being followed are tailored to the individual.

Summary

This chapter has outlined a range of dietary assessment methods and described which tools are most appropriate to use in different circumstances and the limitations associated with those methods. This chapter has explained food composition databases and described how to select the appropriate database for use in a specific context. An awareness of an athlete's circumstances is vital to their food intake and therefore the use of dietary assessment tools that capture the many related elements including the sport-specific needs is vital.

Chapter highlights

- Dietary assessment methods need to be carefully selected based on the athlete or group whose diet needs to be assessed.
- All dietary assessment methods have advantages and disadvantages (see Table 8.1).
- When translating food information from a dietary assessment, the correct food composition database needs to be selected.
- Dietary guidelines and nutrient reference values may be used as comparative tools when analysing a person's dietary intake to create an awareness of any potential nutrient deficiencies.
- Assessing the dietary intake of an athlete requires consideration of the type of sport being undertaken, as well as lifestyle factors, which can all be addressed by a sports nutrition professional.

References

1. National Cancer Institute. *Dietary Assessment Primer: 24-Hour Dietary Recall (24HR) at a Glance.* https://dietassessmentprimer.cancer.gov/profiles/recall/index.html
2. Salvador Castell G, Serra-Majem L, Ribas-Barba. What and how much do we eat? 24-hour dietary recall method. *Nutricion Hospitalaria.* 2015;31(3):46–48.
3. Tapsell LC, Brenninger V, Barnard J. Applying conversation analysis to foster accurate reporting in the diet history interview. *J Am Diet Assoc.* 2000;100(7):818–824.
4. National Cancer Institute. *Dietary Assessment Primer: Food Frequency Questionnaire at a Glance.* https://dietassessmentprimer.cancer.gov/profiles/questionnaire/index.html
5. Perez Rodrigo C, Aranceta J, Salvador G. Food frequency questionnaires. *Nutricion Hospitalaria.* 2015;31(3):49–56.
6. Food Standards Australia New Zealand. *Australian Food Composition Database.* 2022. https://www.foodstandards.gov.au/science/monitoringnutrients/afcd/pages/default.aspx
7. Probst YC, Cunningham J. An overview of the influential developments and stakeholders within the food composition program of Australia. *Trends Food Sci Technol.* 2015;42(2): 173–182.
8. Food and Agriculture Organisation. *FAO/INFOODS Analytical Food Composition Database.* Version 2.0 – AnFooD2.0. 2007. https://www.fao.org/infoods/infoods/tables-and-databases/faoinfoods-databases
9. Capling L, Tam R, Beck KL, et al. Diet quality of elite Australian athletes evaluated using the Athlete Diet Index. *Nutrients.* 2020;13(1):126–141.
10. Stellingwerff T, Morton JP, Burke LM. A framework for periodized nutrition for athletics. *Int J Sport Nutr Exerc Metab.* 2019;29(2):141–151.
11. Dunne DM, Lefevre-Lewis C, Cunniffe B. Athlete experiences of communication strategies in applied sports nutrition and future considerations for mobile app supportive solutions. *Front Sports Active Living.* 2022;12(4):911412.

Part II

Nutrition for exercise

9 Exercise nutrition

Regina Belski

Athletes need to consume a diet that meets their energy, macronutrient, and micronutrient requirements and maximises their exercise outcomes and recovery. The optimal sports nutrition plan for each athlete will change from day to day to accommodate changes in training, goals, and other factors impacting the athlete. However, there are some broad recommendations for what to eat and drink before, during, and following exercise, and these will be the focus of this chapter. The 2017 International Society of Sports Nutrition position stand[1] is considered in this chapter.

More specific recommendations, where available, are discussed in the following chapters, which focus on sporting categories: Endurance (Chapter 17), Strength and power (Chapter 18). Additionally, the emerging trends of macronutrient periodisation, 'training low', and fat adaptation are discussed in more detail in Chapter 10, and strategies for hydration in Chapter 11.

> **Learning outcomes**
>
> **This chapter will:**
>
> - discuss the current recommendations for nutrient intake and hydration prior to, during, and following exercise;
> - explore practical meal and snack ideas for athletes suitable for before, during, and after exercise;
> - highlight that all individual athletes are different, and there is no one-size-fits-all approach to exercise nutrition.

General eating for training and exercise

As discussed in previous chapters, it is critical that athletes consume appropriate intakes of energy, macro-, and micronutrients for training and competition, to have appropriate energy and **substrate** availability for the exercise that they undertake and to enable tissue growth and repair. This means that it is important to consider their overall diet quality,

DOI: 10.4324/9781003321286-11

and not solely what they eat before, during, and after exercise. There are general macronutrient intake recommendations for athletes, which are summarised below.

Substrate

The substance, in this case, the macronutrients carbohydrates, fats, and proteins, on which enzymes work.

Fat intake recommendations for athletes are consistent with public health guidelines and should be individualised based on training level and body composition goals.

Carbohydrate requirements for general daily fuelling of athletes vary greatly based on the type and intensity of sport/exercise:[2]

- light exercise: 3–5 g/kg of body mass (BM) per day;
- moderate intensity: 5–7 g/kg BM/day;
- high intensity: 6–10 g/kg BM/day;
- very high intensity: 8–12 g/kg BM/day.

Protein requirements also vary, with current data suggesting that the level of intake necessary to support metabolic adaptation, repair, remodelling, and for protein turnover in athletes is likely higher than previously recommended, as studies' previous recommendations were based on methods which are now known to underestimate protein needs. The latest International Society for Sports Nutrition position stand on protein and exercise[2] suggests that:

- daily intakes of 1.4–2.0 g/kg/day should be the minimum recommended amount with higher amounts likely needed for athletes attempting to restrict energy intake while maintaining muscle mass;
- meeting the total daily intake of high-quality protein (containing essential amino acids, especially leucine), preferably with evenly spaced protein feedings of 0.25–0.40 g/kg BM/dose, approximately every 3–4 hours during the day, should be viewed as a primary area of emphasis for exercising individuals. Higher doses may be needed to maximise muscle building for older/elderly individuals;
- consuming 30–40 grams of **casein protein** before sleep can lead to short-term increases in muscle protein synthesis and metabolic rate without influencing fat breakdown.

It is worth noting that while recommendations might be higher than previously thought, most athletes' intake still exceeds requirements.[3]

Casein protein

Casein is a family of related phosphoproteins, which are found in mammalian milk. About 80 per cent of the protein in cow's milk is casein.

Eating and drinking before exercise

The key goal of eating and drinking before exercise is to optimise fuel and hydration levels and to make an athlete feel well-prepared for the exercise ahead. There is also now evidence that the nutrients consumed prior to exercise may impact muscle protein synthesis following exercise.

Timing of meals

The right time to consume foods before training or competition will vary depending on when the exercise is to take place. It is generally recommended that consuming a 'main' meal about 2–4 hours prior to exercise will prevent any gastrointestinal (GI) issues from arising; however, if an athlete is training or competing early in the day, or planning a long exercise session, then a small meal or snack 1–2 hours before exercise may be advised.

When working with individual athletes, it is important to listen to their feedback regarding their preferences and past experience, as some athletes have no digestive issues (see Chapter 15) related to eating even within 15 minutes of commencing exercise, while others struggle if less than two hours have passed since their last meal. This simply emphasises that individual gastric emptying rates, as well as the type of food consumed, play an important role in what the best pre-exercise timing may be for an individual athlete.

Content of meals

It is well-recognised that carbohydrate intake before exercise may provide fuel to allow the athlete to train harder or perform better during training and competition. Therefore, a meal or snack high in carbohydrates is generally recommended, as this enables the body to top up its blood glucose and glycogen stores.

Recommendations vary regarding the amount and type of carbohydrates to consume. Low glycaemic index carbohydrates (see Chapter 4) have been promoted as a good choice since they would be more slowly absorbed and lead to a rise in blood glucose in time for, or during, exercise; however, while some early research suggested this outcome, it has not been consistently supported by research. It appears that athletes can select whichever form of carbohydrates they tolerate best if the amount they can consume is appropriate. It is also recommended that foods consumed should be those easier to digest—namely, foods lower in fat and fibre. The reason for lower fat choices is to minimise the length of time the food sits in the stomach, while the lower fibre also allows for food to transition faster, minimising the risk of GI discomfort (see Chapter 15).

The recommended amount of carbohydrates to consume before exercise sessions lasting more than 60 minutes is 1–4 g/kg BM in the 1–4 hours beforehand. However, for training or events lasting less than 90 minutes, the consumption of a high-carbohydrate diet incorporating 7–12 g/kg BM of carbohydrates in the 24 hours beforehand should be adequate to meet the needs of most athletes.[4]

What about protein?

While the benefits of consuming protein immediately after exercise are well known, the benefits of consuming protein prior to exercise are less clear. Recent research suggests that protein consumption before and/or during exercise may further stimulate post-exercise muscle growth. Researchers working in this space have also suggested that the consumption of protein before or during exercise may offer an even greater benefit during the early stages of recovery from more intense training sessions.[5] The International Society of Sports Nutrition position stand on protein and exercise suggests that the timing of protein ingestion should be based on individual tolerance since benefits will be derived from intake before or after a workout.[2] Although it diminishes with time, the anabolic (muscle-building) effect of exercise lasts for at least 24 hours.[2]

Research also suggests that pre-exercise consumption of amino acids in combination with carbohydrates can achieve maximal rates of muscle protein synthesis.[2]

Fluid

As discussed in detail in the chapter on hydration (see Chapter 11), being well-hydrated prior to commencing exercise is important. The current recommendation is to aim for 5–10 mL/kg BM in the 2–4 hours prior to exercise. Depending on the length of the planned exercise session, and whether food is also being consumed, water or sports drinks may be the best options.

Pre-exercise meals and snacks

Some suggestions for suitable pre-exercise meals and snacks are listed in Box 10.1. These are just ideas and may not be suitable for all athletes. Athletes should be supported in developing individualised plans based on personal preferences, and these should be trialled during training.

Common problems reported by athletes

While being nervous is not uncommon in athletes before exercise, nerves can be particularly problematic prior to competition as they can impact the athlete's ability to fuel up appropriately. Athletes often report a lack of appetite, a feeling of 'butterflies' in their stomachs, and nausea as common symptoms. Such issues can impact an athlete's ability to consume a suitable meal or snack prior to training or competition. Athletes should seek support to develop specific strategies to manage and overcome these challenges. This may include finding foods that might be tolerated even with nausea, such as dry toast or plain pasta, or, if pre-exercise eating is not possible, planning the meal the night before an early session to maximise nutrition and hydration status.

Management of GI discomfort, which may include abdominal pain, flatulence, and diarrhoea, which may be caused by nerves or by some of the foods/fluids being consumed by the athlete will be discussed in more detail in Chapter 15. Athletes should never be encouraged to try a new type, amount, or timing of food/supplement/sports drink during competition and should experiment with new foods and fluids only during training sessions where they have control over the environment and situation. The drinks/foods/gels that will be provided at competitions should be identified and trialled well in advance. If these options are not well tolerated by the athlete, individual nutrition provision needs to be planned, practised, and brought to the competition.

Box 9.1   Examples of suitable pre-exercise meals/snacks

Pre-exercise meal (2–4 hours prior)

Breakfast cereal with low-fat milk
Pancakes with jam/fruit and fruit yoghurt
Sandwiches/rolls with meat filling
Pasta dish with a low-fat, tomato-based sauce
Low-fat rice dish

Pre-exercise snack (1–2 hours prior)

Fruit
Fruit yoghurt
Low-fat fruit smoothie
Sports bar/cereal bar
Toast with honey/jam
Low-fat creamed rice

Pre-exercise snack (<1 hour prior)

Carbohydrate gel
Sports bar
Sports drink
Jelly lollies, for example, jelly babies

Eating and drinking during exercise

There are two key approaches to food and fluid provision during exercise; one aims to replace as much of the fuel and fluid used during the exercise session as possible with the aim of maximising exercise performance, and the other focuses on the concept of 'training low' to enhance adaptation.

Replacing nutrient and fluid loss

For exercise sessions up to 90 minutes, it is generally sufficient to simply replace fluid losses. For most athletes, water will be sufficient; however, for those athletes who are big or 'salty' sweaters, beverages containing electrolytes may be a better choice, particularly as sweat rates can vary considerably (from 0.3 to 2.4 L per hour). Furthermore, if athletes are training without having consumed an appropriate meal or snack containing carbohydrates leading up to the session, the consumption of carbohydrates via sports drinks is also often advised.

Stop-start sports

Sports in which the play is frequently stopped due to the ball going out of play or the referee stopping play because of violations of the rules. This includes sports like basketball and football.

For longer sessions, especially those focused on endurance-type exercise, it is important for athletes to consider their likely fluid and nutrient losses and plan suitable drinks/snacks to maintain their fuel and hydration levels and optimise the exercise session.

The recommended amount of carbohydrates to consume during training/events varies based on length and intensity, with 30–60 grams per hour recommended for endurance sports and **stop-start sports** lasting 1–2.5 hours and as much as 90 grams per hour (mixed-substrate) for ultra-endurance sessions/sports lasting in excess of 2.5–3 hours.[4] More details on the needs of endurance athletes, and strategies for fuelling endurance events, can be found in Chapter 17.

There are also specific recommendations from the International Society of Sports Nutrition based on the latest research.[1]

- for extended bouts of high-intensity exercise lasting over an hour, carbohydrates should be consumed at a rate of 30–60 grams of carbohydrates per hour in a 6–8 per cent carbohydrate-electrolyte solution every 10–15 minutes throughout the entire exercise session;
- when carbohydrate consumption during exercise is inadequate, adding protein (0.25 g of protein/kg body weight per hour of endurance exercise) may help increase performance, minimise muscle damage and improve glycogen resynthesis;
- carbohydrate ingestion throughout resistance exercise has also been shown to promote steady blood sugar levels and higher glycogen stores.

It is important to consider what the athlete will tolerate best, as some athletes have no problems consuming sports drinks and a sandwich during an event while others struggle even to drink water without experiencing GI issues. Nutrition plans should be based not only on the type and length of exercise but also on the individual needs and preferences of the athlete.

As discussed in detail in Chapter 11, the current recommendation is to aim to consume 400–800 mL/hour of fluid during exercise, with the aim of avoiding body-water losses of more than 2 per cent. Cold drinks are recommended for hot conditions.

It is important to note that during exercise sessions exceeding two hours in length, GI tolerance and availability of fluids will restrict what fluids will be accessible and tolerable to athletes. This makes it unlikely that athletes will be able to match sweat fluid losses with fluid intake.[6] Athletes should be encouraged to commence exercise well-hydrated and to replace fluid losses after exercise.

Suitable drinks and snacks during exercise

Some suggestions of suitable snacks to consume during exercise are listed below. These are just ideas and may not be suitable for all athletes. Athletes should be supported to develop individualised plans based on personal preferences.

Convenient snacks/drinks providing 30–40 grams of carbohydrates:

- 600 mL sports drink;
- 1 sports bar;
- 1.5 carbohydrate gels;
- 40 g jelly (gummy) lollies/candies;
- 1.5 cereal bars.

Training low

The concept of 'training low' to enhance adaptation generally refers to training with low carbohydrate availability but may also be practised with other nutrients. The aim of this approach is to integrate specific sessions into a training program where the standard practice of providing nutritional support to promote optimal performance is replaced by deliberately withholding nutritional support prior to and during the session. There is some evidence to suggest that the absence of certain nutrients (for instance, carbohydrates) around exercise leads to an increased training stimulus and/or an enhanced metabolic adaptation to exercise. There are numerous different ways in which athletes can 'train low', with different metabolic outcomes. Refer to Chapter 10 for more details regarding the evidence and recommendations for training low.

Eating and drinking after exercise

The key aim of eating and drinking after exercise is to replenish the body's fluid and fuel stores used during exercise and optimise recovery post-exercise. The provision of nutrients after exercise may also enhance metabolic adaptations to exercise.

Carbohydrates

One of the goals of post-exercise nutrition is to restore glycogen levels; this requires adequate carbohydrate intake and time. The glycogen resynthesis rate appears to be around 5 per cent per hour. The consumption of 1–1.2 g/kg BM/h of carbohydrates early in the recovery period (during the first 4–6 hours) has been shown to be effective in maximising refuelling time between workouts.[4]

Protein

Research has shown that the consumption of high-quality protein sources (0.25 g/kg BM or an absolute dose of 20–40 grams), rich in essential amino acids, within two hours of completion of exercise results in increases in muscle protein synthesis.[2]

What if rapid recovery is needed?

During times of intensive training or competition, rapid recovery and restoration of glycogen stores may be required. Where there is less than four hours of recovery time available, the following strategies—as recommended by the International Society of Sports Nutrition based on current research—should be considered.[1]

- intensive carbohydrate refeeding (1.2 g/kg BM/h) with high glycaemic index carbohydrates (see Chapter 4);
- consumption of caffeine (3–8 mg/kg BM);
- combination of carbohydrates (0.8 g/kg BM/h) with protein (0.2–0.4 g/kg BM/h).

Fluid

Hydration and rehydration are discussed in detail in Chapter 11. After exercise, it is recommended that athletes replace 125–150 per cent of fluid loss. For example, if an athlete has lost 2 kilograms of weight during exercise, they should aim to consume 2.5–3 litres of fluid following exercise to replace the loss. Eating solid food at this time will help maximise fluid retention.

Box 9.2   Snack/meal options for after exercise

Sports drink with low-fat fruit yoghurt
Low-fat chocolate milk
Liquid breakfast substitute drinks
Fruit smoothies made with low-fat milk/yoghurt
Pancakes with fruit and low-fat yoghurt

Summary

This chapter has highlighted that an athlete's general nutrition is important for optimal health and wellbeing and poor general nutrition choices will impact exercise performance. Making appropriate choices throughout the day, as well as optimising food and fluid intake around exercise, will help the athlete undertake quality training sessions. The aim of food and drink consumption prior to exercise is to optimise fuel and hydration levels and enable an athlete to feel prepared for exercise. During exercise, the key objective is to try to manage the fluid loss and refuel with carbohydrates to maintain blood glucose levels and train harder or perform better. Following an exercise session, the aim is to refuel, rehydrate, and enhance recovery or adaptation. Nutrition plans should be developed using the most suitable choices based on athletes' specific requirements and personal dietary preferences.

Chapter highlights

- Athletes' general diets are most important for optimal health and exercise performance.
- Training and competition nutrition should be planned in accordance with the individual athlete's training, goals and preferences.
  - Protein: Daily intakes of 1.4–2.0 g/kg/day should be the minimum recommended amount.
  - Carbohydrates: Requirements vary greatly based on the type and intensity of sport/exercise:[7] light exercise (3–5 g/kg BM/d), moderate intensity (5–7 g/kg BM/day), high intensity (6–10 g/kg BM/day), and very high intensity (8–12 g/kg BM/day).
  - Fat: Recommendations for athletes are consistent with public health guidelines and should be individualised based on training level and body composition goals.
- Nutrition should be provided before exercise to be well hydrated with full glycogen stores.
- During exercise, athletes should aim to top up as much lost fluid and carbohydrates as possible or utilise appropriate 'train low' techniques.
  - Carbohydrates: 30–60 grams per hour recommended for endurance sports and stop-start sports lasting 1–2.5 hours.

- Fluid: 400–800 mL/hour of fluid during exercise, with the aim of avoiding body-water losses of more than 2 per cent.
- After exercise, athletes should aim to rehydrate and refuel in time for the next exercise session, as well as consume the appropriate type and amount of nutrients to support metabolic adaptation and muscle growth.
  - Fluid: Replace 125–150 per cent of fluid loss.
  - Carbohydrates: 1–1.2 g/kg BM/h of carbohydrates early in the recovery period (during the first 4–6 hours).
  - Protein: Consume 0.25 g/kg BM or an absolute dose of 20–40 grams within 2 hours.

References

1. Kerksick CM, Arent S, Schoenfeld BJ. International Society of Sports Nutrition position stand: Nutrient timing. *J Int Soc Sports Nutr.* 2017;14(S2):33.
2. Jäger R, Kerksick CM, Campbell BI. International Society of Sports Nutrition position stand: Protein and exercise. *J Int Soc Sports Nutr.* 2017;14(S2):20.
3. Meyer NL, Reguant-Closa A, Nemecek T. Sustainable diets for athletes. *Curr Nutr Rep.* 2020; 9:147–162.
4. Thomas DT, Erdman KA, Burke LM. American College of Sports Medicine joint position statement. Nutrition and athletic performance. *Med Sci Sports Exerc.* 2016;48(3):543–568.
5. van Loon LJ. Is there a need for protein ingestion during exercise? *Sports Med.* 2014;44(S1): 105–111.
6. Garth AK, Burke LM. What do athletes drink during competitive sporting activities? *Sports Med.* 2013;43(7):539–564.
7. Burke LM, Hawley JA, Wong SH. Carbohydrates for training and competition. *J Sports Sci.* 2011;29(S1):S17–S27.

10 Macronutrient periodisation

Louise M Burke

Although most people now recognise that sports nutrition involves a personalised approach to the specific needs of the event and the individual, there is still a perception that the athlete's goal is to develop an optimal meal plan (e.g. a swimmer's diet or Swimmer X's diet), then carefully repeat it each day to provide consistent support for their training and competition goals. In contrast, contemporary sports nutrition guidelines promote the benefits of a periodised approach to the intake energy and macronutrient intake, with each athlete following a range of different dietary practices, aligned to the different phases of their training cycles, competition calendars, or career progress. Although there is no single or unified definition of the term "dietary periodisation", Table 10.1 summarises four different themes that involve a strategic manipulation of nutrient intake between and within days to optimise athletic performance. Since the principles and practices of arranging nutrient intake around training/event sessions (intake pre-, during, and post-session) are covered in Chapter 9, this review will summarise the evidence and application of the other three periodisation themes.

Learning outcomes

This chapter will:

- outline how an athlete's training/competition schedule involves changes in the type, quantity and goals of exercise sessions, which should be supported by changes in energy and macronutrient intake;
- describe how different dietary strategies can enhance the muscle's capacity to use different fuels (e.g. fat vs carbohydrate), which may play a role in enhancing competition performance;
- explain "metabolic flexibility" and some of the ways in which this concept is currently being used or misused;
- describe an emerging theme in sports nutrition, in which nutrient support around training can be provided to promote performance/recovery or withdrawn to increase the training stimulus/adaptation.

DOI: 10.4324/9781003321286-12

Table 10.1 Examples of themes in which nutrients are periodised to enhance performance

Theme	Description	Explanation or examples
General tracking of energy and nutrient goals	Changing energy and nutrient intake (between days, microcycles, macrocycles, etc.) to meet different needs/goals, according to the specific phases of the training and competition plan	Athletes undertake a carefully periodised calendar involving different training phases which prepare them to meet short-term and long-term competition goals. Changes in the exercise load, physique management goals, environmental conditions and many other factors change the energy cost and nutrient needs. The athlete should manipulate their dietary patterns to meet these changes in needs
Nutrient timing	Arranging nutrient intake over the day, and in relation to training sessions, to enhance the metabolic interaction between exercise and nutrition	Carbohydrate intake before and during exercise may provide fuel to allow the athlete to train harder or perform better in competition. Provision of nutrients after exercise may enhance recovery or adaptation; for example, the optimal spread of protein includes intake soon after exercise and every 3–5 hours over the day.
"Fat adaptation"	Exposure to a high-fat diet for a period, either ketogenic or non-ketogenic, to increase the capacity to use fat as a muscle fuel for exercise. The athlete may maintain this diet or include resumption of carbohydrate intake for additional competition fuelling	Hypothetically, capacity for enhanced fuel utilisation during exercise might occur if adaptations can make use of the athlete's relatively unlimited body fat supplies. If increased fat use can be added to scenarios of high carbohydrate availability and utilisation, such "increased metabolic flexibility" might also enhance endurance performance
"Training low" to enhance adaptation	Integrating specific sessions into the training program in which the standard practice of providing nutritional support to promote optimal performance is replaced by the deliberate withholding of nutritional support for the session.	There is evidence that the absence of some nutrients around exercise leads to an increased training stimulus and/or an enhanced adaptation. At present, this theory is mostly applied to the theme of carbohydrate availability. Athletes may deliberately train with low carbohydrate availability (overnight fasting and the absence of carbohydrate intake during the session, with or without low muscle glycogen content) to increase the cellular adaptation to endurance exercise. In particular, there is an increase in adaptation to increase the number and activity of mitochondria, that enable oxidative production of ATP for muscle contraction. Alternatively, the athlete may avoid carbohydrate intake in the hours after a high-quality training session undertaken with high carbohydrate availability to delay muscle glycogen restoration. This tactic prolongs the post-exercise period of increased cellular signalling, also increasing the adaptive response to the session

Theme 1: Periodising nutrition to track the periodisation of training and competition

An athlete's peak performance is achieved over a number of years during which they undertake various cycles of preparation and competition. Although many athletes may have a long-term program aimed at an Olympic cycle or the years of a college scholarship, the yearly training plan or annual competition calendar provides a useful snapshot of the concept of periodised training. Typically, the plan is centred around the major competition for which the athlete organises a performance peak. Depending on the logistics of the event and the culture/philosophies of the sport, the coach and athlete may plan for a single or double peak for the year (e.g. two major competitions, or qualification for a national team then competition in the international event). The yearly training plan varies considerably between sports according to the athlete's level (e.g. developmental, elite, recreational), the type of competition (e.g. weekly fixtures, tournaments, single events spread over a season), and the type of event (how much recovery is needed). However, there are some common elements. These include:

- a generalised preparation phase;
- a period of training that is more specific to the competitive event;
- competition itself; and
- transition between phases including an off-season or rest period.

Figures 10.1 and 10.2 illustrate a simplistic overview of the typical yearly training plans of a team sport and an individual sport, respectively, noting differences in the exercise load and goals across each phase that create differences in nutritional needs and strategies. The basic unit of each phase is the training microcycle (typically, a 7-day rotation), in which a series of workouts (and in some sports, competition) are sequenced to integrate a range of training stimuli that aim to achieve the various physiological, biomechanical, technical, tactical and psychological characteristics needed for success. Typically, the microcycles are manipulated to gradually increase the important loading characteristics (type, volume, intensity, etc.) and then allow for a lighter "recovery' cycle, before continuing to build. At times, an athlete might undertake a special training block such as altitude or heat training, either to acclimatise to the environmental conditions in which a competition might be held or to gain the benefits from the additional training stimulus provided by thermal or hypoxic exposure. In the pre-competition phase, the increased specificity of training will include opportunities to practice and fine-tune nutritional strategies that are important to performance in the event – for example, fluid and carbohydrate intake during exercise. The taper period prior to competition varies across sports but typically involves a reduction in training volume to allow the athlete to reduce their fatigue levels and reach a performance peak.

The periodisation of training clearly can be improved by a careful periodisation of nutrient intake and dietary practices. Different phases of training – from day to day, within a training block or over the year – will have different requirements for energy and muscle fuel support, as well as differences in the focus on the manipulation or maintenance of physique (e.g. to lose body fat, increase lean mass, meet weight division target), competition practice or importance of key nutrients (e.g. adequate iron status during altitude training). Some of the high-level differences and changes in dietary focus are included in Figures 10.1 and 10.2. Here, the annual training plan for a team sport shows the conditioning phase of the pre-season with a gradual increase in match-specific skills and

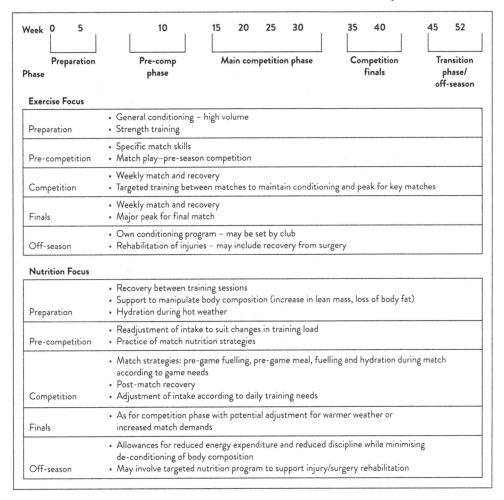

Week	0 5	10	15 20 25 30	35 40	45 52
Phase	Preparation	Pre-comp phase	Main competition phase	Competition finals	Transition phase/ off-season

Exercise Focus

Preparation	• General conditioning – high volume • Strength training
Pre-competition	• Specific match skills • Match play–pre-season competition
Competition	• Weekly match and recovery • Targeted training between matches to maintain conditioning and peak for key matches
Finals	• Weekly match and recovery • Major peak for final match
Off-season	• Own conditioning program – may be set by club • Rehabilitation of injuries – may include recovery from surgery

Nutrition Focus

Preparation	• Recovery between training sessions • Support to manipulate body composition (increase in lean mass, loss of body fat) • Hydration during hot weather
Pre-competition	• Readjustment of intake to suit changes in training load • Practice of match nutrition strategies
Competition	• Match strategies: pre-game fuelling, pre-game meal, fuelling and hydration during match according to game needs • Post-match recovery • Adjustment of intake according to daily training needs
Finals	• As for competition phase with potential adjustment for warmer weather or increased match demands
Off-season	• Allowances for reduced energy expenditure and reduced discipline while minimising de-conditioning of body composition • May involve targeted nutrition program to support injury/surgery rehabilitation

Figure 10.1 Example of a yearly training plan for a team sport (football) with a weekly match fixture.

[adapted from Burke and Jeacocke[1]].

practice matches, the main competition season with a cycle of weekly matches culminating in finals, and an off-season (Figure 10.1). Meanwhile, in Figure 10.2, a swimmer undertakes base training in which 3–4 week cycles of training are integrated, with race-specific training and short race meets being increased towards the major competition. Altitude training may be included in the pre-competition peaking plan, and a significant taper leads into the multiday swimming meet. In the case where a second competition peak is planned (often the most important competition), there is a short transition leading into a truncated preparation cycle. In this sport, there are major differences in the energy and fuel requirements of training, taper and racing, requiring major changes in food intake.

Within the training microcycle/week, different approaches to the optimal nutritional support for each individual training session should lead to changes in daily energy intake, as well as different emphases on the amount and timing of intake of special macronutrients (e.g. carbohydrate and protein) around a workout according to their role in

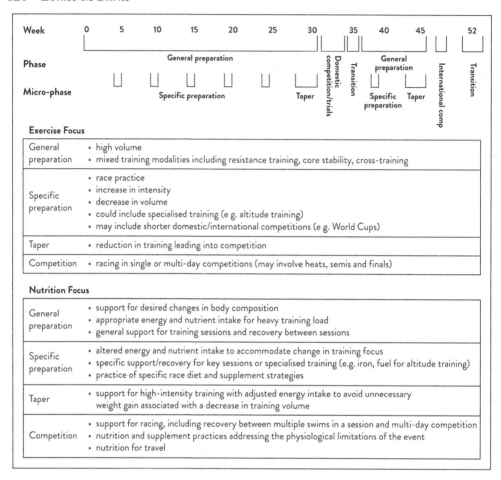

Figure 10.2 Example of a yearly training plan for an individual sport (swimming) with a double peak.

[adapted from Burke and Jeacocke[1]].

"training harder/better" or "training smarter". Some of these issues will be discussed further in Theme 3 and are illustrated by the summary of a typical week of periodised carbohydrate availability in a training study (Table 10.2). Many sports nutrition professionals find it useful to create an athlete's periodised nutrition plan, using an "inside out" approach to build up a series of layers.

1. Identify each key training session for the week and the specific goals of each session. Organise a targeted intake of the most important nutrients pre-, during and/or post each workout.
2. Add the next layer by organising eating occasions for the rest of the day to continue to support these key sessions, but also bearing in mind the athlete's "bigger picture" nutritional needs such as energy (does the athlete need to be in energy balance, or to increase or reduce energy intake to manipulate body composition), key micronutrients (e.g. does the athlete need to increase iron intake? Calcium intake?) and other special issues (e.g. food preferences, finances, food availability, intolerance).

Table 10.2 Dietary strategies that achieve specific goals with carbohydrate availability

Low carbohydrate availability: Strategies undertaken to increase the exercise stimulus and/or to enhance the adaptive response to an exercise bout	
Protocol	*Strategy*
Chronic low carbohydrate availability (achieves low endogenous and exogenous carbohydrate availability)	Ketogenic LCHF diet (<50 g/day carbohydrate, ~80% energy as fat) Non-ketogenic LCHF diet (15–20% energy as carbohydrate; 60–65% energy as fat)
Acute low carbohydrate availability training ("train low") – endogenous	Undertaking prior bout of prolonged sustained or intermittent exercise followed by restricted intake of carbohydrate to limit glycogen resynthesis during a recovery phase. Note that it is the second session that is done as a "train low" session, and the between-session recovery phase can be brief (1–2 hours) or prolonged (e.g. overnight or full day)
Acute low carbohydrate availability training ("train low") – exogenous	Undertaking workout in the morning in a fasted state, and without any carbohydrate intake during the session (Note: could also be done for a session later only water during the session)
Acute post-exercise low carbohydrate availability ("recover low" or "sleep low" – if overnight)	Restricting carbohydrate intake in the hours after a key workout to delay glycogen resynthesis
High carbohydrate availability: strategies undertaken to provide adequate fuel for the exercise session, promoting optimal performance or practising event nutrition strategies	
Protocol	*Strategy*
Chronic high carbohydrate availability	Consuming enough carbohydrate in the everyday diet to consistently meet the fuel needs of training or competition, with intake organised around each exercise session to ensure optimal fuelling
Active refuelling	Consuming carbohydrate in sufficient quantities, starting soon after an exercise session to optimise glycogen resynthesis after the session
Training high – endogenous	Consuming adequate carbohydrate in the recovery between two sessions, including a pre-session snack or meal to provide adequate glycogen for the workout or competition event
Training high – exogenous	Consuming carbohydrate in the pre-exercise meal to ensure high liver glycogen levels as well as carbohydrate during the session to provide an ongoing supply of blood glucose as an additional muscle fuel
Carbohydrate loading	Organising exercise taper in conjunction with high carbohydrate intake to supercompensate muscle glycogen stores prior to endurance/ultra-endurance competition

Adapted from Burke et al.[17]
LCHF = low carbohydrate high fat.

3. Continue by organising menu plans/themes for days with less important sessions, focusing on the bigger picture of nutrition issues. Note that there may be less need to be focused on fuelling for these sessions, and even an opportunity to undertake some "train low" sessions where workouts are deliberately matched up with low carbohydrate eating strategies (see Theme 3). On the other hand, there may be a need to use low-key training days to fuel up for the next day's important workouts.

The sophistication of this approach is likely to lead to daily differences in menus and food intake, or on occasions, similar total intakes that are spread differently between and within days.

The practice of event fluid/fuel intake strategies is an important activity to build into the periodised programs of endurance/ultra-endurance and some team sports. This allows the athlete to individualise and fine-tune a nutrition plan to defend homeostasis and sustain fuel for optimal performance when it is most needed. However, in addition to familiarising with competition eating/drinking behaviours or identifying the foods/drinks that best suit the scenario, targeted intake during training sessions can help to "train the gut".[2] For example, several adaptations may be needed to help the athlete meet the newer targets for aggressive carbohydrate intake during prolonged exercise; these involve increasing gut tolerance or comfort to allow intake of greater volumes of fluid/food as well as enhancing intestinal absorption of glucose via an increase in the number of **SGLT-1** transporters.

SGLT-1 transporter: sodium-dependent glucose transporter

Transport protein found on the walls of cells lining the small intestine, responsible for the transport of glucose and galactose from the small intestine into the circulation.

Theme 2: "Fat adaptation"

In many events, competitive success is determined by the muscle's ability to optimise the production of Adenosine Tri-Phosphate (ATP) to meet the requirements of the exercise task. This reflects both the size of the available fuel stores and the muscle's ability to efficiently integrate their use; a concept termed "**metabolic flexibility**". Depletion of the body's relatively limited carbohydrate stores is a common cause of fatigue or sub-optimal performance during endurance sports (typically defined as events involving prolonged (>90 minutes) continuous exercise). Therefore, it has been proposed that strategies that improve the athlete's capacity to make better use of their larger fat stores will spare the muscle glycogen stores and increase metabolic flexibility. Although training achieves this outcome, the use of fat as a muscle fuel can be further (and more substantially) increased by adapting to a low carbohydrate, high-fat diet (LCHF). Indeed, exposure to a diet providing <20% energy from carbohydrates and >60% from fat undertaking both high-volume and high-intensity training sessions, can achieve a robust retooling of the muscle to increase the mobilisation, transport and oxidation of fat during exercise in as little as 5 days.[3]

Metabolic flexibility

The ability of the muscle to integrate and transition between fuel sources in response to exercise or hormonal stimuli. This is enhanced by training but is decreased in scenarios known as "metabolic syndrome".

If this high-fat diet is further carbohydrate-restricted (<50 g/day carbohydrate plus ~80% energy from fat) while moderating protein intake (and the intake of gluconeogenic precursors), additional benefits from exposure to high levels of circulating ketone bodies are also claimed. This ketogenic version of the LCHF diet has become the more popular version of fat adaptation over the past decade.[4] Despite considerable discussion about this diet being "the future of elite endurance sport" in lay and social media, its effect on high-performance endurance athletes, who compete for prolonged or critical periods at exercise intensities around ~85–90% aerobic capacity, has been consistently observed to be negative.[5] There is no doubt that chronic (>3–4 weeks) adaptation to the ketogenic LCHF diet substantially increases the muscle's capacity for fat oxidation during exercise, providing effective fuel support for moderate-intensity exercise.[6] However, a series of studies undertaken at the Australian Institute of Sport in which highly trained to world-class race walkers were adapted to the LCHF diet, provided recognition of an important biochemical fact: that the oxygen cost of oxidising fat to produce a given amount of ATP is ~5% greater than that of carbohydrate.[7–9] Although these studies have resulted in the highest rates of fat oxidation ever reported in the literature across a range of speeds relevant to the races on the Olympic program, this was associated with a loss of **economy** (a greater oxygen cost to achieve the same speed), that is entirely predictable from the stoichiometry of fat vs carbohydrate oxidation. indeed, in comparison to control groups who undertook the same training whilst consuming diets providing high carbohydrate availability, athletes who trialled the LCHF diets, alone or with the addition of other fuel sources on race day (e.g. restoration of muscle glycogen stores, intake of exogenous ketone supplements) experienced a mean impairment of performance in real-life 10,000 m races of ~7%.[7–10] This suggests that adaptation to LCHF diets may be suited to athletes who compete in events conducted entirely at moderate intensities where the oxygen supply does not become limiting, but actually provides a disadvantage in endurance sports and ultra-endurance sports involving critical passages of higher intensity work, where success is determined by the ability to exercise as economically as possible at the highest sustainable intensity. Indeed, the LCHF diet provides an impairment of the economy of similar magnitude to the improvement in the economy associated with the use of "super shoes": here, the significance of such changes in the economy is demonstrated by noting that every world record in distance athletics has been broken over the past 5 years since the introduction of these shoes.[11]

Exercise economy

In endurance sports, this term is used to describe the oxygen cost of achieving a speed, power or intensity and is highly correlated with competitive performance. Although most high-calibre athletes have a high aerobic capacity (VO_2max), within a group of such athletes, economy of movement – being able to move quickly at a relatively low percentage of this capacity – often determines performance. This is especially important when the duration of the event or critical parts of it are conducted at intensities around the so-called anaerobic threshold.

To overcome the limitations of relying on fat oxidation alone, several studies have tried to integrate the availability of a second fuel source for a competitive event, either by re-establishing high carbohydrate availability (24 h of glycogen super-compensation and carbohydrate intake before and during the event)[8, 12] or by consuming ketone ester supplements.[10] However, these attempts failed to find that fat adaptation-carbohydrate restoration protocols enhance the performance of subsequent prolonged exercise, despite achieving remarkable reductions in muscle glycogen use (for review see Burke[3, 5]). One of the apparent explanations for this outcome is that, rather than sparing glycogen utilisation, fat adaptation impairs the muscle's ability to use it as an exercise fuel. In addition to reducing rates of glycogen breakdown, fat adaptation has been shown to impair muscle carbohydrate oxidation via downregulation of the activity of an important enzyme in the mitochondria – the **pyruvate dehydrogenase** enzyme complex.[13] The consequences of reduced efficiency of carbohydrate oxidation are likely to manifest in a reduced ability to support the ATP requirements for exercise at higher intensities throughout the event,[9] or during sprint efforts within a longer event.[12]

In summary, current evidence suggests that strategies to chronically adapt to high-fat diets achieve a reduction rather than an improvement of metabolic flexibility. Indeed, even when glycogen is available, fat adaptation strategies appear to interfere with the muscle's capacity to use it as an exercise fuel, particularly via oxidative pathways. This is likely to translate into reduced performance in shorter endurance events conducted at these exercise intensities (e.g. half marathon, 40 km cycling Time Trial), as well as an impaired ability to undertake the critical activities within most longer endurance/ultra-endurance sports events – the breakaway, the tactical surge, attacking a hill, the sprint to the finish line – which determine the overall outcome. Therefore, the range of sporting events or scenarios to which they might be suited is small. Furthermore, even in those studies in which reductions in exercise performance in association with ketogenic diets were not apparent, considerable individual variability in response to the diet was reported.[6,14]

Pyruvate dehydrogenase (PDH)

Mitochondrial enzyme complex that commits the breakdown products of glycolysis (the first step in glucose metabolism) into the Citric Acid (Krebs cycle) oxidation pathway. This step is irreversible and is the rate-limiting step in carbohydrate oxidation.

Theme 3: "Training low" to enhance training adaptations

Scientific techniques now allow us to study the cellular responses to exercise and nutrient stimuli. Such techniques have provided the insight that across many areas of sports nutrition, the processes related to muscle adaptation may be opposite to those that promote recovery/performance. Simply stated, many processes that promote recovery from exercise to restore homeostasis and exercise capacity are based on the provision of nutrient support. Meanwhile, the absence or deliberate withdrawal of nutritional support may increase exercise stress and/or promote signalling pathways that remodel the muscle and other physiological systems to enhance the training response. Therefore, the athlete may use some nutritional strategies to compete optimally or to complete key training sessions as well as possible ("train harder"). Conversely, they may implement the opposite strategy to stimulate greater adaptation to the same exercise stimulus (a "training smarter" approach). There is evidence that although fluid intake enhances endurance performance in the heat (see Chapter 14), deliberate dehydration during training sessions may enhance the physiological and cardiovascular processes of acclimatisation.[15] Nevertheless, the area in which most investigation has been undertaken around the theme of strategic addition or withholding of nutritional support involves the manipulation of carbohydrate availability.

Carbohydrate availability

Consideration of the timing and amount of carbohydrate intake in the athlete's diet in comparison to the muscle fuel costs of the training or competition schedule. Scenarios of "high carbohydrate availability" cover strategies in which body carbohydrate supplies can meet the fuel costs of the exercise program, whereas "low carbohydrate availability" considers scenarios in which **endogenous and/or exogenous carbohydrate supplies** are less than muscle fuel needs.

Endogenous carbohydrate fuels

Carbohydrate fuel found inside the muscle cell (glycogen).

Exogenous carbohydrate fuels

Carbohydrate fuel taken up into the muscle from the circulation (blood glucose, which is greatly supplemented by the intake of carbohydrate during exercise).

Dietary practices that promote high **carbohydrate availability** are recommended on days in which competition or high quality/demanding training sessions will benefit from optimal fuelling of muscle and central nervous system function (i.e. optimisation of work rates, perception of effort, skill and technique, concentration and mental processing). As outlined in Theme 1, carbohydrate intake should be integrated with other dietary goals to achieve adequate muscle fuel from glycogen stores supported by additional exogenous carbohydrate supplies as well as support other body processes requiring carbohydrate (e.g. immune system support). Targets will consider both the total amount of carbohydrate and its timing of intake around the workout or event. Competition strategies will need to address the practical considerations for consuming nutrients around exercise (e.g. event rules, opportunity to consume foods/drinks and availability of supplies). On days when training is of lower volume and/or intensity, it may be less critical to meet such targets or practice these strategies.

More recently, it has been shown that glycogen plays important roles in regulating the cellular activities that underpin the muscle's response to exercise. Specifically, undertaking a bout of endurance exercise with low muscle glycogen stores produces a coordinated up-regulation of key signalling and regulatory proteins in the muscle to enhance the adaptive processes following the exercise session.[16] This can be achieved around targeted training sessions, by doing two training sessions in close succession or with minimal carbohydrate intake between them, to enable the second bout to be commenced with depleted glycogen stores. Strategies that restrict exogenous carbohydrate availability (e.g. training in a fasted state) also promote an improved signalling response, although of a lower magnitude than is the case for exercise with low glycogen stores.[16] These strategies enhance the cellular outcomes of endurance training such as increased maximal mitochondrial enzyme activities and/or mitochondrial content and increased rates of lipid oxidation.

Studies in sub-elite athletes, in which these protocols have been superimposed on most workouts in a training block, have shown evidence of enhanced cellular adaptation. Somewhat curiously, however, these "muscle advantages" have not transferred to superior performance outcomes compared with the improvements seen following training with high carbohydrate availability. Although there are always challenges in measuring small but important changes in sports performance, the most likely explanation for the "disconnect" between mechanistic and performance outcomes in these studies is that training with low carbohydrate availability reduced the intensity of the training sessions. In other words, although metabolic benefits were achieved on one hand, they were negated by the sacrificing of training quality. This suggests that "train low" strategies need to be carefully integrated into the periodised training program to carefully match the specific goal of the session and the larger goals of the training period. Indeed, a more recently identified exercise-nutrient interaction adds another strategy to the carbohydrate periodisation options to assist with this integration. Delaying glycogen resynthesis by withholding carbohydrate in the hours after a higher-intensity training session has also been shown to upregulate markers of mitochondrial biogenesis and lipid oxidation during the recovery phase without interfering with the quality of the session.[17]

A practical application of this new strategy is that it allows the sequencing of (1) a "train high" high-quality training session, (2) overnight or within day carbohydrate restriction ("sleep low"), and (3) a moderate intensity workout undertaken without carbohydrate intake ("train low"). This series, demonstrated in two different styles in the case study, supports the important features of each training session while promoting enhanced adaptation. Studies have shown that the integration of several cycles of this sequence into the weekly training programs of sub-elite athletes achieved performance improvements which were not observed in another group who undertook similar training with a similar intake of carbohydrate that was evenly distributed within and between days.[18] Such an approach has been described in the real-life preparation of elite endurance athletes.[19] A summary of strategies that promote high or low carbohydrate availability is provided in Box 10.1.

Finally, it should be recognised that studies of elite athletes appear to show less responsiveness to periodisation of carbohydrate availability than seen in sub-elite athletes. Investigations of the 3-week program of intensified training in world-class race walkers, described earlier, failed to detect any difference in the immediate performance benefits achieved by the group who consumed a periodised carbohydrate diet and another group who consumed an evenly spread distribution of the same total carbohydrate intake to promote high carbohydrate availability for all training sessions.[7, 8] Another study of elite endurance athletes reported no benefits to training adaptation or performance gains from the integration of a within day sequence of a "train high"/"recover low"/"train low" protocol, 3 days a week during a training block, compared with a diet providing more consistent carbohydrate availability.[20] It is uncertain whether the lack of benefits is systematically related to the calibre of the athlete. For example, it is possible that elite athletes have a reduced ceiling for improvements in which differences are harder to detect, or an ability to undertake training of such intensity and volume that the stimulus already maximises the adaptive response. Further investigation is merited but it is likely that most highly trained athletes already integrate some form of periodisation of carbohydrate availability within their schedules, either by design or practicality. The challenge for sports science will be to improve on what athletes achieve through trial and error.

Box 10.1   Case Study: Periodising carbohydrate availability in a training program

Profile and problem

A research project undertaken at the Australian Institute of Sport wanted to implement some strategies for periodising carbohydrate availability into the weekly training schedule of a group of elite race walkers. The training program was set by experienced coaches who explained the purpose of each session as well as the goals of the training block. The research team of sports scientists and sports dietitians examined the potential benefits of organising some sessions to be undertaken with high carbohydrate availability (to promote good performance and practice race nutrition sessions), as well as some sessions with low carbohydrate availability (to increase the training stimulus or increase the adaptive response to the workout). Other nutrition goals for the training week, which were positioned in the base conditioning phase for the season were also considered.

Assessment

Table 10.3 Weekly training schedule for elite race walkers

Day	Monday	Tuesday	Wednesday	Thursday	Friday	Saturday	Sunday
Morning session	15 km walk	10 km recovery walk Gym	Long walk 25 km	15 km walk Gym	Hill session	Long walk – 30 km	Rest
Afternoon session	10 × 1 km interval session at track	10 km recovery walk	5 km walk	10 km moderate Intensity walk	10 km recovery walk	Rest	rest

The following strategies were proposed for implementation around special sessions:

- Wednesday and Saturday am long walks: high carbohydrate availability to support good performance, with practice of race nutrition strategies used in 50 km event
- Monday afternoon interval session: high carbohydrate availability before and during the session to allow good speed to be produced
- Friday morning session: high carbohydrate availability before and during the session to allow strong training performance right throughout the session

- Gym sessions: refuel after the morning walking session before the gym workout; protein intake straight after the session to promote adaptation
- After interval session: restrict carbohydrate intake at dinner and overnight (= "sleep low") to increase the duration of the post-exercise adaptation
- After hill session: restrict carbohydrate intake at breakfast and lunch (= "recover low") to increase the duration of the post-exercise adaptation
- Tuesday morning and Friday afternoon recovery walks: restrict carbohydrate intake before and during the session in concert with delayed glycogen resynthesis to achieve "train low" from both muscle (endogenous) and blood glucose (exogenous) fuels, therefore increasing the training stimulus
- Monday morning and Thursday morning recovery walks: train in a fasted state and with water only during the session to achieve "train low" from blood glucose (exogenous fuels) to increase the training stimulus

Other "Bigger Picture" nutrition goals

- Spread protein intake over each meal and post-exercise snack each day to promote adaptation
- Allow a small energy deficit over the training week to allow a small loss of body fat during the base conditioning phase of training
- Ensure adequate fluid intake during and after each training session, and at meals due to hot weather training
- Ensure meals include nutrient-dense foods to allow good supply of vitamins, minerals and phytochemicals for general health and well-being

Plan

Table 10.4 Summary of weekly eating plan

Day	Monday	Tuesday	Wednesday	Thursday	Friday	Saturday	Sunday
Breakfast and am snacks	CHO-rich breakfast after morning walk	CHO-rich breakfast after morning walk High protein/ CHO shake after Gym	CHO-rich breakfast before long walk Sports drink and gels during walk High protein/ CHO shake after walk	CHO-rich breakfast after morning walk High protein/ CHO shake after Gym		CHO-rich breakfast before long walk Sports drink and gels during walk High protein/ CHO shake after walk Long walk – 30 km	Sleep in
Lunch and afternoon snack	CHO-rich lunch CHO-rich snack pre-interval session and sports drink during	CHO-rich lunch CHO-rich snack in afternoon	CHO-rich lunch CHO-rich snack in afternoon	CHO-rich lunch	Low CHO lunch CHO-rich snack after training session	CHO-rich lunch	CHO-rich brunch

Day	Monday	Tuesday	Wednesday	Thursday	Friday	Saturday	Sunday
Dinner	CHO restricted dinner	CHO-rich dinner CHO-rich dessert for additional fuel for next am session	CHO-rich dinner	CHO-rich dinner	CHO-rich dinner CHO-rich dessert for additional fuel for next am session	CHO-rich dinner	CHO-rich dinner

Notes: All meals include at least 25 g protein and fluids. All training sessions provide access to fluid during and after the session.
(CHO = Carbohydrate).

Summary

This chapter has described how many of the current frontiers in sports nutrition involve the periodisation of nutrient and energy intake – manipulating intakes between and within days to promote specific goals of adaptation, performance and recovery. Each athlete has unique nutritional goals and requirements, which change according to the specific time of their periodised training and competition calendar. The optimal sports nutrition plan will change from day to day to accommodate these changing goals. We await new knowledge about strategies to optimise the muscle's ability to integrate economical use of its available fuel sources as well as the potential for strategic withholding of nutritional support around some training sessions to increase the exercise stimulus and promote greater adaptation. Of course, there is often a disconnect between the hypothetical advantages of a single strategy and the overall effect on performance. Therefore, research must continue to evaluate the overall significance of a strategy rather than focusing on a single perspective. Sports performance involves a complex mixture of whole-body physiology and central drive as well as muscle characteristics. Although in many cases, sports science merely explains or supports practices that athletes and coaches have already found to be valuable, advances in sports nutrition knowledge arising from investigations of cellular changes are likely to lead to new concepts and opportunities to enhance sports performance.

Chapter highlights

- Modern sports nutrition promotes eating practices that are personalised, periodised and specific to the athlete and their event and training schedule.
- Just as athletes have a periodised program of training and competition, nutrition strategies should be strategically organised to maximise the interaction between exercise and key nutrients.
- Energy and macronutrient intake should change from day to day (and even within the day, according to the needs of each training session or competition schedule) according to the specific exercise load, the goals of each session and the athlete's overall nutrition goals.
- An outcome of an athlete's training – especially for endurance sports – is to increase the muscle's ability to store and use carbohydrate and fat fuels. This is known as metabolic flexibility and is particularly important in endurance and ultra-endurance events when the fuel needs of the event may exceed the muscle's normal carbohydrate stores.

- Strategies to consume carbohydrate before, during and after exercise increase carbohydrate availability and are associated with enhanced capacity for prolonged moderate-high intensity exercise, including the ability to increase intensity for critical parts of the event.
- Although a high-fat diet can increase muscle capacity to use fat as an exercise fuel, the adaptations also seem to reduce the capacity for carbohydrate utilisation and may decrease overall metabolic flexibility. Although fat can fuel exercise of moderate intensity, it is associated with reduced exercise economy (a greater oxygen cost to produce the same amount of ATP, and therefore, the same speed or power output). Compared to carbohydrate fuels, it is less able to sustain higher-intensity exercise when the oxygen supply to the muscle becomes limiting.
- Despite the recent renewal of interest, low carbohydrate high-fat diets (LCHF) appear to be less suited to the needs of competitive endurance athletes who need to undertake all or critical of their events at high intensities supported by carbohydrate metabolism. They may be better suited to ultra-endurance events in which the athlete competes at a steady pace of moderate-intensity exercise.
- Endurance athletes may make use of the developing ideas around training protocols that integrate specific strategies of high carbohydrate availability around key training sessions (allowing them to "train harder") alongside strategies that deliberately achieve low carbohydrate availability after or during other sessions to increase the training stimulus and adaptive responses (promoting "a train smarter" outcome).

References

1. Burke LM, Jeacocke NA. The basis of nutrient timing and its place in sport and metabolic regulation. In: Kerksick C, ed. *Nutrient Timing: Metabolic Optimisation for Health, Performance and Recovery.* Boca Raton, FL, CRC Press; 2011. pp. 1–22.
2. Jeukendrup AE. Training the gut for athletes. *Sports Med.* 2017;47(S1):101–110.
3. Burke LM. Re-examining high-fat diets for sports performance: did we call the 'nail in the coffin' too soon? *Sports Med.* 2015;15(S1):S33–49.
4. Volek JS, Noakes T, Phinney SD. Rethinking fat as a fuel for endurance exercise. *Eur J Sport Sci.* 2015;15(1):13–20.
5. Burke LM. Ketogenic low-CHO, high-fat diet: the future of elite endurance sport? *J Phsyiol.* 2021;599(3):819–843.
6. Phinney SD, Bistrian BR, Evans WJ, et al. The human metabolic response to chronic ketosis without caloric restriction: preservation of submaximal exercise capability with reduced carbohydrate oxidation. *Metabolism.* 1983;32(8):769–776.
7. Burke LM, Ross ML, Garvican-Lewis LA, et al. Low carbohydrate, high fat diet impairs exercise economy and negates the performance benefit from intensified training in elite race walkers. *J Physiol.* 2017;595(9):2785–2807.
8. Burke LM, Sharma AP, Heikura IA, et al. Crisis of confidence averted: impairment of exercise economy and performance in elite race walkers by ketogenic low carbohydrate, high fat (LCHF) diet is reproducible. *PLOS one.* 2020;15(6):e0234027.
9. Burke LM, Whitfield J, Heikura IA, et al. Adaptation to a low carbohydrate high fat diet is rapid but impairs endurance exercise metabolism and performance despite enhanced glycogen availability. *J Phsyiol.* 2021;599(3):771–790.
10. Whitfield J, Burke LM, McKay AKA, et al. Acute ketogenic diet and ketone ester supplementation impairs race walk performance. *Med Sci Sports Exerc.* 2021;53(4):776–784.
11. Muniz-Pardos B, Sutehall S, Angeloudis K, et al. Recent improvements in marathon run times are likely technological, not physiological. *Sports Med.* 2021;51(3):371–378.

12. Havemann L, West S, Goedecke JH, et al. Fat adaptation followed by carbohydrate-loading compromises high-intensity sprint. *J Appl Physiol.* 2006;100(1):194–202.

13. Stellingwerff T, Spriet LL, Watt MJ, et al. Decreased PDH activation and glycogenolysis during exercise following fat adaptation with carbohydrate restoration. *Am J Physiol Endocrinol Metabol,* 2006;290(2):E380–E388.

14. McSwiney FT, Wardrop B, Hyde PN, et al. Keto-adaptation enhances exercise performance and body composition responses to training in endurance athletes. *Metabolism.* 2018;81:25–34.

15. Garrett AT, Goosens NG, Rehrer NJ, et al. Short-term heat acclimation is effective and may be enhanced rather than impaired by dehydration. *Am J Human Biol.* 2014;26(3):311–320.

16. Bartlett JD, Hawley JA, Morton JP. Carbohydrate availability and exercise training adaptation: too much of a good thing? *Eur J Sport Sci.* 2015;15(1):3–12.

17. Burke LM, Hawley JA, Jeukendrup A, et al. Toward a common understanding of diet-exercise strategies to manipulate fuel availability for training and competition preparation in endurance sport. *Int J Sport Nutr Exerc Metab,* 2018;28(5):451–463.

18. Marquet LA, Brisswalter J, Louis J, et al. Enhanced endurance performance by periodization of CHO intake: "sleep low" strategy. *Med Sci Sports Exerc.* 2016;48(4):663–672.

19. Stellingwerff T. Contemporary nutrition approaches to optimise elite marathon performance. *In J Sports Physiol Perform.* 2013;8:573–578.

20. Gejl KD, Thams L, Hansen M, et al. No superior adaptations to carbohydrate periodisation in elite endurance athletes. *Med Sci Sports Exerc.* 2017;49(12):2486–2497.

11 Hydration

Ben Desbrow and Christopher Irwin

This chapter explores the role of water as an essential nutrient and the physiological basis of hydration. Firstly, the importance of hydration and the effects of dehydration on performance is discussed. Then, methods of hydration assessment and recommendations for staying hydrated are presented and drinking strategies that promote rehydration during and after exercise are explored. The role of beverage ingredients and how they influence rehydration are also examined. Finally, the impact of drinking alcohol on hydration, recovery, and performance is considered.

Learning outcomes

This chapter will:

- outline the fundamental roles of water in the human body;
- describe the effects of dehydration on performance;
- describe hydration assessment techniques and the strengths and limitations of various methods;
- identify appropriate drinking strategies to optimise hydration for athletes before, during, and after sport;
- introduce the concept of hyperhydration, strategies used to facilitate hyperhydration and the impact of these approaches on performance;
- describe the interaction between food and fluid combinations on rehydration;
- describe the effect of alcohol on recovery and rehydration.

The importance of hydration

Water accounts for approximately 50–70% of body weight (BW) in humans. However, this volume varies with body composition (lean and fat mass) and is therefore generally greater in males (60–70% BW) compared to females (50–55% BW).[1, 2]

Hydrolytic reaction

When the addition of water to another compound leads to the formation of two or more products; for example, the catalytic conversion of starch to sugar.

DOI: 10.4324/9781003321286-13

Total body water

The total sum of water in the body. It is the sum of water within the cells (intracellular) and outside the cells (extracellular).

Water has many important roles in the body. It serves as a chemical solvent, a substrate for **hydrolytic reactions**, a transport medium for nutrients and metabolic waste products, a shock-absorbent, a lubricant (e.g., to the GI and respiratory tracts) and a structural component. Almost every biological process occurring in the human body is dependent on the maintenance of **total body water** (TBW) balance.

Water loss occurs naturally in humans as part of daily living. The majority of daily losses occur through urine (~1–2 litres), faeces (~200 mL), respiration (~250–400 mL), and via the skin (~450–500 mL).[3] In general, this equates to about 2–3 litres per day (L·d^{-1}) for a sedentary adult.[2] However, these amounts are influenced by many factors, such as dietary intake, environmental conditions, and physical activity levels. Individuals exposed to extremely hot climates, and those who are physically active, are likely to have increased losses. But these losses are usually corrected quite rapidly (within 24 hours) provided adequate fluid consumption occurs.[4]

Thermoregulation

The maintenance of the body at a particular temperature regardless of the external temperature.

For athletes, it is the cardiovascular and **thermoregulatory** functions of water that are most critical to performance.[5] The energetic demands of muscular activity (primarily, the demand for oxygen) are met via circulating blood, the major component of which is water. Circulating blood also contributes to thermoregulation, transporting excess heat generated via substrate oxidation from the body's core to the surface of the skin, where it can be lost to the environment. Thus, it is important that athletes are sufficiently hydrated to optimise these processes.

Exercise and dehydration

During exercise, the body cools itself by sweating, but this ultimately results in the loss of body fluid. If this fluid loss is not replaced, it can lead to dehydration. Generally, the body can tolerate low to moderate levels of dehydration (<2% BW loss); however, as levels of dehydration rise (≥2% BW loss), performance (physical and mental) may become impaired.[5] Dehydration can cause:

- increased heart rate;
- increased perception of effort;
- increased fatigue;

- impaired physical performance (e.g., strength, endurance);
- impaired cognitive performance (e.g., concentration, decision-making, skill, and coordination);
- gastrointestinal (GI) issues, such as nausea, vomiting, and diarrhoea;
- increased risk of heat illness.

For that reason, current practical guidelines for athletes encourage the consumption of sufficient volumes of fluid before, during, and after exercise to minimise dehydration.

Exercise can also elicit high electrolyte losses (mainly sodium) through the sweating response, particularly in warm-to-hot conditions. While sweat sodium concentrations vary between individuals (depending on factors such as sweat rate, genetics, diet, and acclimation), in the event of large fluid losses most athletes need to also consider replacing lost electrolytes.

Hydration assessment

There is no general agreement on the most effective method of assessing an individual's hydration status at any single point in time. There are, however, a number of techniques commonly used for the assessment of hydration status. These typically involve either whole body, blood, urinary, or sensory measurements. Some of these methods are only suitable for use in laboratory environments, while others can be used easily in the field. A number of novel techniques have also been developed in an effort to devise ways of accurately measuring changes in hydration status without the need to remove clothing or provide invasive biological specimens. However, these methods are still undergoing experimental testing to determine their validity.

Each method has its own specific strengths and limitations, and the process of selecting the most suitable technique is dependent on several factors that influence practicality, such as cost, the technical expertise required, portability, and efficiency (Table 11.1). In addition, while some methods provide valid assessments of hydration status across acute and chronic time points, others are only valid under specific conditions. For example, most urine markers are not considered to be a valid measure of current hydration status as these values are subject to large variations in response to rapid consumption of fluid.[6] However, they may be used after a standardised period (e.g., on waking) and can serve as a behavioural stimulus to encourage fluid consumption. Monitoring urine colour is a convenient hydration assessment tool and typically indicates prior fluid consumption behaviour. That is, when optimal amounts of fluid are consumed, urine should be pale yellow or clear. If inadequate fluid has been consumed, urine will be dark yellow. Urine colour can be monitored easily by comparing it against the eight-point urine colour chart.[7] However, as with all urine markers of hydration status, urine colour is influenced by rapid consumption of fluid, which facilitates **diuresis**. Therefore, it is best used as an indicator of first-morning hydration status, upon waking and prior to ingestion of any fluid.

Diuresis

Increased or excessive production of urine.

Table 11.1 Summary of commonly used hydration assessment techniques

Measure	Purpose	Practicality					Accuracy	Validity
		Cost	Analysis time	Technical expertise	Portability	Overall practicality		
Field measures								
Urine specific gravity	Fluid concentration	2	1	1	1	M/H	M	C
Urine colour	Fluid concentration	1	1	1	1	H	M	C
Body weight change	TBW change	1	1	1	1	H	M	A
Rating of thirst	TBW change	1	1	1	1	H	L	A
Laboratory measures								
Isotope dilution	TBW content	3	3	3	3	L	H	A & C
Neuron activation	TBW content	3	3	3	3	L	H	A & C
Bioelectrical impedance	TBW content	2	3	2	2	M	M	A
Haematocrit & haemoglobin	Plasma volume change	2	2	3	3	M	H	A
Plasma osmolality	Fluid concentration	3	2	3	3	M/L	H	A&C
Urine osmolality	Fluid concentration	3	2	3	3	M/L	M	C
Salivary osmolality	Fluid concentration	2	1	2	1	M/L	L	A
Experimental measures								
Tear osmolarity	Fluid concentration	3	1	2	2	M	L	A&C

Notes: TBW: Total body water; 1: Small/Little/Portable; 2: Moderate/Intermediate; 3: Great/Much/Not portable; A: Acute; C: Chronic; H: High; L: Low; M: Moderate.

Source: Adapted from Armstrong[6] and Sawka et al.[8]

The precision, accuracy, and reliability of the assessment techniques are particularly important and should be prioritised, within the constraints of technical expertise and cost, when selecting the most appropriate method to monitor the hydration status of athletes.

Before, during, and after sport fluid considerations

An athlete's choice of a beverage (and the volume they consume) can be influenced by many factors, such as availability, palatability, thirst, GI tolerance, temperature, nutrition knowledge, and cost. It is also important to recognise that while fluid consumption may offset the effects of dehydration, it may also facilitate the ingestion of other ingredients (e.g., carbohydrate) known to enhance performance. The timing of consumption relative to the exercise bout has a significant influence on beverage recommendations given to athletes to optimise performance (see Table 11.2).

During exercise ≤ 120 min, GI tolerance (see Chapter 15) and access to fluids restrict the beverages that are likely to be well tolerated by athletes. Water and carbohydrate–electrolyte beverages (sports drinks) are commonly recommended for consumption during events involving high-intensity, short-duration competition (such as netball, football, and basketball). While commercial sports drinks are specifically formulated to be well tolerated and utilised under conditions of physical exertion (containing 6–8% carbohydrate and 10–25% mmol·L^{-1} of sodium), during competition athletes are unlikely to match sweat fluid losses with beverage intakes.[10] This suggests that athletes need to ensure they commence competition well-hydrated and/or aim to replace fluid deficits following exercise.

Pre-event hyperhydration and its impact on performance

When physical or practical barriers prevent optimal fluid intake during exercise that is likely to result in large fluid losses an athlete may consider pre-exercise **hyperhydration**. Hyperhydration typically involves oral ingestion of a large quantity of water (≥10 mL·kg^{-1} body mass) along with an osmotically active agent that prevents the water bolus from triggering post-absorptive diuresis. The most commonly studied osmotic agents are sodium and glycerol, although other oral agents (e.g., sodium bicarbonate, sodium citrate) and intravenous interventions have also been investigated. The effects of hyperhydration

Table 11.2 Summary of fluid recommendations prior to, during, and following exercise to optimise performance

	Recommendation	*Other considerations*
Prior to exercise	5–10 mL·kg^{-1} BW 2–4 hrs before exercise. (hyperhydration guidelines presented separately)	Use urine colour to guide volume. Avoid high-fat fluids.
During exercise	Typically 400–800 mL·h^{-1} Avoid deficit <2% BW	Sweat rates can vary considerably (range 0.3–2.4 L·h^{-1}). Drink cold beverages in hot conditions.
Following exercise	Replace 125–150% of fluid deficit	Food consumption is likely to improve fluid retention.

Source: Adapted from Thomas et al.[9]

(irrespective of the approach employed) are not consistent, and when benefits have been demonstrated, these are typically small.

Hyperhydration

A pre-exercise strategy that aims to increase total body water and/or plasma volume above resting levels, allowing greater fluid deficit to be incurred during exercise before hypohydration occurs and performance is impacted.

Effectiveness of different beverages on fluid retention following exercise

In hydration science, the effect of any beverage on body fluid status is judged by the balance between how much the body retains of any volume that is consumed. Accurately establishing retention rates of different beverages typically involves laboratory research and the prescription of a fixed volume of a beverage under standardised conditions, followed by a period of monitoring fluid losses. The **beverage hydration index** (BHI) has been established to describe the fluid retention capacity of different beverages by standardising values to the retention of still water.[11] The BHI research findings indicate that many beverages are as effective at delivering fluid as water. Only milk beverages and oral rehydration solutions produced superior fluid retention to water (Table 11.3).

Beverage-hydration index

An index system that has been developed to describe the fluid retention capacity of different beverages by standardising values to the retention of still water.

One strength of the BHI is that it recognises that all beverages contribute to total fluid intake (ranking some as more effective than others). In contrast, many fluid recommendations focus on avoiding certain beverages (such as caffeinated beverages or drinks containing

Table 11.3 Summary of fluid retention from commonly consumed beverages when consumed without food

Beverages with inferior fluid retention to water	*Beverages with similar fluid retention to water*	*Beverages with superior fluid retention to water*
Beer (>4%ABV)	Sparkling water	Full-fat dairy milk
	Sports drinks	Skim dairy milk
	Cola	Soy milk
	Diet cola	Milk-based meal replacements
	Tea (hot or iced)	Oral rehydration solutions
	Coffee	
	Beer (≤4% ABV)	

Note: ABV = Alcohol by volume.

Source: Adapted from Desbrow et al.[11, 13] and Maughan et al.[14]

alcohol). However, individuals may respond to this by avoiding and not replacing these beverages, leading to a reduction in total fluid intake. The BHI appears to have a more pronounced impact on fluid retention, than how quickly the fluid is consumed.[12]

Impact of food

Since most fluid consumed by athletes is co-ingested with meals and/or snacks, the influence of food on rehydration has significant practical application. Consuming food may impact on rehydration in a number of ways. Firstly, food may provide nutrients (such as carbohydrate, protein, or sodium) that directly assist with fluid recovery. In addition, the interaction of food and fluid may influence the volume of drink consumed, thereby impacting total fluid intake. To date, only four studies have investigated rehydration in settings where athletes were encouraged to consume food (Table 11.4). Collectively, these studies indicate that the ingestion of food is likely to facilitate rehydration following exercise. Two of these investigations allowed participants to self-select the volume of fluid they consumed (i.e. voluntary rather than prescribed fluid intake), thereby allowing the interaction between food and the volume of fluid consumed to be explored.

Importantly, when drinking and eating voluntarily both males and females appear to achieve similar levels of fluid retention, irrespective of beverage type. However, the consumption of high-energy (kJ) beverages such as sports drinks or milk-based drinks is likely to result in greater total energy consumption and differences in nutrient intakes compared to the consumption of water with food.[15] Therefore, fluid choice post-exercise when food is available should be strategic and considered. Selection should be influenced by immediate post-exercise nutrition requirements, as well as overall dietary intake goals.

Impact of alcohol on hydration, recovery, and performance

Alcoholic beverages (particularly beer and champagne) have a long association with sport. In many countries, athletes commonly consume alcoholic beverages as part of their post-match routine. Clearly, large doses of alcohol have a number of effects (e.g., impairing muscle synthesis, delaying muscle glycogen restoration, and influencing sleep quality) that make it an undesirable recovery agent. However, considering beer may be consumed in large volumes after exercise, researchers have investigated beer's potential to influence rehydration.

Studies on the diuretic impact of beer suggest that the fluid loss associated with alcohol is less pronounced after exercise-induced fluid losses. Additionally, by reducing the

Table 11.4 Studies investigating the interaction of food on rehydration

Study	Food provided	Beverage(s) (method)	Outcome
Maughan et al.[16]	Rice and beef meal	Sports drink (prescribed)	↑ Fluid retention (rehydration) with food
Pryor et al.[15]	Beef jerky	Sports drink (prescribed)	↑ Fluid retention (rehydration) with food
Campagnolo et al.[17]	Selection of foods/snacks	Water Sports drink Milk-based supplement (voluntary)	Rehydration achieved with all beverages
McCartney et al.[18, 19]	Selection of foods/snacks	Water Sports drink Milk-based supplements (voluntary)	Rehydration achieved with all beverages

alcohol concentration of beer (≤4% alcohol by volume) and raising the sodium content, significantly greater fluid retention can be achieved compared to drinking a traditional full-strength beer.[13] A low-alcohol beer with added sodium may provide a compromise to the dehydrated athlete following exercise, in that it is a beverage with high social acceptance that avoids the poor fluid retention observed with full-strength beer.

Summary

This chapter has outlined how water balance can influence the cardiovascular and thermoregulatory responses to exercise and is therefore critical to performance. While a variety of different hydration assessment techniques exist, a single measure that is accurate, valid, and cost-effective in all circumstances remains elusive. General recommendations for fluid intake before, during, and following exercise exist. In addition, athletes anticipating large sweat losses and/or with limited fluid replacement opportunities may consider employing hyperhydration strategies prior to sport. Recovery beverage recommendations should consider the post-exercise environment (i.e. the availability of food), an individual's tolerance for food and fluid pre/post-exercise, the immediate requirements for refuelling (i.e. CHO demands of the activity) and the athlete's overall dietary goals.

Chapter highlights

- Cardiovascular and thermoregulatory functions of water are critical for athletes.
- During exercise, the body cools itself by sweating, but this causes loss of body fluid.
- Performance impairment typically occurs when dehydration exceeds 2% BW loss.
- Hyperhydration may be considered when physical or practical barriers to fluid consumption exist during exercise.
- Hyperhydration studies typically indicate small performance improvements.
- While all beverages contribute to total fluid intake, some fluids (e.g., milk) have superior fluid retention properties (i.e. a higher beverage hydration index (BHI)).
- Ingestion of food is likely to enhance the retention of fluids with lower BHIs after exercise.
- Large doses of alcohol can have a number of negative effects that make it an undesirable recovery agent.

References

1. Oppliger RA, Bartok C. Hydration testing of athletes. *Sports Med.* 2002;32(15):959–71.
2. Jequier E, Constant F. Water as an essential nutrient: the physiological basis of hydration. *Eur J Clin Nutr.* 2010;64(2):115–23.
3. Maughan RJ. Impact of mild dehydration on wellness and on exercise performance. *Eur J Clin Nutr.* 2003;57 Suppl 2:S19–23.
4. Cheuvront SN, Carter R, 3rd, Montain SJ, et al. Daily body mass variability and stability in active men undergoing exercise-heat stress. *Int J Sport Nutr Exerc Metab.* 2004;14(5):532–40.
5. Murray B. Hydration and physical performance. *J Am Coll Nutr.* 2007;26(5 Suppl):542S–8S.
6. Sawka M, Burke L, Eichner E, et al. American College of Sports Medicine position stand. Exercise and fluid replacement. *Med Sci Sports Exerc.* 2007;39(2):377–90.
7. Armstrong LE, Soto JA, Hacker FT, Jr., et al. Urinary indices during dehydration, exercise, and rehydration. *Int J Sport Nutr.* 1998;8(4):345–55.

8. Armstrong L. Assessing hydration status: the elusive gold standard. *J Am Coll Nutr.* 2007; 26(5):575S–84S.
9. Thomas DT, Erdman KA, Burke LM. Position of the Academy of Nutrition and Dietetics, Dietitians of Canada, and the American College of Sports Medicine: nutrition and athletic performance. *J Acad Nutr Dietetics.* 2016;116(3):501–28.
10. Garth AK, Burke LM. What do athletes drink during competitive sporting activities? *Sports Med.* 2013;43(7):539–64.
11. Maughan RJ, Watson P, Cordery PA, et al. A randomized trial to assess the potential of different beverages to affect hydration status: development of a beverage hydration index. *Am J Clin Nutr.* 2016;103(3):717–23.
12. Sayer L, Rodriguez-Sanchez N, Rodriguez-Giustiniani P, et al. Effect of drinking rate on the retention of water or milk following exercise-induced dehydration. *Int J Sport Nutr Exerc Metab.* 2020;30(2):128–38.
13. Desbrow B, Murray D, Leveritt M. Beer as a sports drink? Manipulating beer's ingredients to replace lost fluid. *Int J Sport Nutr Exerc Metab.* 2013;23(6):593–600.
14. Desbrow B, Jansen S, Barrett A, et al. Comparing the rehydration potential of different milk-based drinks to a carbohydrate-electrolyte beverage. *Appl Physiol Nutr Metab.* 2014;39(12): 1366–72.
15. Campagnolo N, Iudakhina E, Irwin C, et al. Fluid, energy and nutrient recovery via ad libitum intake of different fluids and food. *Physiol Behav.* 2017;171:228–35.
16. Maughan R, Leiper J, Shirreffs S. Restoration of fluid balance after exercise-induced dehydration: effects of food and fluid intake. *Eur J Appl Physiol Occ Physiol.* 1996;73:317–25.
17. Pryor JL, Johnson EC, Del Favero J, et al. Hydration status and sodium balance of endurance runners consuming postexercise supplements of varying nutrient content. *Int J Sport Nutr Exerc Metab.* 2015;25(5):471–9.
18. McCartney D, Irwin C, Cox GR, et al. The effect of different post-exercise beverages with food on ad libitum fluid recovery, nutrient provision, and subsequent athletic performance. *Physiol Behav.* 2019;201:22–30.
19. McCartney D, Irwin C, Cox GR, et al. Fluid, energy, and nutrient recovery via ad libitum intake of different commercial beverages and food in female athletes. *Appl Physiol Nutr Metab.* 2019;44(1):37–46.

12 Sports supplements

Martyn Binnie

The preceding chapters have provided an overview of how specific dietary patterns, foods, and nutrients can support exercise performance and adaptations to training as well as enhancing health and wellbeing. While most of the nutritional benefits for an athlete are the result of thoughtfully selected foods and overall dietary patterns, some additional benefits can be gained from specific sports foods and supplements. This chapter will look more closely at the sports foods and supplements used by athletes to enhance performance, promote recovery, and facilitate optimal training adaptation.

> **Learning outcomes**
>
> **This chapter will:**
>
> - define sports foods, fortified/formulated foods, and sports supplements;
> - describe the risks that athletes must consider before supplement use and the resources available to support them;
> - briefly describe the mechanism of action and supplementation protocol of specific supplements that enhance exercise performance;
> - discuss emerging evidence associated with new and potentially beneficial sports supplements;
> - describe the range of factors that influence sports supplementation in real-world scenarios.

Research in sports nutrition has identified how different nutrients can enhance exercise performance, improve recovery, and modulate training adaptation. This knowledge has subsequently led to the development of specific sports foods and supplements. Sports foods refer to food or drink products that provide a more convenient form of nutrients for targeted use around exercise. This includes products such as carbohydrate and electrolyte drinks, sports bars, sports gels, and protein drinks. Outside of these more typical products, there is an increasing prevalence in the availability of protein-fortified foods (PFFs) and other formulated products that aim to enhance or modify the nutritional profile of existing food. This may include protein 'boosted' smoothies, 'health' balls, and calcium-infused orange juice. Conversely, supplements are typically single or multi-ingredient products in powder, concentrated liquid, pill, or capsule form delivering nutrients or other dietary components for a specific health and/or ergogenic benefit (i.e. iron for health and creatine for performance).

DOI: 10.4324/9781003321286-14

The value of convenient nutrition for athletes is high given time-sensitive nutrition targets and often time-poor general environment. Sports food and supplements are effective when there is an increased requirement for high-quality nutrients in response to demanding training schedules and performance goals, and also if there are food intolerances, allergies, limited availability or budget for foods, or to combat food hygiene or contamination concerns. However, athletes are also most at risk of doping violations with strict rules governing the integrity of sport. The World Anti-Doping Authority (WADA) was established in 1999 as an international independent agency to lead a collaborative worldwide movement for doping-free sport. Led by the principles of WADA, countries customarily have their own domestic authorities to help enforce sport integrity, including SIA in Australia, UKAD in the United Kingdom and USADA in the USA. These authorities act to enforce **anti-doping rule violations** (ADRVs), and sanctions can range from a reprimand to a lifetime ban. The basis of ADRVs is guided by the WADA Prohibited List, which is a comprehensive list of prohibited substances (for both in and out of competition) updated annually. This WADA list is also linked to the Global Drug Reference Online (DRO) which allows athletes and support personnel to check the status of a supplement or medication in a specific sport and nation of purchase. In most cases, ADRVs are inadvertent, either from the consumption of a contaminated substance, the inclusion of an ingredient that is not listed, or being misinformed about the status of a supplement. Regardless of intent, the responsibility ultimately falls to the athlete to reduce the risk of an ADRV.

Anti-doping rule violation (ADRV)

An anti-doping rule violation (ADRV) can come with sanctions of up to 4 years or even complete lifetime bans from competitive sport.

Key resources

- Global DRO (https://www.globaldro.com/Home): Provides up-to-date information to athletes and support personnel about the status of supplements and medications based on the WADA Prohibited List.
- Australian Institute of Sport, Sport Supplement Framework (https://www.ais.gov.au/nutrition/supplements): provides guidance for safe and effective nutritional support.
- Informed Sport (https://www.wetestyoutrust.com/) and HASTA (https://hasta.org.au/): Online database of batch tested products to help minimise risk of contamination and ADRVs.

The landscape for the modern athlete is a challenging one, with supplements and sports foods more prevalent and marketing campaigns increasing their global reach and level of impact. This includes a growing risk from the emergence of PFFs and other formulated products where the source of all ingredients is not always clear.[1] To assist athletes, companies such as HASTA and Informed Sport provide batch testing for contamination in commonly used sports foods and supplements. It is critical to reinforce that even with batch testing, no supplement comes with zero risk of ADRVs, and so while the use of batch-tested products is generally considered non-negotiable in competitive athletes, the risk profile for athletes should be established well before the point of purchase. Maughan and colleagues presented a guide to informed decision-making for nutritional ergogenic supplements which encourages the rationale for the specific athlete and situation to be well established.[2] This may include the age and performance level of the athlete, the justification for the specific demands of the sport, and the evidence base to support safe and effective implementation. Along with rules enforced and governed by WADA and domestic anti-doping authorities, it is also common for National Sporting Organisations to enforce their own supplement regulations including rules for specific products (even if WADA approved) or certain levels of athlete (i.e. age or competitive level). Given this complex landscape and the pressures faced in the modern pursuit of athletic performance, athletes, coaches, and their support staff must be well-informed and very calculated when it comes to considering the use of any form of supplementation.

Crucially, the application of nutritional ergogenic supplements for sports must be guided by a strong evidence base and justified for each specific athlete and sport scenario. Current well-established supplements which fall under this category include caffeine, creatine, nitrate, beta-alanine, sodium bicarbonate, and glycerol. The following sections will focus primarily on these supplements with a 'performance' target as this is one of the most common areas that athletes, coaches, and practitioners will be exposed to. A more comprehensive list of associated and evidence-based sports foods and medical supplements can be found in the 2018 review from Maughan and colleagues,[2] and in the shared resources from the AIS Sport Supplement Framework.

Evidence-based performance supplements

Caffeine

Caffeine is the most widely used pharmacologically active substance in the world and improves performance in a variety of exercise tasks.[3] The physiological effects of caffeine occur due to its similarity to the adenosine molecule. Among its many actions, adenosine causes a decrease in alertness and arousal when it binds to receptors on the surface of cells in the brain. Caffeine also binds to these receptors and blocks the effects of adenosine, causing an increased alertness and arousal, and subsequent reduction in the perception of effort during exercise. This can lead to enhanced performance by delaying fatigue and allowing an athlete to exercise at a higher intensity for longer periods of time. These changes may also lead to some additive effects on cognitive functions such as vigilance, memory, mood, and tactical/technical execution in sport-specific scenarios. Doses of 3–6 mg/kg body mass of caffeine consumed 60 minutes pre-exercise are typically reported to be most effective; however, benefits also occur across a broader range of 2–9 mg/kg as well as for shorter timeframes pre-exercise and even during exercise.[4]

Variation in this response to caffeine can be partly explained by the source and mode of administration. Caffeine is present in many commonly consumed foods and in beverages such as coffee, tea, and chocolate- and cola-flavoured beverages. However, the amount of caffeine in these sources can vary significantly, and specifically in the case of coffee, there can be a tenfold difference in the caffeine content of coffee purchased at different retail outlets.[5] Therefore, it is more common for athletes to seek a more known and consistent caffeine content in products such as pills, gels, or even energy drinks.

All these modes of ingestion rely on absorption through the gastrointestinal (GI) system which comes with a delay of 30–60 minutes before caffeine levels peak in the blood and comes with the risk of GI distress around exercise. This limitation has led to emerging support for alternate modes of administration including caffeinated gum and mouth rinses.[4] These methods take advantage of adenosine receptors located in the mouth which lead to a faster rate of absorption (15–20 minutes) for performance benefits, and reduced GI symptoms, making it a more appealing option for certain athletes and sporting situations (i.e. half-time and extra-time in sport).

Another large source of variation in the response to caffeine is from inter-individual factors such as genotype, training status, sex, and habitual caffeine intake. It has been suggested that different genotypes can impact the body's ability to metabolise caffeine, causing some individuals to experience an ergogenic (beneficial) response, some an ineffective response, and others an ergolytic (detrimental) response. Further, training status may impact the response to caffeine, with better-trained individuals potentially having a higher density of adenosine receptors to utilise, as well as a more reliable performance output to benefit from the additive effects of caffeine. There is some research to suggest a diminished response to caffeine in females caused by lower rates of metabolism, however, there is also a relative paucity of research in females. Finally, given the large consumption of caffeine in society (e.g., about 175 mg/day for the average Australian adult), there is interest to determine if there is a diminished response to caffeine in higher habitual consumers. While this does not appear to be the case from the research to date, more studies are needed to examine the higher rate of use and different patterns of intake in the modern population.

Creatine

Creatine is a naturally occurring compound located mostly within the skeletal muscle where it exists in free (creatine) and phosphorylated (phosphocreatine) forms. Small amounts of creatine are endogenously synthesised (~1 g/day), and ingested through the diet (~1 g/day), mostly from animal muscle. Creatine plays a key role in supporting immediate energy supply (~8–10 seconds) through its role in the alactic phosphocreatine system. Supplementation with additional creatine increases skeletal muscle stores of both free and phosphorylated forms, subsequently aiding high-intensity exercise performance. This mechanism may enhance acute high-intensity performance (<30 seconds) and enable a greater adaptation to training, particularly during resistance training which involves repeated, high-force muscle contractions. Accordingly, creatine supplementation augments strength, power, and lean muscle mass gains during such training interventions.[6] Typical creatine supplementation involves consumption of 3–5 g/day of creatine monohydrate for approximately 4 weeks, or longer to support the duration of the specific training phase. Sometimes this protocol is front-ended by a 'loading' period in which a higher dose is taken (~20 g as 4 × 3–5 g doses per day) prior to resumption of a lower 'maintenance' dose to try and fast track the rise in muscle creatine levels, however, this is not an essential practice. Different protocols may be considered for individuals with heightened GI sensitivity (avoid loading), or lower resting creatine stores (i.e. vegetarians who benefit from loading), and dependant on the duration of the training block. Creatine uptake into the muscle is insulin-mediated, and therefore, co-ingestion with a meal (~50 g carbohydrates) may result in a larger increase in muscle creatine. Furthermore, creatine supplementation is commonly associated with an increase in body weight (~1–2 kg) due to water retention that will remain elevated for the supplementation period. After completion, muscle creatine and the associated water retention will dissipate within approximately 4–6 weeks. This may have implications for certain weight-bearing or weight-category sports and athletes.

Nitrate

Dietary nitrate is an increasingly popular supplement due to its capacity to enhance performance across a range of exercise tasks with minimal associated side effects.[2] Once ingested, dietary nitrate can be converted to nitrite by bacteria in the mouth. Circulating nitrite is then converted into nitric oxide (NO) in blood and other tissues. Nitric oxide plays an important role in a variety of functions, including the regulation of blood flow, mitochondrial respiration, and muscle contraction. As such, an increased bioavailability of NO from dietary nitrate ingestion has a positive impact on both endurance (via increased blood flow and enhanced mitochondrial efficiency) and high-intensity (via enhanced function of Type II muscle fibres) exercise performance. The more established benefits of dietary nitrate are in traditional endurance disciplines (i.e. cycling, running); however, there is an increasing body of evidence to also support application in power, sprint, and team sport events.[7] Leafy green and root vegetables (i.e. spinach, rocket, beetroot) are the primary sources of dietary nitrate; however, the average nitrate intake of adults (~60–120 mg/day) is below the threshold suggested to deliver an ergogenic effect (350–500 mg). While it may be possible to reach this target through food alone, products such as the 'beetroot juice shot' have been created to provide a more concentrated and reliable source of nitrate (i.e. *Beet It* contains ~400 mg nitrate). A bolus of 350–500 mg consumed 2–3 hours before exercise is the most effective dosing strategy. There is also evidence to suggest that a prolonged supplementation protocol (3–15 days) may be able to sustain or even augment the ergogenic effect. This may be of interest to the more well-trained athletic population as there is suggested to be a diminished response of nitrate with increasing aerobic fitness levels. Finally, it is also important to avoid the use of antibacterial mouthwashes, confectionery, and toothpaste prior to supplementation with nitrate as this may interfere with the initial breakdown process by mouth bacteria and blunt any subsequent physiological responses.

Beta-alanine

Beta-alanine is the rate-limiting amino acid precursor to the formation of the dipeptide carnosine. Carnosine is found in high concentrations within skeletal muscle, and plays an important role as an intracellular buffer, providing immediate defence against the accumulation of protons and fatiguing acidosis during high-intensity exercise.[3] Supplementation with beta-alanine can increase the levels of muscle carnosine, helping to delay the onset of fatigue and augment performance during sustained high-intensity exercise (30 seconds to 10 minutes). Common supplementation protocols for beta-alanine involve a daily dose of approximately 65 mg/kg body weight (~6.4 g/day) for at least 4 weeks. Time taken to reach maximal carnosine content is variable between individuals, however, the average response is about 18 weeks with most of the change occurring in the first 4 weeks (30–50% above resting levels[8]). With such a prolonged supplementation period compliance can be difficult, but when done correctly, it can help to support training intensity and adaptation as well as acute performance at the end of the supplementation period.

Co-ingestion with food is recommended due to insulin-mediated uptake into the muscle, and it is common for the daily dose to be split with meals (0.8–1.6 g every 4 hours) to help mitigate the acute side effects. The most common side effect is paraesthesia (uncomfortable tingling sensation on skin) which normally peaks around 60 minutes after ingestion and varies in severity between individuals. Washout of elevated muscle carnosine after the supplementation period is reasonably slow (~2%/week), which should be taken into consideration when planning for optimal timing around competition.

Sodium bicarbonate

Sodium bicarbonate acts as a pH buffer in a similar way to beta-alanine, however, it functions within the extracellular environment (i.e. blood). With ingestion of an acute dose of sodium bicarbonate (0.2–0.4 g/kg body weight), the blood content of bicarbonate will typically peak within around 60–150 minutes. An increase in blood bicarbonate concentration is associated with an elevation of blood pH, which in turn increases the pH gradient between the blood and the working muscle, helping to enhance the efflux of fatiguing by-products from the muscle (i.e. $H+$ ions/protons from lactate). This mechanism is effective at delaying the onset of fatigue and augmenting high-intensity performance for durations in which glycolytic flux is high (i.e. 1–10 minutes). While sodium bicarbonate is a well-established ergogenic aid, it is also most associated with GI upset.[2] The most palatable delivery of sodium bicarbonate is found in either tablet or powder form (e.g., Sodibic, ~840 mg/tablet), and strategies to minimise the susceptibility to GI distress include consumption with a carbohydrate-dense meal (~1.5 g/kg body mass) or a split dosing strategy (smaller doses spread out over 30–60 minutes). Current recommendations suggest starting a split dose of sodium bicarbonate (~0.3 mg/kg body weight) 2–3 hours before exercise with a meal. With the ergogenic benefits from elevated bicarbonate thought to last for approximately 3–4 hours, this timing approach may help to mitigate the disruption by any GI symptoms which peak closer to 90 minutes after ingestion.

Glycerol

Glycerol is a supplement that was removed from the WADA Prohibited List in 2018 to be permitted for use as a safe and efficacious substance in high-performance sports. Its previous status as a prohibited supplement was due to its potential ability to mask other banned substances through its influence on plasma volume and parameters of the Athlete Biological Passport. Specifically, glycerol allows for better retention of ingested fluids. This is achieved through modification of the osmotic gradient in the blood enabling greater fluid retention (reabsorption via kidneys) and diminished fluid loss (decreased urine production). Through a similar mechanism, the addition of sodium to a glycerol solution may further enhance this response).[9] When applied pre-exercise, this mechanism can enable a hyperhydrated state which can subsequently offer a range of advantages. Most commonly, pre-exercise glycerol is considered ergogenic in hot and humid conditions in which high fluid losses are expected, and it may also be advantageous when the capacity for fluid intake is low (i.e. marathon swim), limited (i.e. tennis or football matches), or even detrimental to performance goals (i.e. minimising drag forces in a cycling time trial). For its primary application in hot and humid conditions, a pre-exercise state of hyperhydration can reduce the dehydration-driven increase in exercising heart rate and improve the heat storage capacity of the athlete. This has obvious advantages for thermoregulatory function and exercise tolerance in these challenging conditions. Common supplementation protocols for glycerol include the consumption of the more commonly labelled product, glycerine, at a dose of 1.2–1.4 g/kg of body weight with ~25 mL/kg body mass of water between 90 and 180 minutes pre-exercise. As previously mentioned, the addition of 3.0 g/L of sodium may further enhance this response; however, ergogenic benefit has still been demonstrated with glycerol alone. This strategy offers greater fluid retention for up to 4 hours, and importantly for timing considerations (i.e. warm-up planning), peak urine production can be expected about 60–80 minutes after ingestion. The main side effect of glycerol consumption is the associated weight gain with excess fluid; however, some GI discomfort and nausea have also been reported.

Equivocal and emerging supplements

Supplementation for sports performance is constantly changing due to new products and the evolving evidence base. There has been recent interest in antioxidant products that are purported to have beneficial effects on recovery (and indirect effects on performance) through a reduction in exercise-induced oxidative stress or inflammation. This may include food-derived polyphenols (i.e. blackcurrant or cherry) and the amino acid N-acetylcysteine. More contemporary supplements include the 'tastants' which refer to substances that interact with the central nervous system through receptors located in the mouth (i.e. menthol, pickle juice, quinine). Ketone bodies have gained attention as a potential method to improve metabolic efficiency during endurance exercise. Despite these claims, these supplements ultimately exist in this section of the text as they do not have as strong a body of evidence behind them. To effectively navigate this space, it remains critical to stay aware of scientific research as well as the status of supplements within individual sport and global doping regulations.

Real-world considerations

Even with strong evidence from the scientific literature, the translation of knowledge into application in the field is another challenge. Rarely are lab-controlled studies able to fully account for variability experienced by a given individual in a specific sporting scenario. Factors such as the time of day for the event and the environmental conditions may influence choices about the most appropriate supplement choice. Specifically, a later event time may work against the use of caffeine given the possibility of a negative impact on subsequent sleep and recovery (caffeine levels elevated for up to 6 hours). Similarly, if it is a hot event, the choice of hot coffee for the delivery of caffeine would also be contraindicative. It is also typical for athletes to consider a repeat dose for a supplement if they have events spread across the day (i.e. heat and semi-final). The effectiveness of repeat use will be dependent on the **half-life** of the ergogenic effect, and while there is no clear scientific consensus on the matter, it could be suggested that a repeat event within 2 hours does not warrant another dose, while a repeat event within 2–4 hours could benefit from a smaller 'top-up' dose.[10] The other consideration for repeat events is the influence of supplementation to enable a greater workload in the first event, and the negative influence this may have on residual fatigue for a secondary bout. Another common practice is using a combination of multiple supplements with complementary mechanisms to support performance for a single event. For example, beta-alanine and sodium bicarbonate could enhance the intra- and extracellular buffering capacity of the body above the use of one supplement in isolation. Caffeine and creatine could be similarly targeted for additive benefit in high-intensity and repeated exercise bouts. Caffeine may also be additive in combination with sodium bicarbonate for sustained high-intensity exercise performance, however, this specifically has been reported to increase the risk of GI distress. In fact, all these potential combinations come with a relatively unknown ergogenic benefit and risk profile, mostly due to the difficulty in accurately capturing an isolated versus additive effect. Individual responses to supplements must also be considered, and all supplements should be trialled before use in competition.

Half-life

The time required for the concentration of a substance (e.g. caffeine) in the body to reduce by half.

Summary

This chapter has highlighted that the use of sports foods and supplements is a complex area for athletes, coaches, and support personnel to navigate. While there are some clear benefits, a carefully considered approach is needed to maximise benefits while minimising potential risks. An understanding of the mechanisms behind supplement action, as well as practical applications for real-world scenarios, is important in this process.

Chapter highlights

- Sports foods, fortified/formulated foods, and sports supplements may provide convenient sources of nutrients to support performance.
- For the athlete, all ingested products and supplements must come with a risk assessment to minimise the chance of an anti-doping rule violation.
- Sports supplements that have good evidence for enhancing performance include caffeine, creatine, nitrate, beta-alanine, sodium bicarbonate, and glycerol.
- Real-world application of supplements includes repeat dosing for multiple events and the combination of supplements that may have a complementary or additive effect.
- Variation is expected between individuals, and therefore trialling a supplement is essential to maximise benefit and minimise risk.

References

1. O'Bryan KR, Shaw G, Allanson B, et al. Understanding contamination risk associated with protein fortified foods. 2021. https://www.ais.gov.au/__data/assets/pdf_file/0015/1027230/Protein-Fortified-Foods-Report.pdf
2. Maughan RJ, Burke LM, Dvorak J, et al. IOC consensus statement: dietary supplements and the high-performance athlete. *Br J Sports Med*. 2018;52:439–455.
3. Peeling P, Binnie MJ, Goods PSR. et al. Evidence-based supplements for the enhancement of athletic performance. *Int J Sport Nutr Exerc Metab*. 2018;28(2):178–187.
4. Pickering C, Grgic J. Caffeine and exercise: what next? *Sports Med*. 2019;49(7):1007–1030.

5. Desbrow B, Hughes R, Leveritt M, et al. An examination of consumer exposure to caffeine from retail coffee outlets. *Food Chem Toxicol.* 2007;45(9):1588–1592.

6. Kreider RB, Kalman DS, Antonio J, et al. International Society of Sports Nutrition position stand: safety and efficacy of creatine supplementation in exercise, sport, and medicine. *J Int Soc Sports Nutr.* 2017;14:18.

7. Senefeld JW, Wiggins CC, Regimbal RJ, et al. Ergogenic effect of nitrate supplementation: a systematic review and meta-analysis. *Med Sci Sports Exerc.* 2020;52, 2250–2261.

8. Saunders B, Elliott-Sale K, Artioli GG, et al. B-Alanine supplementation to improve exercise capacity and performance: a systematic review and meta-analysis. *Br J Sports Med.* 2017;51(8): 658–669.

9. McCubbin AJ, Allanson BA, Caldwell Odgers JN, et al. Sports dietitians Australia position statement: nutrition for exercise in hot environments. *Int J Sport Nutr Exerc Metab.* 2020;30(1): 83–98.

10. Burke LM. Practical issues in evidence-based use of performance supplements: supplement interactions, repeated use and individual responses. *Sports Med.* 2017;47(S1):79–100.

13 Assessing and changing body composition

Patria Anne Hume

This chapter provides an overview of body composition, anthropometric methods used to assess body composition, and how body composition can be modified through diet and exercise. Understanding how to accurately measure body composition and **anthropometry** changes over time is essential to make meaningful conclusions about interventions aiming to change body composition.

Anthropometry

The comparative study of human body sizes and proportions.

Learning outcomes

This chapter will:

- define and describe body composition;
- outline techniques used to assess body composition;
- describe how body composition can be modified.

What is body composition?

Body composition refers to the amount of fat relative to muscle in a body. However, this technically is total body fat and fat-free mass (FFM), which includes muscle, water, and bone. Body composition is therefore the relative proportions of fat, protein, water and mineral components in the body. Almost 99% of human body mass is composed of six elements: oxygen, carbon, nitrogen, hydrogen (and smaller quantities of their stable isotopes), calcium, and phosphorus.

Isotopes

Elements or atoms that have the same number of protons and electrons but a different number of neutrons.

DOI: 10.4324/9781003321286-15

Body density

The compactness of a body, defined as the mass divided by its volume.

Body composition varies among individuals due to differences in **body density** and degree of obesity. Bone is denser than muscle, which is denser than fat. If there is a relative loss of bone density (osteoporosis) or decrease in muscle mass (with reduced training), the fat mass may be overestimated when using densitometry techniques, i.e., underwater hydrostatic weighing (rarely used now) and air displacement plethysmography (e.g., using the Bod Pod®) to calculate the ratio of fat mass to fat-free mass.

Techniques used to assess body composition

Anthropometry is the comparative study of human body sizes and proportions. Surface anthropometry techniques are commonly used to assess body composition. However, there are a variety of body composition (physique assessment) techniques that can be selected. Assessment of body composition may be conducted using non-imaging (surface anthropometry, air displacement plesthmyography, three-dimensional body scanning, doubly labelled water, bioelectrical impedance), and imaging techniques (dual-energy X-ray absorptiometry, ultrasound, computed tomography and magnetic resonance imaging). Combinations of techniques allow measurement of fat, fat-free mass, bone mineral content, total body water, **extracellular water**, total adipose tissue and its subdepots (**visceral, subcutaneous,** and **intermuscular**), skeletal muscle, select organs, and **ectopic fat depots.**[1] Clinicians and scientists use these techniques to track changes in physique to determine the efficacy of training, nutrition, and clinical interventions.

Extracellular water

Water that is outside the cells, including the water between the cells and the plasma.

Visceral adipose tissue

The adipose (fat) tissue within the abdominal cavity, which is wrapped around the organs.

Subcutaneous adipose tissue

Adipose (fat) tissue directly under the skin.

Intermuscular adipose tissue

Adipose (fat) tissue located within the skeletal muscle.

Ectopic fat depots

Excess adipose (fat) tissue in locations not usually associated with adipose tissue storage, such as in the liver or around the heart.

The selection of technique to employ for assessing body composition will be dependent upon many factors:

- technique precision and accuracy, validity, practicality, and sensitivity to monitor changes in body composition;
- technique advantages and disadvantages for collecting the data, i.e., cost, safety, time available;
- equipment/hardware, calibration requirements, software, skills required, training, and accreditation for techniques;
- client presentation and preparation protocols for techniques.

Athlete presentation for measurement is important, as hydration levels will affect results. Factors such as time of day, prior food or fluid intake, exercise, body temperature, hydration status and gastrointestinal tract contents should be standardised wherever possible prior to any assessment. Given the **diurnal** variation in body mass, fasted early morning assessments, before any food/drink is consumed, following the emptying of an athlete's bladder and possibly bowels are most reliable where practical.

Diurnal

The 24-hour period or daily cycle, such as being active during the day and resting at night.

Surface anthropometry assessment

The International Society for the Advancement of Kinanthropometry (ISAK) provides international standards for surface anthropometry assessment, using skinfolds, girths, lengths, and breadths measurements. Measures include basic ones (e.g., body mass, height), skinfolds (e.g., triceps, biceps, abdominal, calf), girths (e.g., upper arm relaxed, upper arm tensed, waist, hips, calf), breadths (e.g., elbow, knee, wrist), and lengths (e.g., ulna, femur). The advantages of ISAK surface anthropometry assessments are that they take approximately ten minutes for a restricted profile and 30 minutes for a full profile, and equipment is readily available and easily calibrated. The methods are valid and reliable if ISAK training is undertaken to ensure the correct use of callipers and anatomical bony landmarks.[2] The disadvantage is that skinfold callipers compress adipose (fat) tissue, resulting in measurement variation. To help reduce the effects of skinfold compressibility, a complete set of skinfold measurements is obtained before repeating measurements.

Air displacement plethysmography (bod pod®)

Air displacement plethysmography is used to measure body volume and calculate estimates of body density. The Bod Pod® (COSMED USA Inc., Concord, CA) device has a measurement pod of two isolated chambers to measure body volume, calibratable scales, and a computer attached to each measurement device. The Bod Pod® is easy to use, is non-invasive, and suitable for children and pregnant women; however, tight-fitting clothing such as swimwear or underwear must be worn to reduce air gaps. Total test completion including body mass, multiple measures of body volume, and measurement or estimation of lung gas volume, takes approximately ten minutes. The client sits in the measurement chamber, breathing normally and minimising movement. The chamber has a magnetically locking door with a clear window. Within the measurement pod, the technology allows the estimation of lung volume. Two measurements of body volume are undertaken, with a third required if the first two measures are not within 150 mL. From the body volume, the software predicts body fat percentage and absolute values of fat mass and fat-free mass. The Bod Pod® will underestimate fat mass compared to other physique assessment techniques if there are poor standardisation practices in athlete presentation.

Bioelectrical impedance analysis (BIA)

Bioelectrical impedance analysis (BIA) allows measurement of total body water, which is used to estimate fat-free body mass and, by difference with body mass, body fat. BIA assessment devices are readily available, and assessment is quick compared to other methods. A client appointment of 15 minutes is needed for body mass and standing stature measurement, electrode placement and then one minute of data collection. The technique is client-friendly as it is non-invasive and there is low health risk. The procedure is simple and there is good equipment portability. BIA is relatively low cost compared to other methods of body composition analysis. However, precision and validity are low. It is also important to note that there is significant variability between equipment sold/marketed as having BIA functionality and many cheap stand-on scales sold in regular stores with the promise of BIA assessment options are often inaccurate and unreliable and should not be used to assess the body composition of athletes. Higher quality and reliable BIA devices usually have several electrodes that need to be attached to the body, or at least points of contact on several parts of the body rather than just a spot for feet to stand on. It is recommended that a sports professional first review the specific functionality and validity of the equipment they are planning to use with an athlete to see if it is suitable and valid.

Sensitivity to monitor change of physique is low given that variation in client presentation for testing can affect results (e.g., levels of hydration).[3] Data interpretation is impeded given equipment formulas used to calculate body-fat/fat-free mass are not readily available and only final figures are displayed. Client preparation for measurement is important given the effect of hydration on results. Technician training is needed to ensure correct preparation of the skin and reliable electrode placements on the ankle and wrist. Regional body assessment is possible but is invalid.

Deuterium dilution: Doubly labelled water technique

The doubly labelled water technique (known as deuterium dilution) measures body water and total energy expenditure. The client consumes a stable isotope water (known as doubly labelled water) and provides urine samples for several days afterwards. The time commitment for clients is approximately six hours given the repeat samples required. The non-invasive technique measures the rate of carbon dioxide production in clients over seven to 14 days. The most sensitive means of measuring the isotopes of deuterium and oxygen-18 in the samples is by isotope ratio mass spectroscopy. Technique reliability is high. Regional body assessment is not possible; instead, total body water, fat-free mass, and fat mass are calculated. Due to the technical nature, cost, and lack of availability of equipment, the technique's use is uncommon.

Ultrasound

Ultrasound technique for measurement of subcutaneous adipose tissue and embedded fibrous structures employs image capture from any standard-brightness mode ultrasound machine, followed by an image-analysis procedure. The technique avoids tissue compression and movement that occurs when using skinfold callipers. As with skinfolds, the ultrasound technique only samples subcutaneous adipose tissue and does not measure fat stored in deeper depots. It is an accurate and reliable technique for the measurement of subcutaneous adipose tissue provided the practitioner has had certified training in data collection and analysis software use.

All clients must be marked prior to measurement. Measurements are taken from eight standard measurement sites: upper abdomen, lower abdomen, erector spinae, distal triceps, brachioradialis, lateral thigh, front thigh, and medial calf. The operator places the ultrasound probe centre over the marked site to capture an ultrasound image.

Magnetic resonance imaging (MRI) and computed tomography (CT)

Magnetic resonance imaging and computed tomography are imaging techniques that provide accurate measures of body composition at the tissue-organ level. Computed tomography works by measuring the attenuation of X-rays through body tissues, whereas magnetic resonance imaging uses a strong magnetic field to align positively charged protons in the body's tissues which are then digitised to provide an image. Magnetic resonance imaging is a safer method than computed tomography as it does not expose clients to radiation. Due to high cost and low availability, these techniques are generally only used for clients as part of a medical assessment or for research purposes. Both techniques are considered reference methods for body composition assessment due to their high precision and validity.

Dual-energy X-ray absorptiometry (DXA)

Dual-energy X-ray absorptiometry (DXA) is the current gold standard for determining body-fat percentage and lean mass. The DXA machine emits sources of X-ray energies which pass through the body, enabling the determination of bone mineral content, lean mass, and fat mass for the whole body as well as regional areas. Given the exposure to radiation from X-rays, the International Society for Clinical Densitometry has established clinical practice guidelines relating to the collection and analysis of DXA data. Standardisation of how clients present for scanning is important. Ideally, scanning should be conducted in the morning and clients should be well hydrated (urine specific gravity measurements may be taken), glycogen replenished (not having exercised heavily the day before), overnight-fasted, and in minimal clothing (such as singlet and underwear). Clients should be correctly positioned on the scanning bed, being centrally aligned in a standard position using custom-made positioning aids (foam blocks). Following the scan, images should be reviewed so that automatic segmentation of body regional areas can be checked and adjusted manually if required. Body composition assessment using such a protocol will ensure a high level of precision, while still being practical for clients. An assessment can usually be completed within ten minutes.

Three-dimensional body scanning

Three-dimensional body scanning is used to determine surface anthropometry characteristics such as body volume, segment lengths, and girths. Three-dimensional scanning systems use laser, light, or infrared technologies to acquire shape and software to allow manual or automatically extracted measures. Body posture during scanning is important to ensure accurate measures can be made from images. Training is required to ensure the successful use of three-dimensional scanning hardware and software. Hardware for full-body scanning is expensive, so the technique is not commonly available. Three-dimensional body scanning protocols and normative population data are available.[4]

Three-dimensional body scanning systems integrated with other imaging modalities to create multifaceted digital human profiles and artificial intelligence techniques such as deep learning and artificial neural networks, are set to revolutionise the physique assessment landscape over the coming decade. Using computer vision techniques, it is now possible to register an individual's DXA-derived body composition with the mesh exported by the same individual's three-dimensional body scan (Table 13.1).

How body composition can be modified

Body composition changes with growth and maturation, diet, and exercise. Body characteristics such as stature (height), skeletal lengths, and breadths are not adaptable except during growth periods, but body mass, lean mass, and fat mass are modifiable and can be manipulated. A person's genetic profile impacts their **morphology** and their responsiveness to interventions that aim to change body composition and morphology.

Morphology

The body shape.

Morphological prediction

The prediction of adult body shape from a growing child or adolescent.

Table 13.1 Summary of methods used to assess body composition

Technique	Principle	Advantages	Disadvantages
Skinfolds	Uses compression of the surface skin and adipose layer	Simple, quick, easy Inexpensive instruments needed Highly portable	Specialized training required Some athlete discomfort High inter-person variation due to compression of adipose tissue with callipers
Air displacement plethysmography 'BodPod'	Uses air displacement to measure body composition	Suitable for pregnant women and children Minimal training required Simple, quick, and easy Equipment not portable	Some athlete preparation is needed to ensure good standardisation (fasting, fluid intake, bladder emptying, minimal clothing, and body hair) The athlete needs to sit still for 10 minutes Risk of athlete feeling claustrophobic, but there is a viewing window out of BodPod
Impedance	Uses the principle of electrical conductivity with body water	Quick, easy, simple Cheap Portable Minimal technician training	Athlete preparation is needed to ensure good standardisation (fasting, fluid intake, bladder emptying)
DXA	Uses x-ray	Gold standard, highly accurate	Expensive Exposes athletes to small amounts of radiation Athlete preparation is needed to ensure good standardisation (fasting, fluid restriction and minimal clothing) Extensive technician training required
3D body scanning	Uses laser, light, or infrared	Accurate for body volume and surface dimensions	Expensive Not portable Technician training required
Ultrasound	Uses sound to determine adipose tissue	Accurate and reliable for subcutaneous fat	Technician training required Expensive Not portable
Isotope dilution	Athlete consumes stable isotope water	Total body fat evaluated Accurate	High athlete burden and delayed results as urine needs to be collected for several days Expensive Not portable Disease impacts results
MRI + CT	Uses imaging techniques	Small exposure to radiation (especially MRI)	Expensive Technician training required Not portable

Morphological prototype

The best body shape and distribution of soft tissue to maximise performance in a given sport.

Body composition information can be used to monitor the effectiveness of physique manipulation via exercise or nutrition[5] interventions. Physique assessment allows identification of clients who require additional support to restore or maintain physique status (e.g., at-risk clients who have lost or gained weight rapidly). Monitoring the progress of clients in meeting their physique goals (e.g., strength and conditioning goals to increase muscle mass) provides motivation to continue in the intervention.

Dietary approaches to change body composition

Gaining weight

When an athlete is interested in weight gain, in most cases muscle gain is desired. For muscle gain to occur excess energy intake is needed to provide energy for anabolism with a good training program to activate muscle tissue and encourage growth and development.

From a dietary perspective, an excess of 2000–4000 kJ/day (478–957 kcal/day) is usually required to generate consistent muscle gain. This is best achieved by eating regular meals and snacks that are high in energy and nutrients. It is realistic to expect muscle gain of 2–4 kilograms (4.4–8.8 lbs) per month; however, rates of muscle gain vary between individuals and genetics can play a considerable role. Consistency, in terms of both diet and training program, is key for successful muscle gain. Excessive energy intake without appropriate training will result in fat gain instead of muscle gain. As an example, the following food combinations can provide an additional 2000 kJ (478 kcal):

- full-fat fruit yoghurt (200 g) plus 25 almonds plus medium banana; OR
- half a large avocado spread on two slices of toast and an apple.

Eating enough food to obtain the additional energy can be challenging for some athletes, so simple meal and snack ideas can make a big difference. The popularity and ease of 'shakes' and smoothies have been helpful for athletes trying to gain weight. Working with individual athletes to put together a realistic eating plan is important as if a plan is not followed consistently, results are likely to be slow. Prioritising real foods over weight-gain supplements such as protein shakes is recommended due to the superior nutrient density of wholesome real foods compared to commercial protein powder-based products.

Losing weight

Generally, when weight loss is desired it is 'fat' loss people think about; while fat is the most common form of weight athletes may want to lose, there are circumstances—such as in weight category sports—where athletes may not be concerned about what weight type they lose as long as they weigh in below the cut-off (see Chapter 20).

Nutrition professionals generally recommend that weight is lost slowly, aiming for about 500 grams (1.1 lbs) weight loss per week. This can be achieved by reducing energy intake by 2000 kJ (478 kcal) every day below total requirements. This should be based on current dietary intake, the athlete's body composition over the last three months and any planned changes in training. If training is to remain consistent and weight has been stable, then reducing the athlete's usual diet by 2000 kJ (478 kcal) per day can be effective. This can be done by initially reducing discretionary foods and then as needed reducing portion sizes at mealtimes. If weight has not been stable over three months and/or training is about to change considerably, then more care will be needed to determine a suitable total dietary intake to enable healthy weight loss. The best approach will vary by athlete and should be personalised and planned collaboratively.

Protein intake and body composition

The International Society of Sports Nutrition has recommended that high protein intakes (2.3–3.1 g/kg FFM) may be required to maximize muscle retention in lean, resistance-trained athletes.[5] High-protein diets have been defined as intakes ≥ 25% of total energy or 1.2–1.6 g/kg. Higher protein intake can be beneficial for reducing body weight, fat mass, and waist circumference, whilst preserving lean mass in an energy deficit.

Issues to consider for body composition assessment

Data interpretation

Physique assessment provides valuable information; however, taken in isolation physique assessment can easily be misinterpreted or misused. Additional information, such as dietary intake and training load, and input from exercise and health professionals, is required to fully interpret findings and make recommendations.

Physique and sport

Profiling of athletes at all sport participation levels can help determine potential suitability for sport and effectiveness of interventions such as diet and training. Scientists and clinicians want to know what physique characteristics are important for athletes in the sports they work with to help improve performance[6] or reduce injury risk; what should they measure and monitor? Athletes, and their coaches, often ask how the athletes' physique compares to elite athletes in their sport. Accessing normative data for athletes at all levels of participation from development to elite can be difficult. Consideration of population trends for physique characteristics in normative databases is needed. Where possible, current research data should be gained to enable comparisons of physique characteristics for athletes of similar age, gender, ethnicity, and sports participation level.

Large-scale surveys of world-class athletes have been conducted at Olympic Games[7] and world championship events for over 60 years. These data identify unique physique characteristics for selected sports that aim to optimise power, leverage, or have a high metabolic demand. Sports professionals need to understand what physique characteristics are important for athletes to help improve performance or reduce injury risk. As many factors are involved in the physical make-up of a champion sportsperson, there is not necessarily one perfect body shape for a sport. Anthropometric tools have been used in profiling athletes' trajectories to optimise trainable parameters at times that matter most. This is important for weight category sports, where athletes may be at risk of employing unsafe weight control practices to 'make weight'. Rowing and powerlifting are two sports that require body mass to meet weight class categories for competition. Gymnastics is a sport that has pressure for leanness due to aesthetic reasons (see Chapter 20).

Body image

The concept of body image includes how individuals perceive, think, feel, and, ultimately, behave due to their own conception of their physical image. Body-image dissatisfaction is when there is a difference between perceived body image and desired body image. The prevalence of body-image disorders in athletic populations remains worryingly high. Assessment of body image in people may progress with the use of modern three-dimensional scanning technology together with volumetric assessment. The novel iPad SomatoMac application may be useful for estimates of body-image dissatisfaction and distortion, especially in athletes.[8] The SomatoMac application uses male and female **somatotype** photographs that allow more comprehensive estimates of body-image dissatisfaction than existing figural silhouettes and pictorial scales.

Somatotype

Classification of human physical shape according to body build or shape.

Determining if and when body composition assessment of athletes is required/appropriate

Whilst as discussed above, the assessment of body composition can be very useful when working with athletes, it is also important to consider if and when body composition assessment is actually needed and appropriate. In 2020, Ackerman et al. published a conceptual framework on the implementation of body composition assessments within the context of athlete stage of development and their nutritional preparation skills which is summarised in Table 13.2.[9]

Additionally, the 2023 updated IOC REDs consensus statement provides guidelines, aligned to this, for safe and effective body composition assessment to help prevent REDs.[10] To minimise the risk of low energy availability (LEA) and disordered eating (DE) behaviours:

- pre-screening should be undertaken to assess body image and to identify problematic eating behaviours, or DE;
- anthropometric and body composition assessment should only be conducted by trained members of the athlete's health and performance team. They should be trained in the specific methods to be used and should have the skills to support the athlete and coach in making informed 'health first—performance second' decisions relating to body composition;
- consent should be obtained from the athlete before every single body composition assessment and any outcome reports/ information should only be shared with those the athlete authorises to have access to the results.[10]

Table 13.2 Summary of conceptual framework on the implementation of body composition assessments in athletes

Athlete Development Stage	Nutritional Skills	Body Composition Concepts
Developing Athletes	Foundational	Emerging: No body composition assessment should take place unless required for optimal growth, and no focus on body composition in relation to performance outcomes
National/Collegiate level athletes	Developing	Developing: Limited focus should be placed on body composition assessments and discussions, i.e., should **only** be from a health perspective
Elite professional-level athletes	Advanced	Elite: Body composition assessment can take place with a periodised approach only with mature athletes with positive body image.

Source: Adapted from Ackerman et al.[9]

In the case of an athlete where there are indications of disordered eating or poor body image, it may be inappropriate to undertake an anthropometric assessment, as it may compound existing issues. Sports nutrition professionals should consider each individual athlete's circumstances, and the guidelines and framework presented in Table 13.2, prior to undertaking or recommending anthropometric assessment, and discuss it with the coaching/support team where required.

Summary

This chapter has discussed anthropometry and body composition. It has described the different methods available for its measurement in athletes, and the strengths and limitations of each technique. Whilst there are numerous techniques and tools available, sports nutrition professionals should consider if and when body composition assessment is required, and the best-suited approach for the individual athlete. Modification of body composition via the combination of diet and exercise was also discussed, in relation to muscle gain and fat loss, with specific recommendations highlighted below.

Chapter highlights

- Body composition is the relative proportions of fat, protein, water, and mineral components in the body.
- Anthropometry is the comparative study of human body sizes and proportions.
- There are valid and reliable techniques used to assess body composition; however, practitioner training is required and client presentation for assessment can affect results.
- Air displacement plethysmography measures body volume and provides estimates of body density.
- Bioelectrical impedance analysis provides total body water, which is used to estimate fat-free body mass and, by difference with body mass, body fat.
- Doubly labelled water technique measures body water and total energy expenditure.
- Ultrasound enables the measurement of subcutaneous adipose tissue and embedded fibrous structures.

- Magnetic resonance imaging and computed tomography provide accurate measures of body composition at the tissue-organ level.
- Dual-energy X-ray absorptiometry (DXA) is the current gold standard for determining body-fat and lean mass body components.
- Body composition can be modified via growth and development, diet, and exercise.
- Athletes aiming to gain muscle mass need to make sure they consistently have an energy excess of 2000–4000 kJ/day (478-956 kcal/day) and exercise appropriately.
- Athletes aiming to lose fat mass need to make sure they consistently have an energy deficit of 2000 kJ/day (478 kcal/day).
- Physique assessment provides an objective measure of body composition status in relation to physical performance, health status, and diet.
- Sports professionals should use established guidelines and frameworks in determining if and when body composition assessment of athletes is required/appropriate.

References

1. Lee SY, Gallagher D. Assessment methods in human body composition. *Curr Opin Clin Nutr Metab Care* 2008;11(5):566–72.
2. Hume P, Marfell-Jones M. The importance of accurate site location for skinfold measurement. *J Sports Sci.* 2008;26(12):1333–40.
3. Kerr A, Slater G, Byrne N. Impact of food and fluid intake on technical and biological measurement error in body composition assessment methods in athletes. *Br J Nutr.* 2017;117: 591–601.
4. Kolose S, Hume PA, Tomkinson GR, Stewart A, Stewart T, Legg SJ. *Three-Dimensional Physique Assessment in the Military: New Zealand Defence Force Anthropometry Survey Protocols and Summary Statistics.* Hume PA, editor. Auckland University of Technology: Auckland University of Technology; 2021 10th May 2021.
5. Aragon AA, Schoenfeld BJ, Wildman R, et al. International Society of Sports Nutrition position stand: diets and body composition. *J Int Soc Sports Nutr.* 2017; 14: 16.
6. Keogh JWL, Hume PA, Mellow P, Pearson SN. Can absolute and proportional anthropometric characteristics distinguish stronger and weaker powerlifters? *J Strength Cond Res.* 2009;23(8): 2256–65.
7. Kerr DA, Ross WD, Norton K, Hume P, Kagawa M, Ackland TR. Olympic lightweight and open-class rowers possess distinctive physical and proportionality characteristics. *J Sports Sci.* 2007;25(1):43–5.
8. Macfarlane DJ, Lee A, Hume P, Carter L. Development and Reliability of a Novel iPad-based Application to Rapidly Assess Body Image: 3776 Board# 215. *Med Sci Sports Exerc.* 2016;48 (5 Suppl 1):1056.
9. Ackerman KE, Stellingwerff T, Elliott-Sale KJ, et al. #REDS (Relative Energy Deficiency in Sport): time for a revolution in sports culture and systems to improve athlete health and performance. *Br J Sports Med.* 2020;54(7):369–70.
10. Mountjoy M, Ackerman K, Bailey D, et al. The 2023 International Olympic Committee's (IOC) consensus statement on Relative Energy Deficiency in Sports (REDs). *Br J Sports Med.* 2023. In press.

14 Environmental considerations

Alan McCubbin

With the increasing connectedness across the planet, athletes test their physical limits in almost every corner of the globe. A soccer player can walk out into a snow-covered stadium in Europe or the searing heat of an Australian summer. A triathlete can train all winter, then fly halfway around the world to compete at the world championships in the heat and humidity of Hawaii. Some athletes experience environments where oxygen supply is limited—explorers trekking to the peaks of the highest mountains or those training at actual or simulated altitude. Understanding the impact of the environment on exercise physiology and nutrition requirements is crucial in helping athletes stay healthy and perform at their best. This chapter explores the effects of heat and humidity, cold and altitude on the body during exercise, and nutritional strategies used in these environments.

Learning outcomes

This chapter will:

- identify the impact of heat, cold and altitude on the body during exercise;
- describe the effect of environmental extremes on nutritional requirements;
- identify practical challenges maintaining optimal nutritional intake in extreme environments, and strategies to overcome these.

Heat, humidity and exercise

During exercise, additional energy expenditure is accompanied by additional heat production as a by-product, which increases core body temperature. Human body temperature is regulated within a narrow range; less than 35°C (95°F) or greater than 40°C (104°F) places an individual at risk of significant health complications. The heat generated and lost to the environment must therefore be carefully balanced to maintain a stable body temperature. The heat produced by working muscles is transferred to the blood. This blood circulates to the skin, allowing heat exchange with the surrounding environment. Heat exchange mostly occurs via **convection** and **radiation** from the skin, and **evaporation** of fluid from the lungs, and sweat on the skin surface.

DOI: 10.4324/9781003321286-16

Convection

The transfer of heat by the movement of water or air away from the skin. The greater the water or airflow, the greater the heat transfer.

Radiation

The transfer of heat through any medium, without contact, using thermal or infrared radiation. Solar radiation from sun exposure can reverse this effect, resulting in heat gain rather than loss.

Evaporation

Heat loss through the conversion of a liquid to a gas. Sweating secretes water onto the skin surface which is evaporated, transferring heat away from the body.

As environmental temperature increases, the ability to lose heat via convection and radiation diminishes, making evaporation the predominant mechanism of heat exchange. Sweat rate is regulated during exercise to match the need for heat transfer, and maintain a stable, albeit slightly elevated, body temperature (compensable heat stress). If heat production exceeds the body's ability to lose heat, heat balance cannot be maintained and core temperature rises (uncompensable heat stress). In humid environments, the smaller difference between air and skin surface humidity reduces the ability to evaporate sweat from the skin, resulting in less heat transfer away from the body.

Exercise performance in hot and humid environments

Exercise performance in one-off sprint events is usually improved in hot environments, whereas performance in prolonged efforts or repeated sprint efforts (such as team sports) is reduced (see Figure 14.1).[1] Increased core temperature limits performance and increases an athlete's perceived effort for any given exercise intensity. Interestingly, exercising in the heat reduces the activity of working muscles even before the core temperature begins to rise, suggesting an unconscious adjustment occurs in anticipation of heat stress.[2] The significant fluid losses from sweating can result in hypohydration if inadequately replaced and is well established as a performance-limiting factor. Sweat electrolyte losses do not appear to influence performance in hot environments independent of fluid balance.

Unsurprisingly, athletes in sports greater than five minutes duration usually produce better performances in cooler and less humid conditions. The optimal temperature chosen by scientists supporting the Nike Breaking2 Project (to break the two-hour barrier for the marathon) was 7–12°C (45–54°F). Increasing relative humidity from 24 per cent to

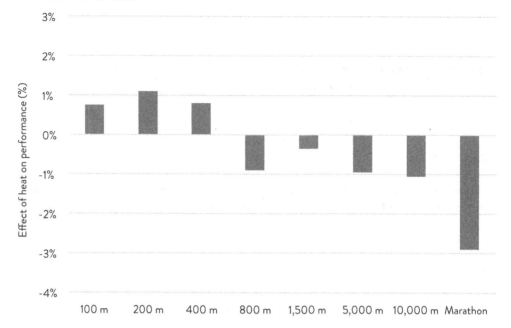

Figure 14.1 Effect of heat (<25°C (77°F) compared to >25°C (77°F)) for running events in IAAF World Championship events held between 1999 and 2011.

Source: Data from Guy et al.[1]

(*Note:* average of male and female data; positive effects indicate faster finish time; negative effects indicate slower finish times).

80 per cent reduced the time cyclists could ride to exhaustion at 70 per cent VO$_2$max by 22 minutes, even though temperature remained constant.[3]

Health consequences of exercising in hot and humid environments

The health consequences of heat stress during exercise are termed exertional heat illness. Although consequences are described on a continuum of severity, each condition can occur independently. Heat syncope, the least severe, occurs because blood is diverted to the skin to maximise heat transfer. During exercise, working muscles in the lower legs compress veins and assist in returning blood to the heart. When exercise ceases, blood return is reduced, resulting in a sudden drop in blood pressure and potential collapse. This effect is exacerbated by hypohydration due to reduced blood volume. Heat syncope is most common in ultra-endurance events held in the heat, whereby athletes collapse just after crossing the finish line.

Heat exhaustion occurs when the heart cannot maintain sufficient cardiac output due to the combination of high demand (exercise intensity) and reduced supply (reduced blood volume from hypohydration). Nausea and vomiting, rapid heart rate, significant fatigue, dizziness or fainting are symptoms and are usually associated with core body temperatures below 40°C (104°F). Exertional heat stroke is a potentially life-threatening condition that usually (but not exclusively) occurs when core temperatures exceed 40°C (104°F). It involves dysfunction of the central nervous system, major organs and skeletal muscles. Rapid cooling and urgent medical attention are required.

Sympathetic nervous system

Often termed the 'fight-or-flight' response. It accelerates heart rate, dilates bronchial passages, decreases motility of the digestive tract, constricts blood vessels and increases sweating.

Exercise-induced gastrointestinal syndrome (EIGS)

Describes the physiological responses (i.e., circulatory-gastrointestinal and neuroendocrine-gastrointestinal) that occur due to exercise, which may compromise GI function (i.e., motility, transit) and GI barrier integrity (i.e., epithelial injury, increased GI permeability, translocation of endotoxins from the lumen into circulation, systemic inflammatory responses) triggering adverse health and performance outcomes.

Exercise in the heat also reduces blood flow to the gastrointestinal (GI) tract and increases the body's **sympathetic nervous system** activity. Both factors increase the risk for **exercise-induced gastrointestinal syndrome (EIGS)** and may contribute to exertional heat stroke risk.[4] Refer to Chapter 15 for more information.

Because of the potential health consequences of exercising in hot environments, many sports have adopted extreme heat policies to shorten, postpone or cancel events in the event of such conditions. The Australian Open tennis tournament reschedules or moves matches indoors and closes the stadium roof where possible to protect player safety. The racewalk and marathon events at the 2019 World Athletics Championships in Qatar were rescheduled to the evening and held under lights to avoid extreme temperatures and solar radiation, and the same events at the Tokyo 2020 Olympic Games were relocated 830 km (515 miles) north to Sapporo in attempt to reduce the level of heat stress. When the weather in Sapporo was hotter than expected, the women's marathon started an hour earlier than originally scheduled.

Effect of heat and humidity on nutrient metabolism and nutritional requirements during exercise

The use of carbohydrate for fuel is increased by 15 per cent or more, and fat therefore reduced, during exercise in the heat. This may occur because of reduced blood flow to muscles, so less oxygen, fatty acids and glucose are delivered, favouring the use of fuels already stored in the muscle—particularly glycogen. There is also increased epinephrine production during exercise in the heat, which increases muscle glycogen use as a fuel compared to fat.

Heat acclimatisation and acclimation

Exertional heat illness and impaired performance are most likely when athletes are not adapted to hot environments. Undergoing heat **acclimatisation** or **acclimation** can significantly improve the body's ability to transfer heat. Developing over one to two weeks of exercise in the heat, these adaptations include:

- blood volume expansion, increased stroke volume and reduced heart rate;
- increased skin blood flow, improving the ability for heat exchange;
- commencement of sweating at a lower core temperature and increased maximal sweat rate.

Heat acclimatisation

The process of adaptation by living and training in a naturally hot environment.

Heat acclimation

The process of adaptation when completing specific training sessions in artificially induced heat, such as a climate chamber or heated room.

One concern raised by sporting organisations, scientists and athletes, is the impact of climate change on outdoor exercise. With heatwaves becoming more common, the risk of exertional heat illness in both training and competition is likely to increase. It seems inevitable that the number of sporting events impacted by extreme heat policies will grow over time. The choice of location for major international sporting events may become geographically limited to ensure they can be run according to schedule. But perhaps the greater challenge is for recreational athletes. With no heat policy or organisation to reschedule, shorten or cancel their training, the recreational athlete needs to decide for themselves whether it is safe or not.

Nutritional interventions for the heat

In addition to increased carbohydrate and fluid requirements, which are outlined in previous chapters, food and fluids have the potential to reduce core body temperature and improve performance in the heat. Pre-cooling involves strategies that lower core temperature prior to exercise. In addition to external cooling with ice vests, ice slushies can be used for internal cooling, with the phase change from ice to water particularly effective at absorbing heat energy. A reduction of 0.25°C in rectal temperature has been observed after consuming 500 grams (17.6 ounces) of ice slushie made from sports drink, with 0.6°C reduction after consuming 1000 grams (35.2 ounces) of slushie.[5] Compared to no ice ingestion, the core temperature remained lower even after competition warm-up in the slushie trials, so the athletes began exercising at a lower temperature (Figure 14.2).

Practical issues affecting nutrition in hot and humid environments

It is easy to keep drinks cold by the side of a team sport field or racquet sport court with an ice chest or electric refrigeration. But when exercise takes place far from a base of support, keeping food and fluids cool becomes more challenging. In multistage desert ultramarathons, for example, sports drinks and gels warming in the sun can make them so unpalatable that athletes no longer consume them. Ensuring foods and fluids are shaded from the sun, and avoiding direct contact with the body will limit heat exchange that warms these products. Where possible, fluids can be frozen prior to prolonged exercise and consumed as they thaw. Care should be taken regarding food safety for non-packaged foods during exercise—storing them refrigerated as long as possible and consuming them early during exercise minimises the risk of microbial contamination.

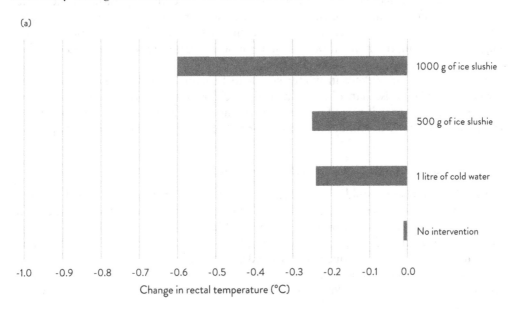

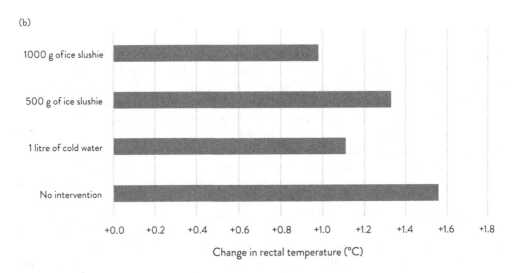

Figure 14.2 Effect of ice slushie ingestion on rectal temperature: (a) 30 minutes after commencing consumption; (b) following a 30-minute warm-up in preparation for competition.

Source: Data from Ross et al.[5]

Cold environments and nutrition requirements during exercise

Exercise in environments near or below-freezing temperatures presents another challenge for athletes, whether snow sports or not. The weight of additional protective clothing can increase energy expenditure and if shivering occurs, this can more than double energy expenditure compared to rest. This is unlikely, however, since exercise produces heat and acts to increase core temperature.

Although sweat rates are often assumed to be lower in cold environments, this is not always the case. Protective clothing can maintain skin and core temperature while reducing heat transfer.[6] In addition, increased fluid losses can occur from the lungs in cold environments, due to reduced moisture present in the air.[6] Thirst sensation is often impaired, reducing the motivation to drink. Good hydration practices should therefore remain a focus, even in cold environments.

It is common for athletes in winter sports to be exposed to less sunlight, and have lower vitamin D status, than athletes who train and compete outdoors in summer months. This is especially true if travelling between the northern and southern hemispheres to train and compete year-round. For more information on vitamin D, refer to Chapter 5.

Practical issues affecting nutrition in cold environments

Many of the impacts of cold environments on nutrition strategies are practical. Athletes in cold environments may be reluctant to drink to reduce the time and inconvenience of removing several layers of clothing to urinate. If thick gloves are worn, dexterity is often impaired, so opening food packages or using drink bottles is more difficult. Wrapping food in foil that can be torn open, and using drink bottles that can be opened with teeth, can avoid these issues. Some sports foods and fluids also become harder to chew or may freeze in cold environments. Practical strategies for accessing nutrition in cold environments are presented in Chapter 28.

Altitude and hypoxia

Altitude exposure is considered to be 2000 metres (6560 feet) or more above sea level. Athletes often exercise at altitude, either for training before competing at sea level or because competition occurs there (as with snow sports). Air is less dense at altitude, reducing oxygen uptake with each breath. Commercial altitude tents or chambers attempt to simulate this by lowering the percentage of oxygen without changing air density.

Fluid losses are greater at altitude compared to sea level, due to both humidity and the increased breathing required to deliver the same amount of oxygen to the blood.[7] Since ATP production from carbohydrate requires less oxygen than fat, there is a shift towards increased carbohydrate and reduced fat oxidation for the same exercise bout at altitude.[8]

Perhaps most importantly, red blood cell production increases as an adaptation to altitude, which is why endurance athletes use altitude training to improve performance at sea level. This draws considerably on iron stores to produce haemoglobin for the new blood cells; iron levels will usually fall after two weeks at altitude. It is recommended that athletes travelling to altitude have their iron status checked beforehand, and supplementation provided as required, before altitude exposure.

Summary

Exposure to hot environments increases physiological strain during exercise, negatively impacting performance in prolonged exercise and increasing the risk of exertional heat illness and EIGS. Heat acclimation or acclimatisation, and providing adequate fluid replacement, is the main strategy for managing hot environments. Ice slushies before exercise may provide an additional benefit in some situations, although is not always practically achievable. Cold environments don't present the same impacts on health or performance, since exercise raises body temperature. Body temperature may drop prior to competition, however, in which case heated foods and fluids may be beneficial. Training or competing at altitude can challenge the body's ability to deliver oxygen for optimal performance. The adaptation to altitude training involves increased red blood cell production, which draws significantly on body iron stores. Supplementation is therefore used in anticipation of such training. In all three conditions (heat, cold and altitude), but for differing reasons, carbohydrate contributes a greater proportion to energy production for the same exercise type and intensity.

Chapter highlights

- Exercise in hot environments causes a greater increase in core temperature compared to cooler conditions.
- Exercise performance in sprint events is often improved or unaffected by heat; however, performance is reduced in prolonged exercise.
- Elevated core temperature can increase the risk of exertional heat illness and EIGS.
- Exercise in the heat increases fluid and sodium losses from sweating and increases the use of muscle glycogen (and therefore carbohydrate) as an energy source.
- Nutrition strategies to improve performance in the heat include pre-cooling with ice slushies, ensuring drinks to be consumed during exercise are kept as cold as possible and ensuring adequate fluid to meet the athlete's needs.
- Exercise in the cold can increase energy and fluid requirements and make the consumption of food and fluids more practically difficult.
- Athletes training and competing in winter year-round are at increased risk of vitamin D deficiency and should be monitored and supplemented as required.
- Altitude exposure increases carbohydrate and fluid requirements and can draw significantly on iron stores.
- Assessing the iron status of athletes prior to prolonged altitude exposure is important to ensure deficiency does not develop, preventing the beneficial adaptations to training at altitude.

References

1. Guy JH, Deakin GB, Edwards AM. Adaptation to hot environmental conditions: An exploration of the performance basis, procedures and future directions to optimise opportunities for elite athletes. *Sports Med.* 2015;45(3):303–311.
2. Tucker R, Rauch L, Harley YX. Impaired exercise performance in the heat is associated with an anticipatory reduction in skeletal muscle recruitment. *Eur J Physiol.* 2004;448(4):422–430.
3. Maughan RJ, Otani H, Watson P. Influence of relative humidity on prolonged exercise capacity in a warm environment. *Eur J Appl Phsyiol.* 2012;112(6):2313–2321.

4. Costa RJS, Snipe RMJ, Kitic CM. Systematic review: Exercise-induced gastrointestinal syndrome-implications for health and intestinal disease. *Aliment Pharmacol Ther*. 2017;46(3):246–265.
5. Ross ML, Garvican LA, Jeacocke NA. Novel precooling strategy enhances time trial cycling in the heat. *Med Sci Sports Exerc*. 2011;43(1):123–133.
6. O'Brien CY, Young AJ, Sawka MN. Hypohydration and thermoregulation in cold air. *J Appl Physiol*. 1998;84(1):185–189.
7. Thomas DT, Erdman KA, Burke LM. American College of Sports Medicine Joint Position Statement. Nutrition and athletic performance. *Med Sci Sports Exerc*. 2016;48(3):543–568.
8. Koehle MS, Cheng I, Sporer B. Canadian Academy of Sport and Exercise Medicine Position Statement: Athletes at high altitude. *Clin J Sports Med*. 2014;24(2):120–127.

15 Gastrointestinal disturbances

Stephanie K Gaskell and Dana M Lis

The importance of good nutrition for health and performance is well established. However, the individuality and personalisation of performance nutrition strategies vary greatly between athletes. In particular, gastrointestinal symptoms (GIS) associated with exercise, related to physiological changes, gut–brain interactions and nutrition intake vary and can impact an athlete's ability to consume a healthy, balanced diet and further deter their capacity to exercise, with more severe symptoms leading to serious impacts on exercise performance. General population awareness of overall gut health and increasing understanding of 'The Athletes Gut' has provided improved strategies and tools to manage GIS. This chapter provides an overview of the prevalence of gastrointestinal (GI) disturbances (e.g. bloating, pain and diarrhoea) among athletes and the physiological, neuroendocrine and nutritional factors involved with exercise-induced gastrointestinal syndrome (EIGS). Nutrition strategies to manage GIS before, during and after exercise will be highlighted.

Learning outcomes

This chapter will:

- describe the prevalence and severity of GI disturbances in athletic populations;
- report the most frequently occurring symptoms of EIGS;
- describe the foundational causes and modulating factors of EIGS;
- outline foundational nutritional strategies that may reduce gastrointestinal symptom frequency and severity.

Prevalence of gastrointestinal symptoms

GIS are common among athletes, with the most severe or frequent reported during endurance exercise, particularly in running as opposed to cycling or swimming. Over 60% of ultra-endurance athletes report GIS during ultra-endurance events (e.g. ultramarathon and ultra-distance triathlon).[1-3] A much lower incidence is reported in shorter duration endurance events (<4 h) and team, power and strength sports (≤10%).[3] GIS vary greatly, and are transient and hard to replicate but three main 'triggers' are usually associated: physiological, mechanical and nutritional. A genetic predisposition is also suggested in those with more consistent GIS occurrences. Research and athlete insight continue to expand the knowledge of training and nutrition strategies that can be implemented to

DOI: 10.4324/9781003321286-17

reduce moderate and severe GIS and the detrimental impact these have on training capacity, nutrient intake and performance.

Common gastrointestinal symptoms

GIS are categorised into two sections: the upper GI section, comprised of the buccal cavity (mouth), pharynx, oesophagus, stomach and duodenum (beginning of small intestine) and the lower GI section, where most of the digestion occurs, and includes the small intestine (duodenum, jejunum, ileum) and the colon (more information on the anatomy and physiology of the digestive system can be found in Chapter 3). Mechanical forces, physiological **and neuroendocrine** changes associated with strenuous exercise and nutritional intake can trigger or augment GIS in both sections, but GIS in the upper section mainly occur in endurance events.

Neuroendocrine

Relating to interactions between the neural and endocrine system, particularly relating to hormones.

Exercise-induced gastrointestinal syndrome (EIGS) is the more recent term used to refer to disturbances of GI integrity and function that are common physiological features of strenuous exercise.[2] Mechanical, physiological and nutritional factors underpin the symptoms associated with EIGS and may be experienced before, during or after exercise, with the direct cause not completely understood. Symptoms range in severity, type and duration. Prevention and reliably reducing symptoms is challenging due to the transient nature, difficulty in replicating, variability of influencing factors (e.g. stress, sleep, climate) and subjective nature of reporting. Most symptom occurrences are reported as mild to moderate in severity and with likely negligible impact on training capacity or performance. Symptoms of greater severity, such as severe nausea, vomiting, diarrhoea or debilitating abdominal pain are more likely to negatively affect athletic performance. The most commonly reported symptoms are:

Upper GI (gastro-oesophageal)

- belching;
- bloating and/or abdominal pain;
- heartburn;
- urge to regurgitate or regurgitation;
- vomiting.

Lower GI

- abdominal bloating and/or pain;
- flatulence;
- urge to defecate;
- defecation with or without abnormalities, i.e., diarrhoea (runner's trots) and/or faecal blood loss.

Other related symptoms

- acute transient abdominal pain;
- low appetite/inability to consume adequate nutrition.

Functional gastrointestinal disorders

Many exercise-associated GIS are like symptoms experienced in functional GI disorders (FGIDs). Although FGIDs are primarily managed by clinical dietitians and other medical professionals, a basic understanding of these conditions is important for sport practitioners because athletes may have these conditions, diagnosed or undiagnosed. It is also suggested that the ongoing physiological stress placed on the gut with strenuous exercise may compromise normal GI system functioning resulting in abnormalities similar to FGID over time.

FGIDs are disorders of gut–brain interaction and are classified by a range of recurrent or persistent GIS. Diagnosis is made by identification of structural and physiological abnormalities, often presenting with a combination of abnormal intestinal contractions, **visceral hypersensitivity** and alterations in the gut lining, **gut microbiota**, immune function and central nervous system functioning. In clinical settings, psychological therapy such as cognitive behavioural therapy may be a part of a universal treatment plan.

Visceral hypersensitivity

Heightened sensation of pain in the internal organs.

Gut microbiota

Microbe population and diversity primarily of the large intestine.

Irritable bowel syndrome (IBS) is one of the most common FGIDs and is estimated to affect 15% of the Western population. More common in females, IBS is a chronic condition occurring at any age, with incidences that vary in frequency and severity. Symptoms of IBS may include abdominal pain, bloating, abnormal/delayed bowel movements, constipation and/or diarrhoea, with no obvious structural or physiological gut abnormalities. Symptoms of IBS overlap with EIGS symptoms.

Pathology of gastrointestinal symptoms

EIGS describes the physiological responses that occur due to exercise and may subsequently impair GI integrity and function resulting in GIS. There are two main pathways in this syndrome: **circulatory-gastrointestinal** and **neuroendocrine-gastrointestinal** pathways and a probable third causal factor, mechanical strain.

Circulatory-gastrointestinal

During exercise, there is a redistribution of blood flow to working muscles and the peripheries consequently resulting in a reduction of blood flow to the splanchnic (GI organs) circulation, termed splanchnic hypoperfusion (i.e., *low* or *decreased* flow of fluid). Splanchnic refers to GI organs such as the stomach, small intestine, colon, pancreas, liver and spleen.

Neuroendocrine-gastrointestinal

Exercise stress activates the sympathetic nervous system and increases the secretion of stress hormones such as corticotropin-releasing hormone, cortisol and catecholamines. As a result of the increased sympathetic drive and stress hormone response, there is a reduction in overall GI functional capacity such as GI motility and transit.

Epithelial barrier

Surface cells lining the GI tract.

Physiological

Exercise intensity, duration and load

Several physiological changes that occur in the GI system during exercise are dependent on the level of exertional stress. A proportionally greater exercise intensity and/or exercise duration will result in greater EIGS and associated GI symptoms. At sustained exercise intensities (≥ 2 h running at 60% VO_2max) disturbances to GI integrity, i.e., epithelial injury, function and systemic responses, and GI symptoms occur. Injury to the **epithelial barrier** increases permeability (also known as leaky gut), allowing bacterial endotoxins to enter the circulation and epithelial injury can further compromise nutrient absorption.[2]

Longer endurance events are associated with a higher incidence and severity of GI disturbances. Athletes competing in ultra-endurance events, compared with relatively shorter events (<4 h) such as the marathon, report up to 85% greater incident rates of GIS.[2]

GI disturbances also occur outside of competition and can compromise athletes' training capacity. Athletes with a high training load and multiple daily sessions may experience recurrent GI disturbances. The reason for this may be that the time between strenuous training bouts is less than the 4–5 days required for intestinal epithelial repair.

Circulatory-gastrointestinal pathway

During exercise, particularly endurance-type exercise at higher intensity, blood flow is redistributed to the working muscles and away from the GI organs which can result in **splanchnic hypoperfusion**. Blood flow to the gut can be reduced by up to 80% during strenuous exercise, i.e., running for 1 h at 70% VO$_2$max.[4] If exertional stress is significant enough, sustained hypoperfusion to the GI epithelium can contribute to injury and inflammation of the epithelium which can lead to increased intestinal permeability and translocation of endotoxins from the lumen into the circulation leading to systemic inflammatory responses.

Factors that contribute to splanchnic hypoperfusion include:

- exercise intensity;
- duration of exercise;
- dehydration during exercise;
- heat stress.

Splanchnic hypoperfusion

Reduction of blood flow to the splanchnic (GI organs) circulation.

Endotoxins

Part of the membrane of the cell wall of Gram-negative bacteria.

Neuroendocrine-gastrointestinal pathway

Exercise stress activates the sympathetic nervous system—this is the part of the nervous system that initiates the fight-or-flight response and reduces the parasympathetic drive responsible for initiating the rest and digest response. In addition, there is increased secretion of stress hormones (e.g. corticotropin-releasing hormone, cortisol and catecholamines). As a result of the increased sympathetic drive and stress hormone response, there is a reduction in overall GI functional capacity, including GI motility and transit.[2] An important interplay between exercise-associated stress response and gut microbiota is increasingly recognised as a contributing factor in exercise-associated GI disturbances and overall GI health.

Environment

The risk of disturbances to the GI system such as intestinal injury, increased permeability and consequently increased systemic response is greater in hot ambient conditions (≥30°C) compared to temperate (22°C) or cooler environments.[3] Exercising in the heat increases total body water loss (see Chapter 14), leading to a decrease in plasma volume, a further reduction of blood flow to the gut and an increase in sympathetic drive. Both heat stress and dehydration appear to increase the risk of exercise-associated GIS. Several high-profile athletes have experienced devasting GIS during exercise in the heat including marathon runner Paula Radcliffe in the 2004 Olympics in Athens.

To minimise the impact of heat on GI stress during exercise, a carefully planned hydration plan should be implemented based on measured sweat rates and calculated fluid requirements. Exercise-associated hyponatraemia (see Chapter 11) has been linked to GIS, particularly nausea and vomiting. Beginning exercise in a euhydrated state and aiming to avoid significant dehydration and/or over-hydration is advised (see Chapter 11).

Mechanical

GIS appear to be more common in exercise with greater mechanical impact (i.e., mechanical strain on the splanchnic area through jarring, jolting, acute impact, friction and/or body position), such as running or triathlon.[2] Upper GIS may be more common in cycling, with its bent-over position, which places pressure on the abdominal area. Technique-related breathing in swimming may result in swallowing air, increasing the occurrence of upper GIS.

Nutrition

Athletes trial various nutrition strategies around training and competition with the aim of individualising and optimising fuelling as well as reducing the risk of GI disturbances. Common pre-emptive nutrition strategies to prevent or minimise GIS include reduced dietary fibre intake, decreased fat and protein intake, adjusting food timing and training the gut to tolerate greater carbohydrate and fluid loads.

Low-residue diet

Diet-limiting foods high in fibre and residue.

Athletes are advised to 'train race-day nutrition'. Ideally, competition nutrition strategies should be like those used in training sessions. Competition-specific strategies aimed at reducing race-day GI disturbances may include a short-term **low-residue diet**, avoiding lactose the day before a competition, or modifying carbohydrates by increasing or reducing intake or changing the carbohydrate type. Research has shown that sport nutrition products with multitransporter carbohydrates (glucose and fructose ratios of 2:1 or 1:0.8) may reduce the occurrence and severity of GIS during exercise. Race fuelling may not always be under the full control of the athletes, as in some events feed stations may offer a variety of unfamiliar foods and fluids to the athlete. A less-experienced athlete may consume fuel options that they have not tested prior or may overfuel due to inexperience or a fear of **'bonking'**. Competition nutrition plans should be tested in training sessions of similar intensity and in similar climatic conditions. Logistical challenges and the additional stress of race situations may alter even the most well-planned nutrition strategies. The following sections elaborate on nutrition strategies to reduce the occurrence and severity of GIS around and during exercise.

Bonking

An athletic term describing a sudden, overwhelming feeling of running out of energy—also termed 'hitting the wall'—during endurance events.

Fibre, fat and protein

Direct links between GIS and dietary fat, protein and fibre have yet to be proven even though numerous studies have attempted to connect exercise-associated GIS with macronutrient quantities and timing. One of the first studies investigating dietary habits and the prevalence of GIS during endurance competition found that athletes who consumed foods high in fibre, fat or protein before competition reported a higher prevalence of GIS, notably vomiting and reflux.[5] More recently, protein hydrolysate ingested before and during exercise was shown to be poorly tolerated and associated with higher rates of GI disturbance.[6] Conversely, a prospective study in triathletes found no association of fibre, fat or protein intake with GIS during the cycle and run leg of a 70.3 triathlon.[5] The individual variability in dietary intake, methodological differences, transient nature and hard-to-replicate characteristics of GIS, make it difficult to draw definite conclusions about the effects of fibre, protein and fat on exercise-associated GIS. However, practitioners generally advise low fibre, low fat and moderate protein intakes around competition alongside individual recommendations.

Meal timing

Similarly, a direct link between meal timing and GIS has not been established. Based on the studies that examined the effects of meal timing on GIS, it is suggested that solid food consumed close to the start of endurance exercise may increase upper GIS. From the limited research and anecdotal evidence, easy-to-digest liquid fuelling options ingested closer to the start of exercise, rather than solids, reduced GIS. Again, repeated testing and individualisation may be needed to determine the best fuelling timing.

Gluten-free diet

Recently, gluten-free diets (GFDs) have grown in popularity among athletes, with a belief that they reduce GIS, improve overall health and even offer ergogenic benefits; however, supportive evidence is lacking. A GFD restricts a family of gluten-related proteins found mainly in food or constituents from wheat, rye and barley. It is interesting to consider that perhaps repeated stress placed on the gut because of strenuous training regimes may compromise gut barrier function and increase susceptibility to dietary triggers, such as gluten; however, this has not been shown in research. Greater awareness and improved diagnostics for clinical gluten-related conditions (**coeliac disease, non-coeliac gluten/wheat sensitivity**) may also influence the increasing number of athletes following a GFD. Self-prescription of a GFD is common among athletes—partly due to the lack of definitive biomarkers to diagnose non-coeliac gluten/wheat sensitivity and looking for solutions to reduce GIS. A clinical need to adhere to a GFD must not be overlooked, but it is also important to be attentive to unnecessary dietary restrictions and subsequent dietary changes that can occur alongside a GFD, as well as the *belief effect*, which may bias GIS perceptions.[5]

Coeliac disease

Autoimmune disease in which the immune system reacts abnormally to gluten, causing damage to the small intestine.

Non-coeliac gluten/wheat sensitivity

A condition characterised by adverse GI and/or extra-intestinal symptoms associated with the ingestion of gluten- or wheat-containing foods, in the absence of coeliac disease or wheat allergy.

FODMAPs

Reported GIS improvement with a GFD may not be due to gluten reduction but the subsequent reduction in some FODMAPs. FODMAPs (fermentable oligosaccharides, disaccharides, monosaccharides and polyols) are a family of short-chain fermentable carbohydrates that are slowly or variably absorbed in the upper intestine and rapidly fermented by colonic bacteria. In the upper intestine, unabsorbed FODMAPs may exert an **osmotic effect**, which means more fluid is drawn into the bowel. Combined with the fermentation of FODMAPs by gas-producing colonic bacteria, fluid and gas distend the bowel. As a result, bloating, abdominal pain, flatulence and alterations in bowel movement occur. A low-FODMAP diet has shown promising results in clinical patients, such as those with IBS.

Many athletes avoid foods high in FODMAPs, such as milk or legumes, with the aim of reducing GIS, with a high rate of reported symptom improvement.[7] Repeated exercise stress placed on the gut, combined with high carbohydrate intakes and high FODMAP loads present in many sports-specific foods, may create the perfect storm for FODMAPs to exacerbate exercise-associated GIS. Short-term dietary FODMAP reduction, 24 h prior to strenuous exercise in a hot climate (2-h running bout, 60% V02max, 30°C (86°F)) found a meaningful reduction in GIS during and after exercise.[8] With ongoing research showing the benefit of acute FODMAP reduction, a 24-h low-FODMAP diet has been suggested for best practice study design for GI research in athletes. Healthy endurance athletes with EIGS do not routinely require a low-FODMAP diet, but it may be helpful to reduce symptoms in susceptible individuals. A trained dietitian should be consulted for FODMAP modification.

Osmotic effect

The movement of water molecules from a higher water potential to a more negative water potential.

Fructose

Endurance athletes may consume more fructose due to increased intake of fruits, juices, honey and sports foods (such as gels and beverages) to meet their energy needs. Fructose is normally absorbed in the small intestine by intestinal transporters, low-capacity facilitated diffusion GLUT 5 and a glucose-activated more rapid diffusion, GLUT 2. Malabsorption of fructose can occur when the activity of one of these transporters, GLUT 5, becomes saturated. Some individuals may have fructose malabsorption, in which fructose is not fully absorbed, exerting an osmotic effect and is then fermented by colonic bacteria and influences GIS. It is possible that athletes ingesting large amounts of high-fructose foods may experience variable fructose malabsorption, resulting in GIS. Fructose absorption can be improved by ingesting smaller doses and consuming it as a component of foods or meals containing other nutrients.

Osmolality, carbohydrate intake and type

Ingestion of carbohydrate solutions with a high osmolality (i.e., having a high concentration of molecules in a solution, also known as hyperosmolar) has been associated with GIS during exercise. Gastric emptying and intestinal fluid absorption are reduced when carbohydrate concentration in solution is greater than 6%.

The ingestion of multiple carbohydrate types increases the oxidation of ingested carbohydrate, improving fuel availability and possibly decreasing GIS. Large amounts of carbohydrate consumed during exercise may be variably absorbed, particularly with a high load of single source carbohydrate (such as glucose). Excessive carbohydrate remains undigested in the intestine and can exacerbate GIS through osmotic actions. Most sports foods that are designed to provide for carbohydrate requirements (e.g. 90 g/h) are formulated with multiple transportable carbohydrate blends such as glucose:fructose at a 2:1 or 1:0.8 ratio, or maltodextrin with fructose, glucose or sucrose. Ingestion of multiple carbohydrate types allows for higher exogenous oxidation rates and therefore fuel availability (Figure 15.1). Feeding tolerance to high carbohydrate intake rates (i.e., ≥ 90 g/h multiple-transportable carbohydrates) during exercise is variable and depends on factors such as exercise scenario (e.g. exercise type, duration, intensity and ambient conditions)

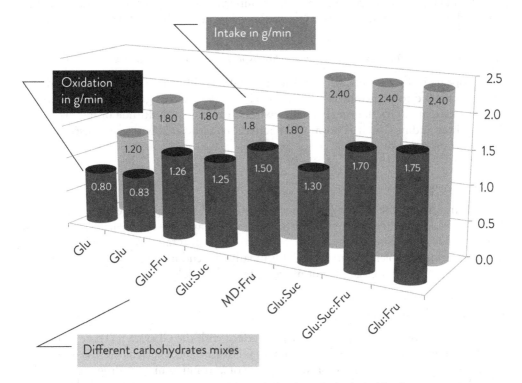

Figure 15.1 Carbohydrate oxidation rates from different carbohydrate blends.

Source: Asker Jeukendrup, SSE#108 Multiple Transportable Carbohydrates and their Benefits (www.gssiweb. org/en-ca/article/sse-108-multiple-transportable-carbohydrates-and-their-benefits).

and fitness status of the athlete. Where exercise demands these upper-end intakes, an individualised approach including gut training strategies is suggested to adapt and minimise the risk of GIS.

Whether carbohydrate is sourced from drinks, gels, bars or gummy chews, it is converted to energy equally as efficiently, though this differs when fibre, fat or protein are added. Therefore, when carbohydrate oxidation is a priority (VO_2max >~50–55%) solids should be low in fat, fibre and protein so delivery of carbohydrate and fluids is not slowed.

Eating during exercise

When GI function is impaired due to the physiological changes explained above, nutrient intake during exercise may increase the risk or severity of adverse symptoms. However, frequent and consistent carbohydrate intake during exercise has been shown to protect the epithelium and reduce the level of gut injury.[1–3]

Training status of athlete and trainability of the gut

GIS are more frequent in novice athletes with a lower training experience. The gut adapts like other body systems to training stress and a feature of this is increased splanchnic blood flow. A seminal study showed that two weeks of a repetitive gut challenge involving ingestion of 90 g/h of carbohydrate during running (2 hrs @ 60% VO_2max) reduced the malabsorption of carbohydrate and incidence of GIS in recreational runners, compared to a placebo.[1] 'Gut training' may be an important tool to increase tolerance to high carbohydrate intakes and the activity of sodium-dependent glucose transporter SGLT-1.

History of gastrointestinal symptoms, genetic predisposition and biological sex

There appears to be a genetic predisposition to GIS, and those with a history of GIS are more susceptible to recurrent GI disturbance. Female athletes generally report greater exercise-associated GIS than male counterparts. However, a multitude of factors underpinning these findings, such as hormonal fluctuations associated with the menstrual cycle, are important to be aware of.

Chronic low energy availability

Clinical and anecdotal data suggest that athletes experiencing low energy availability (LEA) report a higher incidence of GI disturbances. This area has not been well-researched; however, it is reasonable to assume that limited nutrient intake would compromise the ability to absorb or tolerate nutrients. Additionally, depending on the severity and nature of restrictive intake patterns, the gut microbiota may be deleteriously altered.

Medications and supplements

Certain medications and supplements may interfere with the GI system. There is an associated three- to fivefold increased risk of upper GI disturbances such as GORD and gastritis, mucosal bleeding or perforation with the use of anti-inflammatory drugs compared to no medication.[9] It is recommended that prolonged use of non-steroidal anti-inflammatory drugs (NSAIDs) and use prior to exercise be avoided.

Nerve and muscle activity of the large intestine can be affected by supplements such as high-dose iron, leading to constipation. Antibiotics may alter the gut microbiota and cause diarrhoea. Micronutrients, such as high doses of magnesium can cause diarrhoea and high doses of vitamin C can cause abdominal pain/cramps and diarrhoea.

Psychological stress

The interplay between the gut–brain axis is demonstrated with stress, fatigue and mood disturbances frequently linked to GI disturbances. Often, athletes experience GI disturbances only around race situations, where stress, nerves and anxiety levels are higher than in the daily training environment. The psychological demands of intense exercise can initiate a stress response, resulting in the release of hormones initiating a fight-or-flight response. Additionally, a complex interplay between these biochemical changes and GI microbiota is thought to reciprocally influence GIS. In some cases, cognitive behavioural therapy to address stress and coping mechanisms may be part of an athlete's toolbox to treat GI disturbances.

Nutrition advice for athletes with gastrointestinal disturbances

GI disturbances in athletes are multifactorial in nature and there is large individual variation in responses to exertional stress therefore prevention and management strategies require individualisation.[8] More recently, a four-phase GI assessment protocol has been developed for the identification, prevention and management of EIGS and associated GIS.[8] Table 15.1 outlines several dietary and nutritional strategies that may help in the management of GI disturbances in athletes. These tools may be helpful; however, the advice of a sports nutrition professional with specialised training in GI nutrition is recommended. Furthermore, in cases of persistent GIS, both at rest and during exercise, the advice of a medical professional should be sought to determine possible underlying clinical conditions.

Table 15.1 Dietary and nutritional tools in the management of exercise-induced GI syndrome and associated GIS[a]

Dietary and/or other management recommendations	GIS that may be avoided
Avoid gulping fluids during training or competition. Use breathing techniques that avoid swallowing air. Avoid carbonated beverages.	Belching
Avoid agents that relax the lower oesophageal sphincter, such as caffeine, mint, chocolate and alcohol.	Belching GORD
Aim to eat ~2–4 hours prior to training or competition. Shorter times between eating and exercise start may increase the risk of adverse GI effects. As a general rule, the closer nutrition is taken to the start time the smaller the amount of food or fluid that should be ingested. Liquid nutrition options, such as meal supplements, may be better tolerated than solids.	GORD Vomiting Bloating Side ache/cramp Urge to defecate Diarrhoea, runner's trots

(Continued)

Table 15.1 (Continued)

Dietary and/or other management recommendations	GIS that may be avoided
Consume easy-to-digest, low-fibre, low-fat and low- to moderate-protein meals/snacks prior to exercise and as much as 24 hours leading up to competition.	GORD Vomiting Bloating Side ache/cramp Urge to defecate Diarrhoea, runner's trots Flatulence
Choose carbohydrate solutions with a lower concentration or osmolality along with ingesting sufficient water.	GORD Vomiting Bloating Flatulence Nausea
Start exercise euhydrated and aim to minimise body weight loss within individual GI tolerance. Avoid over-hydrating.	Vomiting Bloating Nausea
Avoid over-nutrition prior to and during exercise by having an individualised and tested nutrition plan based on energy and nutrient demands.	Vomiting Bloating Nausea Flatulence
Gut training: The GI system is adaptable and its capacity to uptake fluid and nutrients can be increased with training. Train with carbohydrate and fluids during exercise to improve absorption and identify individual tolerances. A focused carbohydrate challenge protocol, with increasing amounts, may improve GI tolerance and reduce related symptoms. It is best to seek advice on such a protocol from a qualified sports nutrition practitioner.	Vomiting Bloating Nausea Flatulence Belching Side ache/cramp Diarrhoea, runner's trots
Consume low-fibre or low-residue foods for 1–2 days leading up to the event.	Bloating Flatulence Side ache/cramp Urge to defecate Diarrhoea, runner's trots Nausea Vomiting
Allow time for toilet stops before competition or training.	Urge to defecate
Consume a short-term low-FODMAP diet, i.e., 24 hours before strenuous training or competition. High-FODMAP foods eaten before or during exercise may have a detrimental additive effect on GIS though can be protective to GI integrity.	Osmotic diarrhoea BloatingFlatulence
Some may benefit from cognitive behavioural therapy; see an allied health professional trained in this technique.	Diarrhoea, runner's trots, urgency

(Continued)

Table 15.1 (Continued)

Dietary and/or other management recommendations	GIS that may be avoided
Special situations	
Heat	Heat stress is known to increase GI injury, splanchnic hypoperfusion and hypoxia, which may worsen symptoms. Heat acclimation and external and internal pre-exercise/during-exercise cooling may improve gut health, although to date research is limited and conflicting.
ˢ Caffeine	Caffeine can increase colon motility (movement of food), which could be additive to the mechanical impact of running leading to diarrhoea.
Nitrate	May improve splanchnic perfusion.
Other recommendations: Ingesting sufficient water and nutrients during prolonged exercise, i.e., small and frequent intake of carbohydrate, i.e., if the target is 60 g/h carbohydrate, this may be split into doses of 15–20 g/can help maintain splanchnic blood flow and reduce the risk of gut symptoms. Consumption of solutions with multiple carbohydrate types (glucose, maltodextrin, fructose) may reduce the risk of GIS.	

ᵃ Recommendations are based on limited research and may or may not be dietary triggers for individuals.

Summary

This chapter has provided an overview of the GIS that are common among athletes. Most symptoms are mild to moderate in severity but the smaller percentage that are severe can negatively impact performance and potentially the health of the athlete. Exercise-associated GIS can occur during or after exercise and although the cause is not entirely understood symptoms are primarily related to physiological, mechanical and nutritional factors. Nutrition can play an important role in reducing the frequency and severity of the most reported GIS in sport. An individualised and multi-disciplinary approach needs to be taken in managing the athlete's GIS.

Chapter highlights

- Gastrointestinal disturbances are a common occurrence among athletes, particularly ultra-endurance athletes.
- Severe GIS are likely to compromise training capacity and performance.
- Exercise-induced gastrointestinal syndrome (EIGS) describes the physiological responses that occur due to exercise and may subsequently impair GI integrity and function, leading to GIS and/or acute or chronic health complications.
- The main triggers of GI disturbances in athletes are physiological (circulatory-GI and neuroendocrine-GI pathway), mechanical and nutritional.

- Strenuous exercise, particularly endurance-based exercise, influences both a circulatory-GI and neuroendocrine-GI response.
  - There is a redistribution of blood flow to the muscles and peripheries resulting in hypoperfusion to the splanchnic area.
  - The extent of splanchnic hypoperfusion will influence alterations in GI integrity (i.e., epithelial injury, increased intestinal permeability and subsequent systemic response).
  - In addition, there is an increase in sympathetic drive and secretion of stress hormones influencing GI function, i.e., motility and transit.
- An important interplay between the gut–brain axis influences GIS and, in some athletes, may be the reason symptoms are hard to replicate and only occur in race situations or may be influenced by psychological stress.
- Exercise-associated GI symptoms are multifactorial, requiring an individualised and multidisciplinary approach for successful management.

References

1. Costa RJS, Miall A, Khoo A, et al. Gut-training: the impact of two weeks repetitive gut-challenge during exercise on gastrointestinal status, glucose availability, fuel kinetics, and running performance. *Appl Physiol Nutr Metab*. 2017;42(5):547–557.
2. Costa RJS, Snipe RMJ, Kitic CM. Systematic review: exercise-induced gastrointestinal syndrome—implications for health and intestinal disease. *Aliment Therap Pharmacol*. 2017;46(3):246–265.
3. Costa RJS, Gaskell SK, McCubbin AJ, et al. Exertional-heat stress associated gastrointestinal perturbations- management strategies for athletes preparing for and competing in the 2020 Tokyo Olympic Games. *Temperature*. 2020;7(1):58–88.
4. Rehrer NJ, Smets A, Reynaert H. Effect of exercise on portal vein blood flow in man. *Med Sci Sports Exerc*. 2001;33(9):1533–1537.
5. Rehrer NJ, van Kemenade M, Meester W. Gastrointestinal complaints in relation to dietary intake in triathletes. *Int J Sports Nutr*. 1992;2(1):48–59.
6. Snipe RMJ, Khoo A, Kitic CM. The impact of exertional-heat stress on gastrointestinal integrity, gastrointestinal symptoms, systemic endotoxin and cytokine profile. *Eur J Appl Physiol*. 2018;118(2):389–400.
7. Lis D, Stellingwerff T, Shing CM. Exploring the popularity, experiences, and beliefs surrounding gluten-free diets in noncoeliac athletes. *Int J Sport Nutr Exerc Metab*. 2015;25(1):37–45.
8. Gaskell SK, Rauch CE, Costa RJS. Gastrointestinal assessment and therapeutic intervention for the management of exercise-associated gastrointestinal symptoms: a case series translational and professional practice approach. *Front Physiol*. 2021;12:719142.
9. van Wijck K, Lenaerts K, Van Bijnen AA. Aggravation of exercise-induced intestinal injury by Ibuprofen in athletes. *Med Sci Sport Exerc*. 2012;44(12):2257–2262.

16 Injury management and rehabilitation

*Rebekah Alcock, Greg Shaw, Craig Patch
and Alan J Pearce*

Injuries are an unfortunate reality in both recreational and professional sports. At an elite level, the impact of sporting injuries can be significant, often having physical, psychological, professional, and economic consequences for both the athlete and the organisation that contracts them. Injuries range from minor (i.e. cuts, abrasions), to moderate to severe (i.e. musculoskeletal and connective tissue injuries), including the small number that have life-long implications (i.e. concussion), which can lead to cessation of training and competition or even retirement. During rehabilitation of the athlete following injury, nutrition interventions traditionally focused on controlling adverse effects of energy balance issues. However, contemporary nutrition interventions focus on supporting functional tissue maintenance through periods of disuse or reduced training and supporting athletes' return to training and competition in a timely manner. The following chapter will give an overview of nutrition considerations in the management of injuries.

Learning outcomes

This chapter will:

- explain the influence of adequate nutrition in preventing load-related injuries;
- explain the role of specific nutrients in the management of specific injuries;
- describe the timeline of injury rehabilitation;
- discuss nutrition support for assisting the athlete during the rehabilitation timeline;
- describe emerging nutrition interventions related to injury prevention and rehabilitation;
- outline the role of supplementation in injury prevention, mitigation, and management.

Types of injuries

The types of injuries that occur within a sport are related to the characteristics of that sport. For example, contact sports, including football codes commonly result in contact injuries related to collision and/or sudden directional changes, which lead to injuries to the musculoskeletal and/or connective tissues and the brain. Sports such as boxing commonly result in injuries because of a direct 'hit' or 'blow' to the body, or head, and may result in skin lacerations, fractures, dislocations, or concussions. Athletes participating in endurance sports, such as long-distance running and triathlon, are often faced with injuries such as **tendinopathies** or **bone stress injuries**, which may be attributable to poor load

DOI: 10.4324/9781003321286-18

management and overuse of a specific tissue. This chapter will focus on the most common injuries occurring in sport. These include injuries to the bone (stress fractures), soft tissues (including cartilage, ligaments, tendons, and muscle) and 'other' injuries (including injuries to the head and skin). It should be noted that injuries rarely occur in isolation and often involve multiple components of the body.

Tendinopathies

Diseases of the tendons, which may arise from a range of internal and external factors.

Bone stress injuries

An injury that occurs to the bone because of inadequate energy intake to meet energy requirements and/or because of repeated or prolonged force to the bone.

Bone injuries

The term 'fracture' encompasses any injury in which a bone is cracked or broken, and fractures are the most common type of sports injury requiring hospitalisation. Fractures can occur as an acute injury in almost any sport—due to a sudden impact such as contact with another person, obstacle, or a fall—or because of repeated stress to the bone, as is the case for stress fractures. While stress fractures tend to occur over time, they are common in sports where loading can change quickly, such as watercraft sports (rowing, kayaking), running, gymnastics, ballet, basketball, and volleyball. While it is important to focus on the adequacy of key nutrients (i.e. calcium, vitamin D, and vitamin K) that may assist with suitable bone remodelling (healing), preventing nutrient deficiencies and ensuring adequate energy intake (see Chapter 7 for information about low energy availability and relative energy deficiency in sport) is an important consideration for the prevention of bone injuries.

Soft-tissue injuries

Soft-tissue injuries refer to injuries to the musculoskeletal and connective tissues, whether acutely, such as a sprain/strain or tear, or chronically, as in the case of tendinopathies. Soft-tissue injuries are the second most common type of injury requiring hospitalisation. Sports characterised by high-speed movements with or without a quick change of direction, which places significant strain on tissues incapable of handling the load, have a high incidence of soft-tissue injuries resulting from tears, ruptures, and strains. The duration of recovery can range from days to a year, depending on the severity of the injury. However, in sports where athletes increase load rapidly over days or weeks, more chronic conditions like tendinopathies may develop. Specifically, the pain and dysfunction resulting from tendinopathy can significantly interfere with the capacity to train and compete. Tendinopathies are complicated and do not have a common **pathology**, so the treatment of tendinopathies will often be specific to the tendon and the athlete's injury history.

Consequences of soft-tissue injuries can range from reduced load for a period of a few days to inability to complete certain types of exercise for the rest of an athlete's life.

Pathology

A field in medicine which studies the causes of diseases.

Other injuries

Head injuries are frequently reported in contact sports. Symptoms can be as minor as short periods (minutes) of memory loss, to concussion and to further long-term impairment in brain function. Recently, this long-term impairment in brain function has been linked to multiple acute head injuries and **sub-concussive** impacts. Researchers are investigating numerous interventions, including the influence specific nutrients can have on helping the brain regenerate or cope with these injuries. Other injuries, such as skin lacerations (deep cuts) are also common in sport and present significant concern in sports where dietary adequacy may influence wound healing or in events where treatment options may be limited, such as multi-day ultra-endurance running events.

Sub-concussive

A hit to the head that does not produce signs or symptoms of concussion but is hypothesised to have long-term adverse effects.

Special interest area: Concussion

Concussion is a type of mild traumatic brain injury (mTBI) caused by a direct impact to the brain or an indirect impact where the force is transmitted to the brain resulting in temporary disturbance of cognitive functions, such as memory loss, confusion, loss in concentration, and transient amnesia. Other signs include blurred/double vision, bothered by light or noise, irritability/aggression, feeling sluggish, hazy, foggy or groggy, nausea and vomiting, and headache or 'pressure' in the head. Motor signs include loss in equilibrium (balance) problems, slurred speech or ataxia (poor motor control resulting in clumsy movement). Less obvious are mood changes, and some cases have presented with sadness or short-term changes in personality. While loss of consciousness is a clear sign of concussion, loss of consciousness only occurs in about 15–20% of cases. Of note, these signs and symptoms are heterogeneous between individuals. However, due to the nature of signs and symptoms presented that confound with other conditions, a diagnosis of concussion must occur following an observation of physical impact to exclude other potential mechanisms (such as alcohol or drug use).

A concussion produces a short-term physiological cascade contributing to the collection of signs and symptoms. Imbalances between cellular ions (Na^+, K^+, and Ca^{2+}) and an overproduction of free radicals lead to alteration in blood flow in the brain. This is referred to as an 'energy crisis' in the brain, which is the resultant increased demand for energy. This bioenergetic demand versus supply discord results in hypermetabolic events such as hyperglycemia and protein catabolism, and as a consequence, results in an anaerobic cellular state. The intracellular flux of ions (Ca^{2+}) contributes to mitochondrial dysfunction, oxidative stress, neuroinflammation, cellular damage, and, in some cases, apoptosis. Currently, the treatment for concussion is physical and cognitive rest until the acute signs and symptoms dissipate, followed by active rehabilitation involving light but graduated aerobic exercise within symptom thresholds. Nutritional interventions are being trialled, particularly high-dose long-chain omega-3 fatty acids; however, while showing promise, it is not yet accepted in consensus statements or guidelines regarding concussion. Recovery appears to be individual, but emerging evidence suggests that resolution of the symptoms may not indicate physiological recovery,[1] and full recovery may take up to eight weeks.[2,3]

Repetitive sub-concussive impacts, where individuals engaged in activities such as combat/contact sports, or active military engagement, have been linked to progressive degenerative diseases including Alzheimer's disease, motor neurone disease, Parkinson's disease and chronic traumatic encephalopathy or CTE. Usually, symptoms begin a number of years or even decades after the last brain trauma or end of active athletic involvement. Symptoms described include memory loss, confusion, impulsivity, judgment impairment, aggression, mood disorders (depression and/or anxiety), suicidality, parkinsonism, and dementia. However, to date, CTE can only be diagnosed post-mortem.

Docosahexaenoic acid

A long-chain omega-3 fatty acid with 22 carbons and six double bonds, found in fatty fish and breast milk.

Although nutrition interventions for mTBI/concussion are still being explored, a recent systematic review reported positive recovery outcomes for the omega-3 polyunsaturated fatty acids (PUFA), docosahexaenoic acid (DHA) and eicosapentaenoic acid (EPA), vitamin D, magnesium oxide, N-acetyl cysteine (NAC), creatine, and nootropic citicoline.[4]

Animal studies have shown efficacy in high dose (equivalent dosage of 4–10 g/day) omega-3 PUFA post-mTBI in rodents, with a systematic review reporting that high-dose omega-3 PUFA showed improvements across a range of neurological and cognitive performance tests and in molecular and inflammatory markers in animal models.[5] Human trials that have been completed to date show mixed results, which may be due to a dose–response relationship. Studies in vitamin D and magnesium oxide are suggesting positive results, but currently, only one study has been completed in both of these.[6,7]

There is also a growing interest in creatine for the management of concussion/mTBI.[8] While pre-clinical models suggest potential benefits, the evidence to date is limited to a pilot study using an open-label randomised design.[9] Supplementation of creatine following severe TBI (0.4 g/kg/day in an oral suspension) was associated with decreased duration of post-traumatic amnesia, intubation, and hospital stay. They also found improvements in cognition, mood, and social interaction within three months and, continued improvement towards self-care at six months compared to control. Limited evidence has also shown the benefits of creatine supplementation prophylactically in animal models.

While there appears to be promise with some nutritional interventions post-concussion/ mTBI, due to the diversity between study methodologies, prescription doses, and the limited number of studies conducted in humans, definitive recommendations are not yet possible.

Injury prevention

While nutrition support plays a vital role in injury rehabilitation, adequate nutrition plays a critical role in the prevention of injuries. Significant acute changes in training load can lead to a range of injuries. It is not known whether the primary issue is the increase in load or the inability of athletes to change their dietary intake to meet the requirements of the increased load. An International Olympic Committee (IOC) working group has suggested that the inability to match energy intake to account for variations in the energy cost of exercise contributes to injury risk.[10] It is therefore essential that energy intake rises and falls in tight response to training load (see Chapter 10). Adequate intake of protein, carbohydrate, and calcium, timed closely to heavy training, has been shown to positively influence the remodelling process, reducing the breakdown of tissues such as bone that occurs after heavy training sessions. Nutrition recommendations for athletes undertaking increased load should focus on adequate energy availability combined with purposeful nutrient availability, to aid in the prevention of load-related injuries.

Phases of nutrition interventions for injuries

Acute injury begins with the process of acute inflammation, and management begins with a potential period of immobilisation and a varying period of rehabilitation depending on the injury before returning to training and subsequently competition. There are four stages in the rehabilitation program (immobilisation, return to train, train to play, and the final is when the athlete returns to competition) which are outlined in Table 16.1. Nutrition plays a critical role in each phase of this injury rehabilitation process, as outlined below. Although it is tempting to suggest nutrition will have a significant impact on injury rehabilitation, its key role is in supporting the rehabilitation program. Nutrition will boost the repair process, but the interventions will only be as successful as the program they are designed to support; thus, a multidisciplinary approach to support the rehabilitation of the injured athlete is essential.

Periods of injury rehabilitation can have athletes exposed to an environment which increases their risk of developing disordered eating behaviours, over time potentially escalating to more severe eating disorder symptoms and behaviours (refer to Chapter 7 for more information on eating disorders). Practitioners need to be acutely aware of this risk and ensure any nutrition interventions are focused on the maintenance of functional mass and not solely focused on minimising the accumulation of adipose tissue. If immobilisation is expected for extended periods (>5 days) athletes are advised to implement nutrition strategies that help offset muscle wasting associated with disuse.

Nutrition to support collagen synthesis

Recently, novel nutrition interventions such as gelatin, hydrolysed collagen, or collagen-specific peptide formulations, have been suggested to improve the regeneration of connective tissue post-exercise and during a period of injury rehabilitation.[11-13] The exact

Table 16.1 Overview of rehabilitation and nutrition planning for the injured athlete

Phases	First phase: Immobilisation Disuse 1 day to 12 weeks	Second phase: Return to train 3 days to 10 weeks	Third Phase Train to play: 2–10 weeks	Return to Competition Have completed rehabilitation program and are ready to compete
Physical	Immobilization reduces energy expenditure. Athletes often reduce energy intake, however, energy requirements may be increased due to tissue repair and remodelling. Muscle atrophy needs to be minimised.	Retrain & rebuild muscle and connective tissue. Optimise physique. May include full-load resistance training and aerobic training using uninjured muscles and limbs.	Enhance adaptation to training	Train for competition intensity
Fitness	Minimise loss of aerobic fitness	Re-develop aerobic fitness	Retrain aerobic/anaerobic capacity	Injured limbs or muscles should be returned to similar, if not enhanced, muscle size and function prior to return to competition and should not require ongoing nutritional support.
Nutrition	Avoid severe energy restrictions leading to poor nutrient availability (especially protein). **Energy availability:** 146–188 kJ/kg **CHO intake:** lower end of the guidelines (~3 g/kg BM/day) **Protein intake:** >2 g/kg BM/day HBV protein sources high in leucine (>3 g) evenly distributed every 2–3 hrs in meals and snacks **Supplements:** Fish oils: 4 g/day	**Energy availability:** 188 kJ/kg **CHO intakes:** matched to training requirements on a day-to-day basis **Protein intake:** 1.4–2 g/kg BM/day HBV protein sources high in leucine (>3 g) (every 2–3 hrs) CHO: to meet training requirement 3–8 g/kg BM Supplements: creatine (load 20 g/day × 5 days, then 5 g/day for return to train) **Supplements:** Creatine, caffeine, beta-alanine	**Energy availability:** 146–188 kJ/kg FFM **Protein:** 1.8–2.4 g/kg BM/day CHO: vary **CHO intakes:**Matched to training requirementsavailability Supplements: to increase work completed/physiological adaptation include creatine, beta-alanine, nitrates, and caffeine	As per traditional sports nutrition guidelines for healthy athletes

Notes: BM: body mass, HBV: high biological value, CHO: carbohydrate.

mechanism by which these improve collagen remodelling remains unclear. However, it has been suggested that the availability and integration of non-essential amino acids predominant in collagen protein, including glycine, proline, and lysine may improve the synthesis and integration of new collagen fibrils into the injured tissue. Recently, it has been shown that food and supplemental sources of collagen result in improved amino acid availability.[14] This may lead to increased incorporation of collagen into the muscle tissue; however, this has only been seen after exercise.[15,16] This illustrates that increased amino acid availability does not independently increase the collagen protein synthetic response and that supplementation needs to be specifically timed and targeted to support collagen-containing tissue remodelling in relation to exercise.

Nutrition for chronic inflammation

While acute inflammation is a necessary and natural process of the body's immune system in response to initial tissue injury, chronic inflammation can lead to persistent pain and has the potential to contribute to long-term damage within the tissue. Dietary sources of anti-inflammatory nutrients are highly effective at maintaining inflammatory processes. Increasing the intake of omega-3 fatty acids through the intake of fish oil supplements or oily fish is recommended. There is also an increasing focus on the bioactive components of plant-based foods that may assist in reducing inflammation, such as **polyphenols**. Polyphenols of interest include epigallocatechin (EGCG) (found in green tea), curcumin (found in turmeric), and rutin (found in a wide variety of plants, including apples and citrus fruits). While research is continuing to develop on the bioactive components of food, athletes may be able to help manage inflammation by consuming a diet rich in plant-based foods.

Although whole foods provide an opportunity for the athlete to meet multiple goals simultaneously and should always be the first choice, supplements may be required in circumstances where dietary intake is inadequate, and/or a therapeutic dose is necessitated. However, the source and quality of any supplement should be carefully considered by athletes. Additionally, the risk of contamination with the use of supplements should always be prioritised by athletes governed by the WADA (World Anti-Doping Authority) code (refer to Chapter 12).

Polyphenols

A large group of naturally occurring bioactives found in plants, and provide protection against chronic diseases.

Summary

This chapter has outlined how strategic and targeted nutrient and energy intake has the potential to support the rehabilitation process of the injured athlete for a range of injuries. This is achieved by minimising wasting and supporting the rehabilitation of essential tissue during disuse. Once this has been achieved the fast-tracking of redevelopment, and training of injured tissue back to pre-injury levels can be achieved by the addition of timely nutrients and optimised energy availability. Recently, the role that nutrition can play in the management of concussion and mTBI in sporting populations is an area nutrition professionals should continue to stay abreast of. Furthermore, there is a significant role that nutrition professionals can play in reducing the risk of ongoing health implications post injury and preventing the occurrence of future injuries.

Chapter highlights

- Injuries are a significant economic cost, both locally, and internationally, and may result in long-term health implications for athletes, post their athletic careers.
- Injuries range from moderate to severe and are related to the characteristics of the sport.
- There are emerging nutrition-focused interventions that may reduce the impact of injuries, result in improved rehabilitation periods, and mitigate ongoing risk.
- It is important to consider the different phases of the injury/rehabilitation process, from prevention through to 'return to play', when considering nutrition interventions.
- It is important to achieve a balance between consuming adequate energy to support the body in the healing and regeneration process and preventing unwanted changes in body composition.
- Practitioners need to be cautious to focus on supporting the body's capacity to heal, and maintaining functional body mass, rather than focusing on body composition as this may contribute to disordered eating risk.
- The purposeful timing of macro- and micronutrients can significantly influence the adaptations achieved during the rehabilitation process.
- Supplements are warranted in specific circumstances, such as when a therapeutic dose is necessitated; however, meeting nutrient goals should be achieved through the intake of whole foods where possible.

References

1. Pearce AJ, Hoy K, Rogers MA, et al. Acute motor, neurocognitive and neurophysiological change following concussion injury in Australian amateur football. A prospective multimodal investigation. *J Sci Med Sport*. 2015;18:500–6.
2. Broglio SP, McAllister T, Katz BP, et al. The natural history of sport-related concussion in collegiate athletes: findings from the NCAA-DoD CARE Consortium. *Sports Med*. 2022;52(2): 403–15.
3. Kara S, Crosswell H, Forch K, et al. Less than half of patients recover within 2 weeks of injury after a sports-related mild traumatic brain injury: a 2-year prospective study. *Clin J Sport Med*. 2020;30(2):96–101.
4. Finnegan E, Daly E, Pearce AJ, et al. Nutritional interventions to support acute mTBI recovery. *Front Nutr*. 2022;9:977728.
5. Patch C, Hill-Yardin E, Lewis M, et al. The more, the better: high dose Omega-3 fatty acids improve behavioural and molecular outcomes in preclinical models in mild brain injury. *Curr Neurol Neurosci Rep*. 2021;21:45.
6. Lee JM, Jeong SW, Kim MY, et al. The effect of vitamin D supplementation in patients with acute traumatic brain injury. *World Neurosurg*. 2019;126:e1421–e6.
7. Standiford L, O'Daniel M, Hysell M, et al. A randomized cohort study of the efficacy of PO magnesium in the treatment of acute concussions in adolescents. *Am J Emerg Med*. 2021;44: 419–22.
8. Forbes SC, Cordingley DM, Cornish SM, et al. Effects of creatine supplementation on brain function and health. *Nutrients*. 2022;14(5).

9. Sakellaris G, Kotsiou M, Tamiolaki M, et al. Prevention of complications related to traumatic brain injury in children and adolescents with creatine administration: an open label randomized pilot study. *J Trauma Acute Care Surg.* 2006;61(2):322–9.

10. Mountjoy M, Ackerman K, Bailey D, et al. The 2023 International Olympic Committee's (IOC) consensus statement on Relative Energy Deficiency in Sports (REDs). *Br J Sports Med.* 2023. In press.

11. Khatri M, Naughton RJ, Clifford T, et al. The effects of collagen peptide supplementation on body composition, collagen synthesis, and recovery from joint injury and exercise: a systematic review. *Amino Acids.* 2021;53(10):1493–506.

12. Shaw G, Serpell B, Baar K. Rehabilitation and nutrition protocols for optimising return to play from traditional ACL reconstruction in elite rugby union players: a case study. *J Sports Sci.* 2019;37(15):1794–803.

13. Tack C, Shorthouse F, Kass L. The physiological mechanisms of effect of vitamins and amino acids on tendon and muscle healing: a systematic review. *Int J Sport Nutr Exerc Metab.* 2018; 28(3):294–311.

14. Alcock RD, Shaw GC, Tee N, et al. Plasma amino acid concentrations after the ingestion of dairy and collagen proteins, in healthy active males. *Front Nutr.* 2019;6:163.

15. Holwerda AM, Trommelen J, Kouw IWK, et al. Exercise plus presleep protein ingestion increases overnight muscle connective tissue protein synthesis rates in healthy older men. *Int J Sport Nutr Exerc Metab.* 2021;31(3):217–26.

16. Trommelen J, Holwerda AM, Senden JM, et al. Casein ingestion does not increase muscle connective tissue protein synthesis rates. *Med Sci Sports Exerc.* 2020;52(9):1983–91.

Part III

Applied sports nutrition

17 Endurance athletes

Gregory Cox

Endurance sport encompasses a variety of activities (running, swimming, cycling, paddling), sometimes in combination (adventure racing, triathlon), across a range of distances and intensities (5-km ocean swim, 10-km run, ironman triathlon, or multi-day stage cycling race). Other activities, while not considered endurance sports as the actual competition lasts 3–6 minutes (e.g., sprint canoe, rowing, middle-distance running), routinely incorporate endurance training sessions. Endurance sport athletes have unique requirements to maximise favourable responses to training, assist recovery, maintain health and well-being, and facilitate daily training and competition performance. Given the daily complexity of endurance training and the interaction with nutrition, alongside the unique nutrition strategies for endurance competition, purposeful dietary planning is required. Understanding the sport culture, individual athletes' food preferences and beliefs, dynamics of weekly training, environmental conditions, and the logistics for nutrition support when racing will define the effectiveness of nutrition support to endurance sport athletes. This chapter will explore daily training needs of endurance sport athletes and outline various nutrition considerations for endurance competition.

Learning outcomes

This chapter will:

- outline the nutrition challenges faced by endurance athletes in daily training;
- describe and subsequently interpret daily energy and carbohydrate requirements for endurance athletes;
- describe an athlete's daily food and fluid intake requirements and identify key areas to support daily training performance, recovery, and the favoured metabolic adaptations to training;
- identify important considerations for racing and the need to customise nutrition support across the wide variety of endurance events;
- explain how to manipulate fluid intake advice according to an athlete's likely requirements.

Nutrition principles for daily training

Endurance athletes (recreational and elite) commit considerable effort, time, and finances to training and racing. Yet few invest in the services of experienced, qualified sports

DOI: 10.4324/9781003321286-20

nutrition practitioners to assist in individualising their daily food and fluid intakes or in developing a race nutrition plan. Rather, endurance athletes rely heavily on information from other athletes, online forums, sport-specific magazines, supplement company websites, and coaches. A common mistake for recreational endurance athletes is to model their daily and/or race nutrition choices on an elite athlete. Social media is commonly used by endurance athletes to inform the broader community about their food and fluid preferences. Daily training, physiology, and annual race calendars vary considerably between endurance athletes and ultimately dictate daily nutritional needs and race-day nutrition tactics. Given the delicate balance involved in maintaining health and well-being while optimising daily training performance and recovery, expert nutrition advice should be sought by endurance athletes.

Elite and recreational endurance athletes alike are time-poor. Elite endurance athletes can train up to five sessions daily while juggling sponsor commitments, travel, and performance support appointments. Recreational endurance athletes, while not training at the same level, are required to balance lifestyle commitments such as work, study, and family in between daily workouts. Careful planning of daily meals and snacks that provide nutritious options aligned with the training goals, while offering convenience and taste is a high priority for endurance athletes. Further, consideration of the annual training plan is required, as the emphasis changes throughout the year (see Chapter 10).

Matching daily energy needs

Dietary surveys of endurance athletes commonly report dietary intakes that fall below recommendations for energy (kilojoules or calories), carbohydrate, and iron. This mismatch of daily energy intake with the daily energy requirements for training is likely due to a combination of issues. Firstly, there is no strong biological drive to match energy intake to activity-induced energy expenditure. Hunger is often suppressed in endurance athletes following intense training, particularly in activities such as running which can cause gastrointestinal (GI) discomfort and upset. Secondly, given the perceived importance of maintaining a light and lean physique to optimise endurance performance, many endurance athletes adopt an overly restrictive approach with their food and fluid choices in an attempt to minimise body fat levels and/or body mass. Finally, endurance athletes may be unaware of the energy expended during training or may not be sufficiently organised to ensure appropriate foods and fluids are available on heavy training days, creating a practical barrier to meeting their daily energy needs. Interestingly, when athletes are well supported and organized – such as cyclists contesting the Tour de France – research has demonstrated that they are able to match energy intake with daily energy expenditure even on the most strenuous of cycling stages.[1]

Given daily fluctuations in training, endurance athletes should be educated so that they possess the necessary food knowledge and skills to customise daily food and fluid intakes to manipulate daily energy, and subsequently nutrient intakes. Athletes need to be well organised to include additional extras in the way of training food and fluids, between-meal snacks, and/or main meal extras on heavy training days to increase their daily energy intake. Additional foods and fluids included throughout the day should be determined by the additional energy cost of training, the primary goal of individual training sessions, the time for recovery between training and individual food and fluid tolerance, as well as logistics. Conversely, on rest days or lighter training days when daily energy requirements are reduced, food and fluid intake should be adjusted accordingly.

An important consideration when supporting elite endurance athletes is their increased ability to burn energy (fuel) during training and competition. Elite endurance athletes work at higher absolute intensities, often for longer durations than their less-trained counterparts, so despite being accustomed to the exercise, elite athletes burn more fuel. While elite athletes improve their 'economy' of movement in response to high volume (intensity, duration, and frequency) of training, their daily exercise energy expenditure is increased. Further, as athletes build fitness over a training year, daily energy expenditure increases, namely due to an increase in exercise energy expenditure.[2] This is true for elite and recreational athletes, alike. Endurance athletes, their coaches, and performance support staff should be vigilant to ensure daily food and fluid intake is aligned with daily training, particularly on days when athletes are undertaking strenuous, extended training sessions.

Endurance athletes, male and female, are at increased risk of 'problematic' low energy availability.[3] This is not surprising, given the high daily training loads common to many endurance training programs coupled with an emphasis on maintaining light and lean physiques. Low energy availability occurs with a reduction in energy intake and/or an increased exercise load, leading to the disruption of hormonal and metabolic systems. Low energy availability is central to **relative energy deficiency in sport (REDs)**, which affects numerous aspects of health and performance, including metabolic rate, menstrual function, bone health, immunity, protein synthesis, and cardiovascular and psychological health.

Relative energy deficiency in sport

Relative energy deficiency in sport, a syndrome of impaired physiological function caused by 'problematic' low energy availability.

Disordered eating and eating disorders

Athletes are more likely to present with disordered eating (DE) than a clinical eating disorder (ED). DE and ED involve eating behaviours that are not healthy and may include skipping meals, compulsive or binge eating, fasting, active and passive dehydration, compulsive or excessive exercise, and use of laxatives, diuretics, vomiting, and diet pills.[4]

Disordered eating is common in cases of low energy availability; however, mismanaged attempts to quickly reduce body mass or fat mass or acute increases in daily training loads may result in low energy availability. Performance support staff and coaches should be vigilant of DE and communicate regularly to discuss the health and well-being of the athletes in their care. Communication around the annual plan and weekly training load is central and allows the sports nutrition professional to adjust messaging around daily fuel requirements. The inclusion of assessment tools such as resting energy expenditure, dietary intake, exercise energy expenditure, hormone profiling, body composition, and bone health are useful tools in managing endurance athletes to better understand their health and well-being. The reader is directed to the Australian Institute of Sport (AIS) and

National Eating Disorders Collaboration position statement on disordered eating in high-performance sport.[4]

Exercise energy expenditure

The long-term training and competition plan (i.e., Olympic Cycle) clarifies key nutritional strategies that align with the physical development of an endurance athlete; the annual training plan provides insights into the nutrition logistics and focus throughout the year (i.e., travel, heat, and altitude exposures); whereas the weekly training plan and individual training session metrics provide the specifics of daily nutritional needs and challenges. Sports nutrition professionals should work closely with athletes, coaches, and sports physiologists to understand daily exercise energy expenditure (EEE). The frequency, intensity, time (or duration), and type of training will guide adjustments to daily nutrition strategies to ensure athletes manipulate daily energy intake to accommodate changes in EEE. Using available training information via training platforms (i.e., Training Peaks, Strava) for estimates of EEE or manually calculating (using Metabolic Equivalents (METs) or indirect calorimetry) EEE provides important information to understanding dietary adjustments required to assist athletes in meeting daily energy requirements.

Carbohydrate intake guidelines for daily training

For endurance athletes training strenuously, daily carbohydrate demands can exceed the body's capacity to store carbohydrate. Thus, the availability of carbohydrate as fuel to support training performance and assist recovery is crucial. During intense sustained or intermittent exercise typical of endurance events or high-intensity endurance training sessions, carbohydrate is the primary fuel to support exercise performance. Carbohydrate intake should be modified in response to fluctuations in daily training load. Further, the intake of additional carbohydrate should be strategically coordinated around training to optimise training performance, facilitate recovery, and enhance the adaptation to training.

Current carbohydrate intake guidelines should be carefully interpreted which requires sports nutrition practitioners to understand daily training patterns to customise carbohydrate intake recommendations for individual athletes on a daily basis – see Table 17.1. No longer are carbohydrate guidelines provided generically to athletes based on body size or type of sport. In assessing daily carbohydrate needs when managing endurance athletes, practitioners should consider:

- daily training intensity, frequency, and duration;
- body weight and body composition of the athlete;
- body composition adjustments, whether it be weight loss, lean body mass gain, or additional requirements associated with growth;
- subjective feedback from the athlete (or coach) relating to training performance and recovery;
- sex;
- training state and training age;
- changes in the training environment, such as altitude and heat.

Table 17.1 Daily carbohydrate intake recommendations for endurance athletes

	Situation	Carbohydrate targets	Comments on type and timing of carbohydrate intake
Daily carbohydrate needs to support training and recovery: These general recommendations should be fine-tuned with individual consideration of total energy needs, body composition, daily training loads, and feedback from training performance.			
Light	Low-intensity or skill-based activities	3–5 g/kg/d	Timing of carbohydrate intake around training should support the primary goal for each session. Convenience, athlete tolerance, individual preferences, and logistics are important considerations. Nutrient-rich carbohydrate food/fluids assist the athlete in meeting overall nutrition goals and should be prioritised.
Moderate	Moderate exercise program (i.e., ~1 hr per day)	5–7 g/kg/d	
High	Endurance program (i.e., 1–3 hr/d moderate- to high-intensity exercise)	6–10 g/kg/d	Timely intake of a carbohydrate-containing food/fluid immediately after training should align with overall nutrition goals and consider the timing of the next training session and scheduled meal.
Very high	Extreme commitment (i.e., >4–5 hr/d moderate- to high-intensity exercise	8–12 g/kg/d	
Acute fuelling strategies: These guidelines promote high carbohydrate availability to support optimal performance in endurance competitions or key training sessions. Event demands and logistics should be carefully considered when interpreting these guidelines.			
General fuelling up	Endurance events <90 min	5–10 g/kg/d	Athletes may choose compact carbohydrate-rich sources that are low in fibre/residue and easily consumed to ensure that fuel targets are met while avoiding issues relating to GI discomfort.
Carbohydrate loading	Endurance events >90 min	36–48 h of 8–12 g/kg/d	
Pre-event fuelling	Before exercise	1–4 g/kg consumed 1–4 hr before exercise	Timing, amount, and type of carbohydrate food and drinks should be chosen to suit the practical needs of the event and individual preferences/experiences of the athlete. Choices high in fat/protein/fibre may need to be avoided to reduce the risk of GI issues. Low glycaemic index choices may provide a more sustained source of fuel for situations where carbohydrate cannot be consumed during exercise, although being familiar with these foods is important. Liquid-carbohydrate-containing options provide a convenient option, particularly for athletes unable to tolerate foods due to 'pre-race nerves'.

Source: Modified from Burke et al.[5]

Box 17.1   Case study: 25-year-old elite female triathlete

Consider a 25-year-old elite female triathlete. As background, while growing up swimming, she found a love for running in her late teenage years before transitioning to triathlon 4 years ago. She has always strived for excellence at school and sport and applies healthy diet principles to her everyday food and fluid intake. She is currently injury-free, although she suffered a bone stress injury shortly after transitioning from running into triathlon. She has a regular menstrual cycle, although, at a similar time last year, her menstrual cycle was absent for three months.

She is conscious of her appearance and is currently 55 kg and 168 cm and weight-stable. She is in the competitive phase of the year – so she is fit and capable of undertaking sustained, high-intensity training.

Questioning begins with her overall training week, then focuses in on a key training day which includes two key sessions:

7:30 am to 9:00 am – 4.2 km swim (10 × 200 m efforts ~ 30 min); remaining ~ 50 min, moderate intensity

3:30 pm to 5:00 pm – 16 km run (8 × 1 km efforts @ 3:30 min/km ~ 28 min); remaining ~ 60 min, light intensity

She has been provided nutrition support throughout her career and has good nutrition knowledge; however, the coach is concerned she is reluctant to 'eat beyond athlete normal' to meet the daily demands of training.

Elite triathletes need to be well organised to meet daily energy, carbohydrate, and nutrient needs to maintain training performance, health, and well-being. Timing appropriate snacks around training and including nutritious foods at meals that provide antioxidants in addition to carbohydrate, protein, and healthy fats will assist training performance and recovery.

1. The first step, is to estimate her daily energy expenditure. It's time-consuming to do this for each day of the week, so focusing on a key performance day is a time-efficient strategy. Use an energy prediction equation to calculate her resting energy expenditure REE and add an activity factor (1.3 – light) to account for daily living, exclusive of exercise (training):

Harris Benedict Equation (Women):

$$REE = 2741 + \left(40.0 \times \text{weight}\right) + \left(7.7 \times \text{height}\right) - \left(19.6 \times \text{age}\right)$$
$$= 5745 \text{ kJ/day or } 1375 \text{ kcal/day}$$
$$= 5745 \times 1.3$$
$$= \sim 7470 \text{ kJ/day or } 1785 \text{ kcal/day}$$

During hours when exercise is performed (in this case, 3 hours), the energy expenditure is removed as exercise energy expenditure (EEE), which includes the resting energy expenditure, will be added.

Adjusted BEE $= 7470 - \left(\left(7465/24 \right) \times 3 \right)$

$= 6535$ kJ/day or 1565 kcal/day

2. She doesn't have a Garmin or similar device that estimates EEE, so an estimate for both sessions can be calculated using Metabolic Equivalents (MET – see https://sites.google.com/site/compendiumofphysicalactivities/home). The following table provides an example calculation of EEE using MET calculations for the two training sessions.

Total energy expenditure = Adjusted BEE + EEE

$= 6535 + 6935 = 13470$ kJ/day or 3220 kcal/day

Exercise Energy Expenditure (EEE) calculations using Metabolic Equivalents (METS)	
Swim (kcal/min): 0.0175 × **MET** × weight (kg)	**Run (kcal/min):** 0.0175 × **MET** × weight (kg)
High-intensity Efforts = 0.0175 × **9.8** × 57 = 9.78 kcal/min	High-intensity Efforts = 0.0175 × **16.0** × 57 = 15.96 kcal/min
Lower intensity swimming = 0.0175 × **5.8** × 57 = 5.79 kcal/min	Lower intensity running = 0.0175 × **10.5** × 57 = 10.47 kcal/min
Swim: 9.78 × 30 min = ~293 kcal 5.79 × 50 min = ~290 kcal ~ 583 kcal or (2440 kJ)	**Run:** 15.96 × 28 min = ~447 kcal 10.47 × 60 min = ~628 kcal ~ 1075 kcal or (4495 kJ)
Exercise Energy Expenditure ~ 1660 kcal or 6935 kJ	

3. A dietary recall specific to the day of training, reveals the following dietary intake – see Initial Dietary Recall in the table below.

When taking a dietary recall specific to a day of training, it's important to establish the athlete's typical dietary intake for a rest or non-exercise day and then understand the foods/fluids they have strategically added to accommodate for the additional training. In this case, the athlete identifies that the only additions to support training are the inclusion of a pre-training snack and half-strength sports drink during morning training.

Estimated daily energy intake is 2145 kcal (8975 kJ) and carbohydrate intake is 237 g/day or when expressed relative to body weight, 4.3 g/kg/day. Estimated energy and carbohydrate intakes fall below estimated values for energy intake and recommended intakes for carbohydrate (6–10 g/kg/d when undertaking an endurance program (see Table 17.1).

Schedule	Initial Dietary Recall	Energy intake kcal (kJ)	CHO (g)
Pre-training 5:30 am	1 × slice of sourdough toast with nut butter	155 (645)	**16**
Quality swim 6:00 am	Half strength sports drink – ~ 400 ml @ 3% carbohydrate	50 (205)	**12**
Immediately post-swim			
Breakfast 8:00 am	1 cup of mixed flake cereal + banana (sliced), blueberries + ¾ cup of milk	440 (1840)	**77**
Mid-morning snack 10:30 am	Sliced apple with nut butter	170 (710)	**22**
Lunch 12:30 pm	Flour tortilla wrap with hummus sliced leg ham and fetta cheese and salad	405 (1700)	**38**
Pre-training snack 2:00 pm to 2:30 pm			
Post-training snack 5:00 pm	Apple	95 (400)	**20**
Dinner 7:00 pm	Salmon Steak – medium fillet (150 g); medium sweet potato & beetroot – baked, olive oil spray; steamed vegetables; drizzle of garlic aioli- Following Dinner:2 squares of 78% dark chocolate	830 (3475)	**52**
Daily energy intake		**2145 (8975)**	**237**

4. In a planned progression of changes to her dietary intake over 2–3 dietary consultations with a sports nutrition professional, daily energy and carbohydrate intakes are increased to 3250 (13580 kJ) and 420 g, respectively (see Adjusted Dietary Intake in the table below). The overall increase in energy intake aligns closely with estimated energy expenditure; and carbohydrate intake (7.6 g/kg/day) relative to body weight falls within current recommendations for an endurance program.

Suggested dietary modifications:

a) The addition of honey to pre-training snack and switching to full strength sports drink throughout the performance component of the morning swim session will promote high carbohydrate availability to assist with high-intensity swimming efforts.

b) A fruit smoothie immediately post-training is high in energy and carbohydrate to promote rapid glycogen repletion. Further, it's a nutrient-rich choice, providing a timely intake of protein post-exercise.

c) Mid-morning snack and lunch include added compact, carbohydrate-rich options, that can be easily tailored into the snack or meal.

d) A pre-training snack is introduced for the afternoon session, again to promote high carbohydrate availability for a performance training session.

e) Additional nutrient-rich carbohydrate foods are added to dinner, to further consolidate daily energy intake to match requirements on a high-volume training day.

5. The sports professional should continue to work closely with the athlete, coach, and other support team members to fine-tune daily dietary intake and modify it according to changes in daily training loads throughout the week and the remainder of the year. Sports nutrition advice is not static and should be modified alongside the annual training plan. This is particularly important for endurance athletes as daily training varies considerably throughout the year.

Dietary Recall and food and fluid adjustments to align dietary intake with daily training.

Schedule	Initial Dietary Recall	Energy intake kcal (kJ)	CHO (g)	Adjusted Dietary Intake	Energy intake kcal (kJ)	CHO (g)
Pre-training 5:30 am	1 × slice of sourdough toast with nut butter	155 (645)	16	ADD honey	175 (740)	22
Quality swim 6:00 am	Half strength sports drink – ~400 ml @ 3% carbohydrate	50 (205)	12	CHANGE to full-strength sports drink – ~400 ml @ 6% carbohydrate	100 (410)	25
Immediately post-swim				ADD banana and honey smoothie with yoghurt immediately post-swim	325 (1370)	55
Breakfast 8:00 am	1 cup of mixed flake cereal + banana (sliced), blueberries + ¾ cup of milk	440 (1840)	77		440 (1840)	77
Mid-morning snack 10:30 am	Sliced apple with nut butter	170 (710)	22	ADD tub berry yoghurt	320 (1330)	46
Lunch 12:30 pm	Flour tortilla wrap with hummus sliced leg ham and fetta cheese and salad	405 (1700)	38	ADD wrap (double wrap)	620 (2580)	70
Pre-training snack 2:00 pm to 2:30 pm				ADD pre-training snack – 2 rice cakes with jam	120 (500)	25
Post-training snack 5:00 pm	Apple	95 (400)	20		95 (400)	20
Dinner 7:00 pm	Salmon Steak – medium fillet (150 g); medium sweet potato & beetroot – baked, olive oil spray; steamed vegetables; drizzle of garlic aioli Following Dinner: 2 squares of 78% dark chocolate	830 (3475)	52	ADD slice of breadADD glass of milk	1055 (4410)	80
Daily energy intake		2145 (8975)	237		3250 (13580)	420

Source: Gregory Cox.

Refuelling strategies employed after exercise should reflect the likely glycogen used in the session, the timing of the next session, the next meal time, and the broader nutrition goals of the athlete (see Box 17.2). Hence, the approach taken to refuelling strategies should be periodised throughout the week and over the training year, depending on the key training goals. An integrated training and nutrition strategy will allow preparation before, and recovery after, key training sessions and competition. It may not matter that lower-intensity sessions are undertaken without full refuelling – in fact, there may actually be some advantages to this.

Box 17.2   How much glycogen do endurance athletes use?

An intense high-quality endurance cycling session consisting of 8 × 5-minute maximal efforts will deplete muscle glycogen stores by about 50%.[6] A sports nutrition professional should be familiar with the specific carbohydrate requirements of the athletes they manage when providing advice regarding strategies for carbohydrate intake around daily training and racing.

In the 1–2 hours after hard exercise, the muscle is primed to absorb and store carbohydrate – this is referred to as the **window of opportunity**. While early feeding promotes refuelling at the high end of the storage range, the muscle will continue to take up carbohydrate in response to food consumed at meals throughout the day. It is worth taking advantage of this window when recovery time is short (i.e., < 8 hr) and refuelling needs are particularly important (e.g., after an early morning session with the next session scheduled later that morning (as would likely be the case for an elite triathlete). The overall carbohydrate intake, not the timing in close proximity to the training of carbohydrate intake, will be the driving force behind how much muscle glycogen is restored during recovery periods that extend over longer periods such as 24–48 hours.

Window of opportunity

In sports nutrition, this refers to the 1–2 hour period after hard exercise in which the muscle is primed to absorb and store carbohydrate at high rates.

Training with low carbohydrate availability and ketogenic low-carbohydrate, high-fat diets

In recent times, much has been written about purposely training and/or sleeping with low muscle glycogen stores to accelerate favourable adaptations that occur in response to aerobic exercise. Training when fasting, withholding carbohydrate during extended sessions, limiting carbohydrate during recovery between training sessions, and sleeping with low muscle glycogen stores have all been investigated to determine the likely benefits of 'training low'. Whether to strategically incorporate *training low* techniques into the weekly training schedule should be discussed with the athlete support team as there are several performance and health implications to consider.

Ketogenic, low-carbohydrate, high-fat (K-LCHF) diets have attracted significant social media attention, particularly amongst ultra-endurance athletes. K-LCHF can promote substantial increases (~200%) in maximal fat oxidation rates during exercise in endurance-trained athletes at moderate intensities (~70% VO_2 peak). However, in high-level athletes, performance of higher-intensity (>80% VO_2 peak) endurance exercise is comprised, most likely due to the increased oxygen cost of energy production from fat. The optimal adaptation period for K-LCHF diets; the value of altering periods of high carbohydrate availability with K-LCHF diets; and the influence of K-LCHF diets on bone and iron metabolism are topics worthy of future research and consideration by sports nutrition practitioners. In practice, K-LCHF diets create practical barriers to meeting daily energy and nutrient requirements, as it is particularly difficult to limit carbohydrate to low absolute intakes (<50 g) while achieving a high energy intake. Training low, and K-LCHF diets are discussed further in Chapter 10.

Protein to promote recovery and gains in lean body mass

While much of the research focus on endurance athletes has centred on carbohydrate, protein plays a particularly important role for endurance athletes. While protein requirements for endurance athletes are increased, they are typically met as the athlete increases their daily energy intake in response to daily training. However, strategic timing of protein-containing foods and/or fluids immediately after training and/or during extended training sessions can assist in maintaining or increasing lean body mass as well as enhancing favourable metabolic responses to endurance exercise. Sports nutrition practitioners should be purposeful in their planning by including protein-containing foods and fluids immediately following targeted endurance training sessions (see Box 17.3).

Box 17.3 Achieving lean physique goals with gains in lean body mass

Endurance athletes commonly strive to manipulate body composition to achieve a lean physique by implementing strategies that promote fat loss. This requires athletes to restrict energy intake to create an energy deficit. While this may be tolerable for short periods, it is important to consider the longer-term physique goals of the athlete. An alternate approach is to implement nutrition strategies that promote gains in lean body mass (i.e., muscle mass) alongside inherent strength elements that exist within most endurance training schedules such as strength-focused cycling sessions, hill running, swimming with resistance (i.e., swim paddles), and/or integrated strength and conditioning sessions in the gym. In this instance, an athlete may remain weight stable, decrease body fat stores and increase muscle mass, creating a more capable physique aligned to the demands of endurance competition.

Iron is an important micronutrient for endurance athletes

Endurance athletes are prone to having low iron status caused by inadequate dietary intake in combination with increased iron losses (e.g., through **gastrointestinal bleeding,**

Table 17.2 Components in food that affect the bioavailability of iron

Iron enhancers	Iron inhibitors
Vitamin C-rich foods (ascorbic acid)	Phytates
• salad, lightly cooked green vegetables, some fruits, and citrus fruit juices or vitamin C-fortified fruit juices	• found in cereal grains, wheat bran, legumes, nuts, peanut butter, seeds, bran, soy products, soy protein, and spinach
Some fermented foods	Polyphenolic compounds
• miso, some types of soy sauce	• strong tea and coffee, herb tea, cocoa, red wine, and some spices, for example, oregano
Meat enhancer factor	Calcium inhibits both haem and non-haem iron absorption as iron and calcium co-compete for absorption across the gut (milk, cheese)
• found in beef, liver, lamb, chicken, and fish	
Alcohol and some organic acids	
• very low-pH foods containing citric acid, tartaric acid, for example, citrus fruit	Peptides from partially digested plant proteins
Vitamin A and beta-carotene	• soy protein isolates, soy products
• liver, animal fats, carrots, sweet potato	

sweating, and haemolysis), increased iron needs (e.g., when training at altitude), and reduced iron absorption (which occurs during the post-exercise window, particularly when exercise is undertaken with low glycogen stores). Regardless of the stage of iron depletion, all types of iron deficiency should be carefully managed.[7] A planned assessment schedule for iron status should be considered within the annual training, competition, and travel plans of endurance athletes. Athletes will benefit from education that highlights dietary sources of iron as well as ways to improve iron absorption (Table 17.2). The use of iron supplements may be necessary at specific times for certain athletes and should be managed by the sports medicine physician and sports nutrition professional.

Gastrointestinal bleeding

Bleeding that occurs from any part of the GI tract, but typically from the small intestine, large intestine, rectum, or anus. Gastrointestinal bleeding is not a disease but is a symptom of many diseases. For athletes, bleeding may occur due to the sloughing of the intestinal lining as a result of the continual jarring that occurs when running on hard surfaces.

Race-day nutrition strategies

Optimal performance during competition is achieved by targeting the factors that would otherwise cause fatigue or a reduction in work output and/or skill. Common nutritional factors that can cause fatigue in endurance events include depletion of glycogen stores, low blood glucose levels (**hypoglycaemia**), dehydration, GI upset, and less commonly low blood sodium levels (**hyponatraemia**). Eating strategies in preparation for the race and during the race should be implemented to avoid or reduce the impact of these problems.

Hypoglycaemia

Low blood glucose levels.

Hyponatraemia

Low blood sodium levels.

Carbohydrate loading for endurance racing

Carbohydrate is stored within the muscle as glycogen. Carbohydrate loading, if done appropriately, increases muscle glycogen stores – thereby delaying the point of fatigue, commonly referred to as 'bonking' in endurance circles. Carbohydrate loading emerged in the late 1960s when Scandinavian researchers found that 3–4 days of carbohydrate deprivation, followed by three days of high carbohydrate eating resulted in a supercompensation of muscle glycogen and a subsequent improvement in endurance exercise capacity.[8] This method was later refined with current guidelines suggesting 24–72 hours of high carbohydrate eating and rest without the pre-depletion phase.

Despite a greater reliance on muscle glycogen when pre-exercise concentrations are elevated with carbohydrate loading prior to exercise, carbohydrate loading is generally associated with enhanced performance when exercise duration exceeds 90 minutes. In shorter duration endurance events (e.g., 10-km (6 mile) road runs, a 40-km (25 mile) cycling time-trial or a 2–3-km open water swim), suitable fuel stores in the muscle are achieved by a combination of tapered exercise or rest, plus adequate carbohydrate intake (5–10 g per kg body mass) over the 24–36 hours before the event. For many athletes, this dietary prescription is already achieved in the everyday training diet, so no extra effort or planning is required. However, for some athletes (i.e., women or athletes restricting energy intake to facilitate weight loss) increasing total dietary energy and carbohydrate above their normal intake may be needed to achieve these fuelling-up goals.

For longer duration events, such as marathon, 70.3, or ironman triathlon, achieving a high carbohydrate intake (8–12 g per kg body mass) for 24–72 hours before an event will require athletes to modify their typical daily food and fluid intake. It is unlikely that an athlete's typical carbohydrate intake will fall within this range to super-compensate muscle glycogen stores. A well-structured and considered carbohydrate loading plan will ensure an athlete increases their carbohydrate intake while avoiding GI issues. Box 17.4 provides some common practice considerations for sports nutrition professionals.

Box 17.4   Carbohydrate loading practice considerations

- Athletes should be provided with adequate information regarding the carbohydrate content of foods. Many athletes have a limited understanding of the carbohydrate content of everyday foods and fluids or formulated supplementary sports foods such as carbohydrate gels, sports drinks, and energy bars. Providing a carbohydrate-ready reckoner will assist the athlete in achieving the required carbohydrate intake (see the suggestions in Box 17.6).
- Low-fibre foods should be included within a carbohydrate loading plan to help maintain a typical fibre intake for the athlete.
- When devising a carbohydrate loading plan, it is important to understand the athlete's likely exercise routine for the final 2–3 days before competition. Additional training should be considered in dietary planning to ensure adequate energy is available to allow additional carbohydrate consumed to be available for glycogen storage rather than used to meet daily energy needs.
- When formulating a carbohydrate loading plan, it is important to consider the likely glycogen storage capacity of the athlete when determining the subsequent amount of carbohydrate to be consumed. For well-trained elite athletes with a long training history and low body fat stores, higher amounts of carbohydrate within the guidelines should be considered. For recreationally engaged endurance athletes and those with lower relative lean body mass (higher body-fat levels), carbohydrate intake goals should be modified to the lower end of the suggested intake range.
- If formulating a carbohydrate loading meal plan that includes low-nutrient foods such as confectionery, soft drinks, and sports drinks, it is worthwhile including a disclaimer such as *The food suggestions and volumes specified in the carbohydrate loading meal plan are specific to carbohydrate loading and should not be misinterpreted to reflect everyday healthy eating habits or strategies. Many of the above suggestions are contrary to everyday healthy eating guidelines and are specific to pre-race endurance competition nutrition requirements.*

Pre-race meal

A carbohydrate-rich meal or snack scheduled 1–4 hours before a race has a role in fine-tuning competition preparation by topping up muscle glycogen stores and restoring liver glycogen stores (following an overnight fast). Including fluid (~400–600 mL) with the pre-exercise meal will maximise fluid retention and ensure the athlete is well-hydrated, especially where a fluid deficit is likely to occur during the event. The pre-race meal should be carbohydrate-focused, relatively low in fat and contain moderate amounts of protein. Above all, the pre-race meal should be familiar to the athlete to achieve gut comfort throughout the event, preventing the athlete from either becoming hungry or suffering GIdisturbance or upset. Liquid meal alternatives that contain carbohydrate and protein provide an excellent option for athletes who cannot tolerate solid foods immediately before the race start. Given the variety of endurance races, scheduling of events, food availability, and environmental conditions, athletes are best advised to plan and subsequently rehearse their pre-race meal. Fine-tuning may require input from a skilled sports nutrition professional to avoid GI upset and optimise the readiness to compete. Box 17.5 provides some examples of carbohydrate-rich pre-race meals.

Box 17.5   Examples of pre-race meals

Early morning race start. Choices need to be simple and easy to prepare and consumed 1½–2 hours before race start. Water should be included and varied according to anticipated fluid requirements, environmental conditions, other fluids contained within the meal and the athlete's thirst level.

- Cooked oats + low-fat milk with honey, + banana + glass of fruit juice
- ¾–1½ cups of cereal + low-fat milk + slice of toast with savoury spread + milk coffee
- Toasted muffin/s or crumpet/s or bread + jam or honey + banana with 400–600 mL of sports drink + ½–1 sports bar
- 1–2 pancakes with syrup + liquid meal supplement
- 400–600 mL of sports drink + sports bar
- Fruit smoothie (banana, low-fat milk, yoghurt, and honey) or fruit smoothie

Late race start. A normal schedule of meals should be consumed before the pre-race meal. Timing of pre-race meals can be varied to suit athlete preference (1–3 hours pre-race). Water should be included and varied according to anticipated fluid requirements, environmental conditions, other fluids contained within the meal and the athlete's thirst level.

- Roll(s) or sandwich(es) + 400–600 mL of sports drink
- Spaghetti with tomato or low-fat sauce + glass of fruit juice
- ½–1 cup of creamed rice + 2 slices of toast with savoury spread and 400–600 mL of sports drink

Important considerations for carbohydrate intake during racing

Reported race-day carbohydrate intake rates vary considerably between athletes undertaking endurance exercise. This is not surprising, as some events or disciplines within a multidiscipline event provide better access to and tolerance of the intake of food and fluids. For example, Kimber et al.[9] found that 73% of the total energy consumed during an ironman triathlon was consumed during the cycle leg of the race. One interesting finding from this study was that overall finishing time was inversely related to carbohydrate intake during the run for male competitors. Pfeiffer et al.[10] also found that high rates of carbohydrate intake were usually observed in faster athletes; however, high rates of carbohydrate intake are associated with increased rates of GI upset, such as nausea and flatulence. While there are obvious benefits to exercise performance of providing carbohydrate during endurance sports,[11] it is important that carbohydrate intake suggestions are well tolerated by the athlete. Many athletes do not consume carbohydrate routinely during training, which may partly explain why they suffer GI upset and discomfort when they compete and ingest carbohydrate-containing fluids and foods.

Researchers at the AIS were the first to demonstrate that athletes are able to increase their use of ingested carbohydrate during a simulated race if they routinely consume carbohydrate during daily training for four weeks.[12] It appears that athletes can train their gut to increase absorption and subsequent delivery of the ingested carbohydrate to the working muscle. The practical significance of this research highlights the importance of 'training the way you race'. In preparation for endurance racing, athletes should rehearse their race carbohydrate intake strategies in race-like training sessions that mimic the demands of competition.

The amount, timing, type, frequency of intake, and form of carbohydrate should be considered when advising endurance athletes in relation to carbohydrate intake during training and racing (Table 17.3). In brief, in high-intensity endurance sports lasting less than 45 minutes, there appears to be little benefit to consuming carbohydrate during exercise. While the athlete should start exercise with normalised muscle glycogen stores, there is little to gain by consuming carbohydrate in these brief endurance events or training sessions. However, consuming small amounts of carbohydrate – even rinsing the mouth with carbohydrate – provides a performance advantage in endurance exercise

Table 17.3 Carbohydrate intake recommendations for endurance athletes during exercise

	Situation	*Carbohydrate targets*	*Comments on type and timing of carbohydrate intake*
During brief exercise	<45 minutes (e.g., 10 km track event)	Not needed	
During sustained high-intensity training sessions or races	45–75 minutes (e.g., half marathon, road cycling time-trial)	Small amounts including mouth rinse	Carbohydrate-containing drinks, including sports drinks and carbohydrate gels, provide practical options for athletes undertaking high-intensity endurance sports.
During endurance events or extended training sessions	1–2.5 hours (e.g., marathon)	30–60 g/h	Most endurance events require athletes to refuel/rehydrate while they are actually racing. The availability of foods and fluids varies according to the race. Race organisers may provide selected foods and fluids from feed/aid stations on the course, whereas some athletes may carry their own supplies. A range of everyday foods/fluids and specialised sports supplements, including sports drinks and gels, provide convenient, well-tolerated options. Athletes should practice in training to find a refuelling plan that suits their individual goals, including hydration needs and gut comfort.
During ultra-endurance exercise	>2.5–3 hours (e.g., ultramarathons, ironman triathlons, cycling stage races)	Up to 90 g/h	As above. Higher intakes of carbohydrate are associated with better performance. Specifically designed sports foods and fluids providing multiple transportable carbohydrates (glucose:fructose mixtures) will achieve high rates of oxidation of carbohydrate consumed during exercise. Including a variety of tastes and textures during longer or multi-day endurance races is important to avoid 'flavour fatigue'.

Source: Adapted from Burke et al.[5]

lasting 45–75 minutes.[13] Consuming carbohydrate in these events provides a central stimulus, altering the perception of effort and allowing for greater work outputs. The frequency of exposure, not the amount of carbohydrate consumed, is central to planning carbohydrate intake strategies for these events.

As the duration of the endurance event extends beyond 90 minutes, providing carbohydrate during exercise will provide an alternate fuel for the exercising muscle while maintaining high rates of carbohydrate oxidation. Furthermore, carbohydrate intake will assist in maintaining blood glucose levels within normal ranges.

For extended-duration endurance events, there is a dose-response benefit to consuming carbohydrate.[14] The maximal amount tolerated and available for oxidation will be increased by consuming multiple transportable carbohydrates (glucose and fructose), as they are absorbed across the gut on different transporters. Further, as previously mentioned, rehearsing race-day carbohydrate intakes, particularly high rates of carbohydrate, will improve tolerance.

There is a myriad of sports foods, fluids, and everyday food items that can be incorporated into a race-day plan for an endurance athlete. The combination of everyday food items and specialised sports foods should be based on the ease of intake and the athlete's food and fluid preferences. Box 17.6 provides various suggestions for race-day food and fluid intakes.

Box 17.6   Carbohydrate food and fluid suggestions for endurance racing

High-intensity endurance events 45–75 minutes

- small quantities (exposures) of carbohydrate;
- mouth rinse or frequent intake of carbohydrate-containing drinks (e.g., sports drink) if practical and tolerated + water as tolerated.

High-intensity endurance events 90–150 minutes

- carbohydrate intake target of 30–60 g of carbohydrate per hour;
- water should be consumed to alleviate thirst in addition to fluids listed to top-up fluid intake.

Hourly suggestions for 30–60 g/h

- 200–300 mL of sports drink ± sports gel (25–30 g CHO per gel); OR
- ~200–300 mL of cola soft drink ± sports gel (25–30 g CHO per gel); OR
- 400–600 mL of sports drink; OR
- 1–2 × sports gel (25–30 g CHO per gel).

Endurance events >2½–3 hours

- carbohydrate intake target is up to 90 g of carbohydrate per hour;
- for ultra-endurance races a variety of tastes (sweet and savoury) should be considered to avoid flavour fatigue;
- the amount of carbohydrate consumed should reflect the nature of the event and specific requirements of the athlete;

- the combination of solid vs liquid forms of carbohydrate should be modified to reflect the intensity of exercise and the duration of the event;
- intake of carbohydrate-containing fluids should be managed to control hourly carbohydrate intake;
- water should be consumed alongside carbohydrate-containing fluids to align with hourly fluid requirements.

Hourly carbohydrate suggestions for 40–60 g/h

- 300–400 mL of sports drink + 1 × sport gel (25–30 g CHO per gel); OR
- 2 × sport gels (25–30 g CHO per gel); OR
- 400–600 mL of sports drink + banana; OR
- 600 mL of sports drink + granola bar; OR
- 400–500 mL of cola drink.

Hourly carbohydrate suggestions for 70–90 g/h

- 600 mL of sports drink + 2 × sport gels (25–30 g CHO per gel); OR
- 500–600 mL of sports drink + sandwich (savoury or sweet spread); OR
- 200 mL of sports gel concentrate – 8 × sports gels (~25 g CHO per gel) added to a 600 mL drink bottle topped up with water to 600 mL; OR
- 600 mL of cola drink + ½ sports bar (40 g CHO per bar); OR
- 250 mL of liquid meal supplement + cereal bar or granola bar; OR
- 400–600 mL of sweetened iced tea + 40 g of dried fruit and nut mix + ½–1 sandwich (savoury spread); OR
- 300–500 mL of sports drink + 60 g chocolate bar + 20 g packet of potato crisps (chips); OR
- 40 g of confectionery or sports confectionery + 2 pikelets (small pancakes) and jam + fun-size chocolate bar.

Source: Gregory Cox.

Fluid intake considerations for endurance athletes

In many endurance sports, sweat losses are considerable, resulting in significant loss of fluid and dehydration. This is magnified in hot, humid environments and in sports where there are practical barriers to drinking (e.g., mountain bike racing and marathon running). While the effect of dehydration or hypohydration on exercise performance has been extensively investigated, it's still a hotly debated topic amongst researchers.[15] The point of contention is the tolerable fluid loss where the effects on exercise performance become apparent, which is likely dependent on the individual – their level of training and fitness, their starting hydration status and their acclimation, the environment (effects are greater in the heat or at altitude) and clothing.

Race and/or training fluid intake advice should be individualised to ensure athletes use available opportunities to drink fluids at a rate that prevents thirst and keeps their accumulating fluid deficit below 2% of body mass. Figure 17.1 provides an insight into the complex nature of providing individualised fluid intake advice. For instance, an elite male triathlete racing at high speeds in a hot Olympic-distance triathlon should create opportunities to maximise fluid intake and take visual cues from other athletes as a reminder to

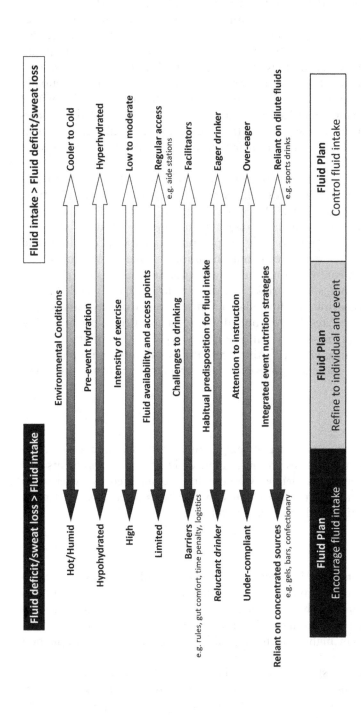

Figure 17.1 Fluid intake advice.
Source: Adapted from Burke.[16]

drink as sweat losses will be high and opportunities to drink limited. Further, the speed of racing will impact tolerance and gut comfort when ingesting fluids. In contrast, a recreational female runner who runs/walks a marathon in cool weather can expect lower sweat rates, while having ample opportunity to slow or stop at aid stations. For this athlete, controlling her opportunities, rather than drinking as much as tolerated, should underpin her fluid intake advice to minimise the risk of over-drinking. While not common, overzealous fluid intake combined with low sweat losses may lead to the potentially fatal condition of hyponatraemia (low blood sodium concentration, often known as water intoxication). The development of a race fluid intake plan can be assisted by undertaking fluid balance assessments during race-like training sessions in similar environmental conditions so that the athlete can gauge their typical sweat rates in comparison to their opportunity/ability to rehydrate.

The most suitable drink choices and delivery methods will depend on the sport and the need to address other nutritional goals. Fluids need to be palatable (temperature, taste) and available to encourage intake. Other characteristics to consider include the beverage temperature, which can be manipulated both to improve palatability in the specific environment and to contribute to body temperature regulation; cold fluids and ice slushies can reduce core temperature in hot conditions, while warm fluids may increase body temperature in cold environments. Many endurance events offer a range of fluids, most commonly, water, sports drink, cola soft drinks, and, in extended races, warm broths or soups. Sports drinks are formulated to meet a range of needs and simultaneously provide fluid, electrolytes, and carbohydrate. Cola soft drinks provide additional carbohydrate and small amounts of caffeine which, when included later in exercise, may provide a performance benefit.[17] Above all, athletes should be familiar with the sports drink on offer at the endurance event and/or plan to provide their preferred choice.

Summary

This chapter has highlighted the importance of being familiar with the training and competition demands of endurance athletes to understand daily energy requirements and interpret daily carbohydrate intake guidelines. Carbohydrate requirements vary based on event durations and intensities, so nutrition plans should be tailored based on these requirements with consideration of the individual athlete.

Chapter highlights

- As a sports nutrition practitioner, it is important to understand daily training schedules and intended outcomes of training to appropriately plan food and fluid intakes for endurance athletes. Importantly, nutrition strategies that promote health and wellbeing should be prioritised in endurance athletes due to the risk of underfuelling. This is particularly important in high-performance athletes, who undertake the highest daily training loads.
- Sports nutrition practitioners should use available technologies to estimate exercise energy expenditure given the variability in daily training observed in endurance athletes. This requires interaction and discussion with coaches and sports physiologists to explore daily training.

- Carbohydrate intake guidelines should be carefully interpreted to ensure daily recommendations align with the athletes' overarching nutrition-related goals. Importantly, timely intake of nutrient-rich foods and fluids containing carbohydrate and protein will facilitate speedy recovery following daily training, particularly when several sessions are planned.
- Sports nutrition practitioners should be vigilant in monitoring dietary intake, markers of health and well-being, and daily training performance as endurance athletes are susceptible to problematic low energy availability. This requires input from the coach and other performance support staff.
- Endurance athletes commonly suffer from low iron status and, as such, should be carefully monitored and managed.
- Carbohydrate loading offers a particular advantage to endurance athletes competing in events longer than 90 minutes. Dietary strategies should be employed to achieve high carbohydrate intakes while avoiding high intakes of fibre.
- The pre-race meal should be carbohydrate-focused and customised to suit the athlete and race schedule. Above all, food and fluids should be familiar to the athlete.
- Carbohydrate intake for racing should be scaled according to the duration and intensity of the event. For athletes consuming high rates of carbohydrate, race-day nutrition plans should be rehearsed to minimise the risk of GI discomfort during the race.
- Race-day carbohydrate and fluid intakes should be adjusted to suit individual athlete preferences, race demands, and environmental conditions. Given the variety of endurance events, sports nutrition practitioners should become familiar with the practical challenges faced by athletes in meeting their race-day nutrition goals.

References

1. Saris WH, Van Erp-Baart MA, Brouns F. Study on food intake and energy expenditure during extreme sustained exercise: the Tour de France. *Int J Sports Med.* 1989;10(Suppl1):S26–S31.
2. Heydenreich J, Kayser B, Schutz Y, et al. Total energy expenditure, energy intake, and body composition in endurance athletes across the training season: a systematic review. *Sports Med Open.* 2017;3(1):8.
3. Mountjoy M, Ackerman K, Bailey D, et al. The 2023 International Olympic Committee's (IOC) consensus statement on Relative Energy Deficiency in Sports (REDs). *Br J Sports Med.* 2023. In press.
4. Wells KR, Jeacocke NA, Appaneal R, et al. The Australian Institute of Sport (AIS) and National Eating Disorders Collaboration (NEDC) position statement on disordered eating in high performance sport. *Br J Sports Med.* 2020;54(21):247–1258.
5. Burke LM, Hawley JA, Wong SH, et al. Carbohydrates for training and competition. *J Sports Sci.* 2011;29(Sl):S17–S27.
6. Stepto NK, Martin DT, Fallon KE. Metabolic demands of intense aerobic interval training in competitive cyclists. *Med Sci Sports Exerc.* 2001;33(2):303–310.
7. Sim M, Garvican-Lewis, LA, Cox GR. Iron considerations for the athlete: a narrative review. *Eur J Appl Physiol.* 2019;119(7):1463–1478.
8. Bergstrom J, Hermansen L, Hultman E. Diet, muscle glycogen and physical performance. *Acta Physiol. Scand.* 1967;71:140–150.
9. Kimber NE, Ross JJ, Mason SL. Energy balance during an ironman triathlon in male and female triathletes. *Int J Sport Nutr Exerc Metab.* 2002;12(1):44–67.
10. Pfeiffer B, Stellingwerff T, Hodgson AB. Nutritional intake and gastrointestinal problems during competitive endurance events. *Med Sci Sports Exerc.* 2012;44(2):344–351.

11. Stellingwerff T, Cox GR. Systematic review: carbohydrate supplementation on exercise performance or capacity of varying durations. *Appl Physiol Nutr Metab*. 2014;39(9):998–1011.
12. Cox GR, Clark SA, Cox AJ. Daily training with high carbohydrate availability increases exogenous carbohydrate oxidation during endurance cycling. *J Appl Physiol*. 2010;109(1):126–134.
13. Rollo I, Williams C. Effect of mouth-rinsing carbohydrate solutions on endurance performance. *Sports Med*. 2011;41(6):449–461.
14. Smith JW, Pascoe DD, Passe DH. Curvilinear dose-response relationship of carbohydrate $(0–120 \text{ g.h}^{(-1)})$ and performance. *Med Sci Sports Exerc*. 2013;45(2):336–341.
15. James LJ, Funnell MP, James RM, et al. Does hypohydration really impair endurance performance? Methodological considerations for interpreting hydration research. *Sports Med*. 2019;49(2):103–114.
16. Burke LM. Nutritional approaches to counter performance constraints in high-level sports competition. *Exp. Physiol*. 2021;106(12):2304–2323.
17. Cox GR, Desbrow B, Montgomery PG. Effect of different protocols of caffeine intake on metabolism and endurance. *J Appl Physiol*. 2002;93(3):990–999.

18 Strength and power athletes

Gary Slater and Lachlan Mitchell

The ability to generate explosive muscle power and strength is critical to success in Cross-Fit, Olympic weightlifting, and powerlifting, throwing events including javelin, discus, shot put, and hammer, and 100- and 200-metre sprints in track and field. The athletes competing in these events will typically incorporate some form of resistance exercise into their overall training program, as well as diverse sport-specific training. Given the disparity between the sport-specific training programs of strength and power athletes and their subsequent metabolic implications, this chapter will focus on the nutritional implications of resistance training among strength and power athletes. The sport of bodybuilding will also be addressed given the focus on resistance exercise in the overall training program prescription.

Learning outcomes

This chapter will:

- describe the training nutrition needs of strength and power athletes, including macronutrient needs over the day;
- identify appropriate nutrition strategies to facilitate recovery;
- identify issues regarding supplement use in this population;
- describe the competition demands and translate them into specific nutrition guidance;
- appreciate the impact of physique traits on competitive success among this athlete population and how to manipulate these through dietary interventions.

Training programs

Athletes participating in throwing events typically undertake periodised training programs that aim to develop maximum strength and power of the major muscle groups. Training involves a range of modalities including **plyometric exercises**, sprinting, power lifts, Olympic lifts, and weighted throwing drills to complement technical throwing training. Periodisation of resistance training typically involves a transition from high-volume, high-force, low-velocity movements requiring less coordination characteristic of traditional powerlifting to more **explosive**, lower-force, low-repetition training using Olympic lifts in preparation for competition. The focus on explosive Olympic lifts over more traditional strength-based lifting results in more favourable power and strength gains,

DOI: 10.4324/9781003321286-21

derived primarily from neural rather than skeletal muscle **hypertrophy** adaptations. Consequently, this style of training enhances traits important to athletic development and is common among other explosive athletics disciplines like sprinting and jumping events, as well as increasingly being incorporated into the training practices of powerlifters.

Plyometric exercises

Exercises in which muscles exert maximum force in short intervals of time, with the goal of increasing power—for example, jump training.

Explosive

Requiring a maximum or near maximum power output from the athlete in a short amount of time.

Hypertrophy

An increase in skeletal muscle size through growth in the size of its cells.

Unlike other sports that use resistance exercise to complement sport-specific training, CrossFit, powerlifting, Olympic lifting, and bodybuilding use resistance training as a primary mode of training. While Olympic and powerlifting athletes are primarily concerned with enhancing power and strength respectively, bodybuilding training primarily aims to induce skeletal muscle hypertrophy. Consequently, the training programs of bodybuilders are unique, typically of greater volume than those of other athletes, using higher repetition ranges with multiple sets per muscle group and little rest between sets.

Training nutrition

Nutrition plays an important role in three aspects of training for strength and power athletes: (1) fuelling of sport-specific and strength training, (2) recovery from this training, and (3) the promotion of training adaptations, including skeletal muscle hypertrophy. Resistance exercise requires a high rate of energy supply, derived from both the phosphagen energy systems and glycogenolysis (see Chapter 2),[1,2] with the contribution of each dependent upon the relative power output, the work-to-rest ratio and muscle blood flow.[2] The source of fatigue during resistance exercise is likely multifactorial, including neuromuscular and peripheral metabolic factors such as a decline in intramuscular pH,[3] the latter somewhat dependent on the intensity and volume of training undertaken as well as the time point within a resistance training session. Metabolic fatigue during the earlier part of a workout may be due at least partly to reductions in phosphagen energy system stores and mild acidosis, while subsequent fatigue may result more from acidosis and impaired energy production from glycogenolysis.[3]

Given the extreme muscularity of these individuals and the association between muscle mass and total energy expenditure, it is not surprising that these athletes have generous energy intakes.[4] However, when expressed relative to body mass the energy intakes of strength and power athletes are generally unremarkable relative to those reported for athletes in other sports but lower than current strength athlete guidelines of ~185–210 kJ/kg BM/day.[5] This likely reflects the fact that taller and/or more muscular individuals have lower resting and total energy requirements relative to body mass. Given this, traditional sports nutrition guidelines for macronutrients may need to be adjusted for larger athletes, reflective of their lower relative energy requirements. Consideration should also be given to the distribution of nutrient intake,[6] with limited information available on the daily distribution of energy and nutrient intake, making it difficult to infer compliance with guidelines relating to key periods of nutrient intake, including before, during, and after exercise.

Carbohydrate

A single resistance training session can result in reductions in muscle glycogen stores of as much as 40 per cent,[2,3] with the amount of depletion depending on the duration, intensity, and overall work accomplished during the session. Higher-repetition, moderate-load training characteristic of programming prescribed to promote skeletal muscle hypertrophy results in the greatest reductions in muscle glycogen stores. Reductions in muscle glycogen stores have been associated with performance impairment and, therefore, lower training capacity, although this effect is not always evident and may be dependent on the method used to induce a state of glycogen depletion. Nonetheless, it is possible that impaired training or competition performance could occur in any session or event that relied on rapid and repeated glycogen breakdown.

Given that resistance training is merely one component of the overall training program of sprint and throwing event athletes, and that the skeletal muscle damage that accompanies resistance training impairs muscle glycogen resynthesis, it would seem pertinent to encourage strength-trained athletes to maintain a moderate carbohydrate intake. Guidelines proposing an intake within the range of 6 g/kg BM/day for male strength athletes,[1] and possibly less for females,[7] have been advocated. Lifters and throwers typically report carbohydrate intakes of 3–5 g/kg BM/day, while bodybuilders maintain daily intakes equivalent to 4–7 g/kg BM/day, independent of gender.[4] While this may appear low relative to endurance athletes, conclusive evidence of benefit from maintaining a habitual high carbohydrate intake among strength athletes remains to be confirmed. Given the lower relative energy expenditure of larger athletes and their requirements for other nutrients, plus the impact of adjusting carbohydrate on total energy intake, recommendations for carbohydrate intake at strategic times, including before, during, and after exercise, may be more applicable to the strength athlete, ensuring carbohydrate availability is optimised at critical time points. Thus, a range of daily carbohydrate intakes of 4–7 g/kg BM would be considered reasonable for these athletes, depending on their phase of training and daily training loads.

Protein

Strength-trained athletes have advocated high-protein diets for many years. While the debate continues on the need for additional protein among resistance-trained individuals, general guidelines now recommend athletes undertaking strength training ingest approximately twice the current recommendations for protein of their sedentary counterparts, or as much as 1.2–1.6 g protein/kg BM/day.[8] Given the relatively wide distribution of protein in the meal plan and increased energy intake of athletes, it should not be surprising that most strength-trained athletes easily achieve these increased protein needs.[4] Exceeding the upper range of protein intake guidelines offers no further benefit as excess protein is broken down and excreted. Furthermore, there is evidence that an intense period of resistance training reduces protein turnover and improves net protein retention, thus reducing the relative dietary protein requirements of experienced resistance-trained athletes.

Simply contrasting an athlete's current daily protein intake against guidelines does not indicate whether dietary intake has been optimised to promote gains in muscle mass or enhance the repair of damaged tissues. Rather, consideration should be given to other dietary factors, including total energy intake, the daily distribution of protein intake (especially as it relates to training), and the source of dietary protein.[8] While there is very little information available on the eating patterns of strength athletes, available literature suggests the majority of daily protein intake is ingested at main meals from an even mix of animal- and plant-based sources, with a skewed pattern of intake towards the evening meal, indicating a significant proportion of athletes fail to achieve optimal protein intake at breakfast and lunch. Thus, rather than focusing on total daily intake, athletes are encouraged to focus more on optimising protein quality and distribution throughout the day. Given muscle protein synthesis becomes less efficient in response to persistently high levels of amino acids in the blood, it has been suggested that 4–5 evenly spaced feedings of 0.4–0.5 g/kg BM) high biological value protein should be recommended for strength athletes.[8]

Fat

The dietary fat intake of strength and power athletes is generally greater than that recommended for healthy individuals and is often derived from sources rich in saturated fat, presumably from an emphasis on animal foods in the pursuit of a higher protein intake. While it is unclear what the impacts of such dietary practices are on athletes' blood lipid profiles, it may explain in part the lower dietary carbohydrate intakes reported among strength and power athletes. Given that replacing fat with **isoenergetic** amounts of carbohydrate has a favourable effect on protein balance, it is tempting to recommend a reduction in dietary fat intake, especially for those individuals exceeding current guidelines. However, consideration must be given to the practical implications of substituting a high energy-density macronutrient with a lower energy macronutrient and the impact this may have on energy balance, especially among strength and power athletes with very high energy needs. Conversely, there may be situations in which a higher intake of foods rich in unsaturated fats may be advocated for strength and power athletes struggling to achieve energy needs because of an emphasis on the selection of lower energy-density foods in the meal plan.

Isoenergetic

Containing the same number of calories/kilojoules.

Pre-exercise and during exercise

Athletes are encouraged to pay particular attention to dietary intake in the hours before exercise, on the assumption that pre-exercise nutritional strategies can influence exercise performance. While this is a widely accepted practice prior to endurance exercise to enhance work capacity, evidence is also emerging for a beneficial role of carbohydrate consumed immediately prior to strength training.[9] For example, Lambert et al.[10] reported that supplemental carbohydrate ingestion prior to and during resistance exercise (1 g/kg before, 0.5 g/kg during) increased total work capacity, a response which has been replicated elsewhere. However, not all studies have shown a benefit from consuming carbohydrate prior to exercise; it is proposed that the ergogenic potential for carbohydrate ingestion is most likely to be observed when undertaking longer-duration, high-volume resistance training. At present, a specific recommendation for an optimum rate or timing of carbohydrate ingestion for strength and power athletes before and during any given training session cannot be determined. Given the lower relative energy expenditure of resistance exercise to endurance exercise, the lower range of existing exercise carbohydrate intake guidance for endurance athletes (for instance, 1 g/kg before and 0.5 g/kg carbohydrate during exercise) may be a reasonable proxy until more specific resistance training research is undertaken. As with all athletes, strength and power athletes should be encouraged to initiate training in a euhydrated state given that even moderate hypohydration can impair resistance-training work capacity.

Recently, there has been interest in combining carbohydrate and essential amino acids both before and during resistance exercise, presumably to increase substrate availability and thus exercise performance, to promote a more anabolic (muscle-building) hormonal environment, to stimulate muscle protein synthesis and to reduce muscle damage and soreness. Some initial research found that greater muscle protein synthesis occurred when nutritional support was provided before rather than after resistance exercise, but this has not been replicated elsewhere. Consequently, current guidelines recommend that protein be consumed after exercise because this is when there is maximal stimulation of muscle protein synthesis.

Recovery

Given that resistance training typically forms only one component of an athlete's training schedule, recovery strategies proven to enhance the restoration of muscle glycogen stores, such as eating carbohydrate after exercise, should be routinely implemented following resistance training. General sports nutrition guidelines recommend carbohydrate should be consumed at a rate of 1.0–1.2 g/kg BM immediately after exercise. However, this has no influence on muscle protein metabolism. In contrast, consuming protein after exercise results in an exacerbated elevation in muscle protein synthesis at the same time as a minor suppression in muscle protein breakdown, resulting in a positive net protein balance. The ingestion of approximately 30–40 grams (0.4–0.5 g/kg BM) of high biological-value protein after resistance exercise appears to be sufficient to maximally stimulate muscle protein synthesis, with higher doses recommended following resistance-training sessions engaging the whole body and among elderly or injured athletes. So, eating both carbohydrate and protein immediately after resistance training results in more favourable recovery outcomes, including restoration of muscle glycogen stores and muscle protein metabolism, than consuming either nutrient alone. Eating protein after exercise also reduces the amount of carbohydrate required in the acute recovery period, with an energy-matched intake of 0.8 g/kg BM/hour carbohydrate plus 0.4 g/kg BM/hour protein resulting in similar muscle glycogen resynthesis over five hours compared to 1.2 g/kg BM/hour carbohydrate alone following intermittent exercise, with a similar response evident following resistance exercise. Preliminary evidence also suggests that consuming both carbohydrate and protein after exercise may reduce muscle damage often seen in strength-trained athletes; whether such a change has a functional benefit is unclear.

Supplementation practices

Supplement use is reported to be higher among athletes than their sedentary counterparts, with particularly high rates of supplement use among weightlifters and bodybuilders. The high prevalence of supplement use among bodybuilders, Olympic weightlifters, track and field athletes, and those who frequent commercial fitness centres is not unexpected, given the range of products targeted at this market. While multi-vitamin and mineral supplements are very popular among all athletes, other products such as protein powders and specific amino acid supplements, caffeine, and creatine monohydrate are also frequently used by strength-trained athletes.

Recognising the nutritional value of food sources of protein and essential amino acids, creatine monohydrate appears to be the only supplement that has been reported to enhance skeletal muscle hypertrophy and functional capacity in response to resistance training. However, liquid meal supplements rich in carbohydrate and protein may be valuable in the post-exercise period to boost total energy and specific nutrient intake at a time when the appetite is often suppressed. There is also evidence that caffeine enhances muscular strength. While other dietary supplements such as individual amino acids and their metabolites have been advocated for use among bodybuilders, preliminary literature and research supporting their ergogenic potential is limited, and thus cannot currently be recommended.

Strength-trained athletes continue to seek supplement information from easily available sources, including websites, social media, magazines, fellow athletes, and coaches. The accuracy of this information may vary, leaving the athlete vulnerable to inappropriate and/or ineffective supplementation protocols and an increased risk of inadvertent doping. The presence of muscle dysmorphia, a body dysmorphic disorder characterised by a preoccupation with a sense of inadequate muscularity common among bodybuilders, may also influence supplementation practices and lead to anabolic steroid use.

Anabolic steroids

Drugs which help the repair and build of muscle tissues, derived from the male hormone testosterone.

Competition

Competition demands of strength sports are characterised by explosive single efforts where athletes have a given number of opportunities to produce a maximal performance, with significant recovery between each effort. This recovery time means that muscle energy reserves are unlikely to be challenged, even in the face of challenging environmental conditions of competitions like the Summer Olympic Games. Consequently, nutrition priorities should focus on more general goals like optimising gastrointestinal tract comfort and preventing weight gain during the competition taper.

Olympic weightlifting, powerlifting, and bodybuilding are unique among strength and power sports in that competition is undertaken via weight categories or, sometimes in bodybuilding by height class. As such, these athletes are likely to engage in acute weight-loss practices common to other weight-category sports including short-term restriction of food and fluids, resulting in a state of glycogen depletion and hypohydration. While performance is typically compromised in sports requiring a significant contribution from aerobic and/or anaerobic energy metabolism (Chapter 2), activities demanding high power output and absolute strength are less likely to be influenced by acute weight loss. Furthermore, the weigh-in is typically undertaken two hours prior to the commencement of weightlifting competition, affording athletes an opportunity to partially recover, from any acute weight-loss strategies undertaken prior to weigh-in. The body mass management guidelines for other weight category sport athletes would also appear applicable for Olympic weightlifters.[11]

Given the association between lower body-fat levels and competitive success, bodybuilders typically adjust their training and diet several months out from the competition to decrease body fat while maintaining or increasing muscle mass. While a compromise in muscle mass has been observed when attempting to achieve the extremely low body-fat levels desired for competition, this is not always the case. The performance implications of any skeletal muscle loss are unknown given the subjective nature of bodybuilding competition. In female bodybuilders, such dietary restrictions are often associated with compromised micronutrient intake and menstrual dysfunction, presumably because energy availability falls below the threshold of ~125 kJ/kg fat-free mass/day required to maintain normal endocrine (hormonal) regulation of the menstrual cycle (refer to Chapters 7 and 25 for more information).

If muscle protein breakdown is experienced by an Olympic weightlifter or power-lifter as they attempt to 'make weight' for competition, a compromise in force-generating capacity, and thus weightlifting performance, is theoretically possible. More details on weight-category sports and weight-making can be found in Chapter 20.

Physique

Within the lifting events, physique traits influence performance in several ways. While the expression of strength has a significant **neural** component, lifting performance is closely associated with skeletal muscle mass. Excluding the open weight category, weightlifters also tend to have low body-fat levels, enhancing the development of strength per unit of body mass. Successful weightlifters also have a higher sitting height-to-stature ratio with shorter limbs, creating a biomechanical advantage. An association between physique traits and competitive success in the Olympic throwing events has been recognised for some time, with successful athletes heavier and taller than their counterparts and growing at a rate more than general population trends. In contrast to other strength sports, bodybuilding is unique in that competitive success is judged purely based on the size, symmetry, and definition of musculature. Not surprisingly, bodybuilders are the most muscular of all the strength athletes. Successful bodybuilders have lower body fat, yet are taller and heavier with wider skeletal proportions, and are much broader across the shoulders than the hips.

Neural

Relating to a nerve or the nervous system.

While it is reasonable to presume that the nutritional focus of strength and power athletes remains on skeletal muscle hypertrophy throughout the year, this is rarely the case, except perhaps during the 'off-season' for bodybuilders or specified times of the annual **macrocycle** of other strength and power athletes. Furthermore, significant changes in body mass among bodybuilders, Olympic weightlifters and powerlifters will likely influence the weight category they compete in and those they compete against. Thus, the intention to promote skeletal muscle hypertrophy must be seriously considered by athletes and their coaches before being implemented.

Macrocycle

Refers to the overall training period, usually representing a year.

Summary

This chapter has described the important role nutrition plays for athletes competing in sports where the expression of explosive power and strength are critical to competitive success. While the total energy intake of strength and power athletes tends to be greater than endurance-focused athletes, intake relative to body mass is often unremarkable, with less known about the distribution of nutrient intake over the day. Strength and power athletes will benefit from a greater focus on the strategic timing of nutrient intake before, during, and after exercise to assist them in optimising resistance-training work capacity, recovery, and body composition. Strength and power athletes create unique challenges for the nutrition service provider given their reliance on readily accessible sources of information, susceptibility to sports supplement marketing, potentially distorted body image and challenges associated with achieving a specified weight category in some sports plus the general void of scientific investigation in recent years relating specifically to this unique group of athletes.

Chapter highlights

- Strength and power athletes tend to consume more total energy, but less energy relative to their body mass, than endurance-focused athletes.
- Strategic timing of nutrient intake before, during, and after exercise will help to optimise training work capacity, recovery, and body composition.
- Strength and power athletes are recommended to consume daily carbohydrate intakes of 4–7 g/kg body mass, and daily protein intakes between 1.0 and 1.2 g/kg body mass in the form of 4–5 evenly spaced feedings of ~30–40 grams (0.4–0.5 g/kg body mass) high biological-value protein.
- Athletes should consume carbohydrate at a rate of 1 g/kg before and 0.5 g/kg during training and focus their protein intake after training during maximal stimulation of muscle protein synthesis.
- Recovery should include consumption of 30–40 grams (0.4–0.5 g/kg body mass) to stimulate muscle protein synthesis, and 0.8 g/kg BM/hour carbohydrate plus 0.4 g/kg BM/hour protein to promote glycogen repletion.
- Athletes' dietary practices may be influenced by inaccurate nutrition information, sports supplement marketing and distorted body image.
- Creatine and whey protein isolate may be considered for strength and power athletes after they have optimised their dietary intake.

References

1. Lambert CP, Flynn MG. Fatigue during high-intensity intermittent exercise: Application to bodybuilding. *Sports Med.* 2002;32(8):511–522.
2. Tesch PA, Colliander EB, Kaiser P. Muscle metabolism during intense, heavy-resistance exercise. *Eur J Appl Physiol Occupat Physiol.* 1986;55(4):362–366.
3. MacDougall JD, Ray S, Sale DG. Muscle substrate utilization and lactate production during weightlifting. *Can J Appl Physiol.* 1999;24(3):209–215.
4. Slater G, Phillips SM. Nutrition guidelines for strength sports: Sprinting, weightlifting, throwing events, and bodybuilding. *J Sports Sci.* 2011:29(S1):S67–S67.
5. Manore MM, Barr SI, Butterfield GE. Joint position statement: Nutrition and athletic performance. American College of Sports Medicine, American Dietetic Association, and Dietitians of Canada. *Med Sci Sports Exerc.* 2000;32(12):2130–2145.
6. Thomas DT, Erdman KA, Burke LM. Position of the Academy of Nutrition and Dietetics, Dietitians of Canada, and the American College of Sports Medicine: Nutrition and athletic performance. *J Acad Nutr Diet.* 2016;116(3):501–528.
7. Volek JS, Forsythe CE, Kraemer WJ. Nutritional aspects of women strength athletes. *Br J Sports Med.* 2006;40(9):742–748.
8. Witard OC, Garthe I, Phillips SM. Dietary protein for training adaptation and body composition manipulation in track and field athletes. *Int J Sport Nutr Exerc Metab.* 2019;29(2):165–174.
9. King A, Helms E, Zinn, C, et al. The ergogenic effects of acute carbohydrate feeling on resistance exercise performance: A systematic review and meta-analysis. *Sports Med.* 2022;52(11): 2691–2712.
10. Lambert CP, Flynn MG, Boone JBJ. Effects of carbohydrate feeding on multiple-bout resistance exercise. *J Strength Cond Res.* 1991;5(4):192–197.
11. Burke LM, Slater GJ, Matthews JJ, et al. ACSM expert consensus statement on weight loss in weight-category sports. *Curr Sports Med Rep.* 2021;20(3):199–217.

19 Team sport athletes

Brooke L Devlin, Sarah L Jenner and Stephen J Keenan

Team sports are popular at a variety of levels, ranging from amateur social competitions for health and fitness to Olympic, national, and international elite competitions. The physical demands of team sports are multifaceted and, as such, a thorough understanding of the physiological demands, duration, and intensity of each team sport is required to ensure appropriate nutrition strategies are in place. Furthermore, team sports present unique challenges with regard to nutrition. The first section of this chapter covers the differences between team sport athletes and individual athletes and the importance of individualised nutrition advice in a team setting. The second section focuses on the structure and characteristics of competition and the demands of travel influence and impact on nutrition strategies and practices. Finally, the chapter will conclude with a discussion of food service provision for team sport athletes, why this is important, and some of the issues nutrition professionals need to consider when catering to large groups of athletes including a case study as an example.

> **Learning outcomes**
>
> **This chapter will:**
>
> - present the differences between team sport athletes and individual athletes and the importance of pack mentality in team sports;
> - explain the importance of individualised nutrition advice and why blanket-style nutrition recommendations are not advised;
> - identify challenges nutrition professionals need to overcome when working with team sport athletes;
> - describe how each sport presents unique nutritional challenges related to the game and outline food service provision and catering for team sport athletes.

What is different about team sport athletes?

Popular team sports for men and women include basketball, cricket, volleyball, rugby, hockey, soccer, and football. These sports differ in their competitive seasons, game lengths, skill requirements, and movement patterns. Additionally, the time of year each sport is played differs. Some sports are played predominantly in the warm summer months, and others in the winter. Some sports are played indoors where the climate may be controlled,

DOI: 10.4324/9781003321286-22

while others are played outdoors and subject to environmental conditions. These factors need to be taken into consideration when preparing nutrition recommendations.

As with individual athletes, the nutritional requirements of team sport athletes depend on the physiological demands, predominant energy systems, duration, frequency, and intensity of the sport. Within a team sport, there are a number of different positions that athletes can play (such as offensive or defensive) and the position an athlete plays may influence their nutritional requirements. For example, in a sport such as soccer (football), the nutrition requirements of the goalkeeper will be different to a position such as a midfielder due to differences in the distance, frequency, and intensity of movements.

Unlike many individual sports and events, team sports require athletes to repeat regular short, high-intensity efforts interspersed with longer periods of rest and low- to moderate-intensity efforts, such as jogging and walking. Therefore, team sports are typically both anaerobic and aerobic (Chapter 2) in nature and, consequently, athletes are required to develop speed, agility, muscular strength, and power as well as endurance. Furthermore, technical and tactical elements are incorporated into the games, with the skills required dependent on the game and position played.

While sports nutrition principles and practices will be similar between individual athletes and team sport athletes, additional issues must be considered regarding nutrition practices of team sport athletes. These issues are discussed throughout this chapter.

Pack mentality

Depending on the sport, the number of athletes in a team can vary from five up to groups as large as 50. Regardless of the size of the team, group dynamics can have a major influence on nutrition practices of athletes.

Pack mentality

For team sport athletes, a pack mentality occurs when individual athletes within the team act in a similar manner to others in the group.

In team sport, it is common for there to be a '**pack mentality**' that influences athletes' behaviours, including their nutrition practices. In the case of nutritional intake, if there are some athletes within the team who follow suboptimal practices or have extreme dietary behaviour, this can influence the overall nutrition practices of the team.

While pack mentality may be seen to negatively influence nutritional intake in some cases, it can also be used to assist in improving nutrition practices of athletes and make positive changes to the nutritional intake of the team.[1] As with any team environment, there will be natural tendencies for some individuals to be leaders. Working with leaders in a team environment who follow optimal nutrition practices is an effective strategy to influence the nutrition practices of other athletes in a team and improve the culture. For example, drinking alcohol after a game is common due to the social nature of team sports. However, when a key team member limits their alcohol consumption, it can positively influence the overall alcohol intake of the team. To improve and influence the nutritional intake of athletes in team sports it is vital to consider the team environment, culture, and natural tendency for a pack mentality to occur.

Blanket approaches to nutrition advice

There are a range of factors that influence the performance of an athlete including fitness, strength, and game tactics amongst others. As such, high-level competitive team sports have a large team of coaching and support staff. Despite its ability to influence performance, nutrition is not always a priority due to budget constraints and competing pressures.

In these high-pressure and simultaneously time-and resource-poor environments, it is common for blanket nutrition advice to be provided to a team of athletes. Blanket nutrition advice can be described as nutrition advice that is the same for all the athletes, and delivered in the same manner, regardless of individual differences. It groups all athletes together (under one blanket), and assumes the information and nutrition advice required is the same. This is problematic. It is well established that individual athletes within a team are unique and will respond differently to nutrition interventions and advice. For example, caffeine has been found to improve athletic performance,[2] but not all athletes respond to caffeine in the same way and athletes also vary in their tolerance of caffeine-containing beverages and supplements. Therefore, athletes require specific, individually tailored, personalised nutrition advice that takes into consideration a range of individual health, social, and sport-specific factors.

Group nutrition education and nutrition knowledge

Although desirable to receive individualised nutrition advice, it is common for team sport athletes to receive group nutrition education. Group nutrition education sessions are advantageous as a time- and cost-effective method to educate and influence nutritional practices. They can also assist in building a positive team environment and culture. However, education provided in a group setting often employs 'blanket' advice and does not cater for the differing nutrition needs or learning preferences of athletes.

Group nutrition education sessions are used to improve nutrition knowledge, and sometimes also food and cooking skills, with the aim of positively influencing nutrition practices of a group of athletes at one time. Evaluation of such sessions is important to identify areas for improvement, their effectiveness in improving nutrition knowledge, food skills, and dietary practices, and to advocate for increased nutrition services.

Food and fluid provision for team sports

The implementation of nutrition strategies in team sports is often subject to rules and regulations that restrict opportunities for intake of food and fluids. While sports such as basketball or Australian football include numerous breaks in play that allow delivery of food or fluids to players, opportunities in other codes, such as soccer (football) and cricket, are much more limited. Often substitutions, treatment of injured players, and half-time breaks are the only times players can access food and fluid, and to do this, they may need to dash to the sidelines. This can pose challenges when trying to replace large fluid losses or provide large quantities of carbohydrate; providing these in large volumes at half-time breaks may lead to gastrointestinal (GI) disturbance. Studies that have informed fluid and carbohydrate intake guidelines have often used protocols that involve providing small amounts periodically, which is impractical in team sports. Therefore, nutrition support needs to be customised to both the sport and the individual.

Competition structure and access to food/fluid during the game

The structure of competition varies between sports and can create difficulties when trying to optimise fluid and food ingestion. For some sports, a greater emphasis may need to be placed on ensuring athletes take every opportunity to rehydrate or ingest carbohydrates. Cricket, for example, may be played in extreme heat, with some formats of the game lasting 6–7 hours per day for five days. Although originally developed in temperate English weather, it is now also played in the harsh Australian summer, the severe heat of Dubai and the extreme humidity in India, with temperatures occasionally reaching over 40°C (104°F). While those in the outfield may have access to drinks on the boundary line, batsmen—who are generally also wearing heavy pads, gloves, and a helmet—may have much more limited access to fluids, with drinks breaks generally scheduled only once per hour (though they break for meals over the course of the day). In Australia, soccer is also played in the summer, with drinks generally only available at the break between 45-minute halves or if there is an extended stoppage in play. In circumstances such as these, it is important to think strategically about providing athletes with optimal nourishment. In cricket, for example, if there is a break in play for injury, to change the ball or if the batsman calls for a new bat or gloves, a drinks runner should be sent out to the players at the same time if possible. In soccer, placing drink bottles around the ground, allowing players to access fluids quickly during stoppages or substitutions, will allow them to maintain a better hydration status. For events lasting 90 minutes or more, it is important to provide fluids such as sports drinks that contain carbohydrate and electrolytes, with added flavours to promote greater intake (see Chapter 11 for more information on hydration).

Whilst important to ensure that opportunities are created for athletes to ingest food and fluid during play where possible, the importance of designated breaks should not be ignored. Sports drinks, along with food or supplements such as fruit, gels, or lollies (candies), should be presented as easily accessible for athletes. Often athletes will have treatment or presentations from the coaching staff during their designated breaks. Setting up their food and drinks on a table just inside the door to the changing rooms may increase opportunities to consume and reduce the risk of missing an opportunity to refuel. For those who have more individualised refuelling strategies, placing the appropriate amount of food and drink in, or in front of, their locker may allow them to adhere to this more easily. While structured breaks such as half-time allow greater opportunity for food and fluid intake, it should also be stressed that trying to achieve recommended intakes needs to be balanced with GI comfort, and force-feeding athletes may actually lead to poorer performance.

Catering for the team

Catering for athletes in the team environment ranges from individual to team-wide provision of food, all of which provide unique challenges. Food provision may be influenced by training and competition schedules, personal preferences, and body composition goals. Addressing all concerns at once can be difficult, and while in-house catering staff could be utilised to accommodate each player's different requirements (as is the case in some larger organisations around the world), smaller organisations may need to bring in outside catering to ensure adherence to budget.

On-site, team-wide catering offers a cost-efficient method of providing nutritious food to athletes. This can be particularly important when the training schedule runs over normal mealtimes. It is not uncommon for players to complete two training sessions each day and this may involve long days with limited opportunities to seek food.

Providing a meal can help players refuel to train and compete at the intensity required; however, it is not as simple as providing sufficient carbohydrate, protein, and fat. In one team, there are differing taste preferences as well as nutrition priorities. The first player in the lunch line may be trying to add muscle mass, while the second is looking to reduce body fat, and the third is recovering from injury. On top of this, each player is a different size and may have a different training load. How then can each player be catered for with one generic meal? To allow each individual to customise their meal, education, and presentation of food is critical; these are discussed below.

Education

While group education may be cost-effective, individual nutrition knowledge is important to help athletes make appropriate food choices, especially when faced with buffet-style catering. Each player should be aware of their own goals, and how nutrition contributes to them, to enable appropriate food choices. Putting up posters or noticeboards in the food provision area may help create an environment that reinforces education. Having the team dietitian and/or other nutrition support staff present occasionally during food service will allow the players to confirm their food choices.

Presentation

Presentation of the food is critical to allow players to customise their own meals. Mixed-meal dishes such as stir-fries and casseroles may not be ideal, as players may have differing protein, carbohydrate, and fat requirements. Separating the protein, carbohydrate and, potentially, the fat (although most meals provided are likely to have low to moderate fat content), allows the athlete to pick and choose ingredients and portion sizes to suit their needs. For example, instead of a stew, it may be more appropriate to offer roast meat, separate starchy and non-starchy vegetables, and a jug of gravy or sauce. Some options, such as burgers, may not need separation, as the athlete can pull them apart to consume what they require. Options such as pasta may not allow easy separation of components but are often very popular among teams, especially in the lead-up to the competition. In such circumstances, it may be worthwhile offering multiple options to accommodate players with lower loads who may be periodising carbohydrate intake (see Chapter 10).

Catering for the individual within the team

Ideally, players will gain the skills necessary to prepare appropriate food that matches their nutrition goals. Occasionally, however, due to lack of time, motivation, or available facilities, this will not occur. In this case, it may be worthwhile exploring catering options for the individual. There are many food service companies that provide meals appropriate for the athlete and are often able to customise meal plans.

Post-game meals

Post-game meals pose some unique challenges. Not only are there many athletes who subscribe to the idea that they can 'eat whatever they want' post-game due to their workloads, some will have large appetites while others will have none at all. Providing foods that meet their nutritional needs for recovery in several different forms can help work around these issues if the athlete is well-educated on suitable choices. Liquids such as flavoured milks are a popular post-match recovery option for those with smaller appetites, while fruit, sandwiches, wraps, protein shakes or bars, muesli/granola bars, and hot meals such as pasta and rice dishes all provide nutritious recovery options. While all of these can be great choices, logistics often preclude offering all of them at once, meaning there will often be some athletes who miss out on their preferred option. A good compromise can be organising a smaller range of more portable foods (such as milk, fruit, sandwiches, shakes, and bars) in the changing rooms post-match with a subsequent meal at a nearby restaurant, depending on the timing of the match.

Travel

Teams that travel for competition or training need to consider several factors relating to nutrition. These vary depending on whether the travel is domestic or international in nature, with domestic travel posing fewer challenges than international travel. When travelling anywhere via air, consideration should be given to food and fluid provision; this is discussed in Chapter 27.

When travelling to a country where the types of foods consumed are significantly different from those in the athletes' home country, efforts should be made to educate players on appropriate food choices. Topics to cover may include avoiding food from areas that have a high risk of food contamination, such as street stalls, and ensuring athletes drink bottled water in areas that do not have safe tap water. Where possible, it is ideal to contact the accommodation or restaurants in which the team will be eating before they travel. Organising a menu of suitable, familiar foods will help reduce the risk of GI issues, or players not eating. Again, having a stockpile of suitable snacks for players will also help them achieve their nutritional goals.

Summary

This chapter has discussed that although 'pack mentality' is common among teams of athletes, each individual athlete is likely to have different goals, taste preferences, learning styles, and motivations. Each of these needs to be taken into consideration, along with the intricacies of each sport, including training schedules and competition structures, when providing food for teams or advising athletes on what to consume. Education is key to empowering individual athletes to make appropriate food choices, and while a blanket approach to nutritional advice may seem tempting, a customised approach is likely to be much more effective. To enable athletes to put their training into practice, it is important to ensure that their food environment is conducive to making good choices. Pre-planning by the nutrition and catering staff will help make the good choice the easy choice.

Chapter highlights

- The different game factors (game length, skill requirements, position played, movement, game breaks, and season played) must all be considered when formulating nutrition advice for individuals in team sports.

- 'Pack mentality' can be used in a positive way to influence the nutrition intake of team sport athletes.
- Ideally, blanket nutrition recommendations need to be avoided and individualised nutrition advice provided in a team sport setting.
- Providing appropriate food and fluid during competition can be complicated by game structure.
- Thinking strategically will ensure athletes have a maximum number of opportunities to refuel.
- Team-wide catering is a valuable tool, but individuals need to receive education to make the right choices.
- When travelling, differences in culture and hygiene standards need to be considered.

References

1. Jenner S, Belski R, Devlin B, et al. A qualitative investigation of factors influencing the dietary intakes of professional Australian football players. *Int J Env Res Public Health*. 2021;18(8): 4205.
2. Burke LM. Caffeine and sports performance. *Appl Physiol Nutr Metab*. 2008;33(6):1319–1334.

20 Weight category and aesthetic sport athletes

Regina Belski

Weight category and aesthetic sport athletes have some additional nutrition considerations that are not strictly linked to performance. For weight category sports, which include sports like boxing and lightweight rowing, athletes are required to be under a certain weight. If an athlete is over the cut-off during the weigh-in, they cannot compete. This can lead to suboptimal practices to 'make weight', including severe fluid and food restriction, use of laxatives and diuretics, and extreme use of saunas. Timing of weigh-ins also varies from sport to sport and even among competitions, with some being immediately before an event and others several days beforehand, so it is vital to understand the rules and processes of the sport and competition in which the athlete is competing.

For aesthetic sports, which include sports like gymnastics, ballet, and diving, there is a strong focus on appearance as part of the way performance is assessed. Problems relating to nutrition can result, as this focus on aesthetics can lead to problems with body image and suboptimal dietary practices to try to control body size or shape.

This chapter discusses the common challenges faced when working with weight category and aesthetic sport athletes and provides some practical strategies on how best to support these athlete groups.

Learning outcomes

This chapter will:

- describe the additional challenges faced by athletes competing in weight category sports;
- describe the additional challenges faced by athletes competing in aesthetic sports;
- present two different approaches to managing the weight-making behaviours of athletes.

Weight category sports

Weight category sports are those sports where athletes are required to compete in weight categories or classes—for example, boxing, lightweight rowing, wrestling, and judo—and sports such as horseracing, where jockeys are weighed prior to every race.

Weight categories were introduced to these sports as additional weight leads to accompanying increases in strength if that weight is derived from muscle mass and puts athletes at a competitive advantage. To create a fair competition, a maximum weight limit is set. Some examples of weight categories used in a selection of sports can be seen in Table 20.1.

DOI: 10.4324/9781003321286-23

Table 20.1 Weight categories for selected sports (International Olympic Committee (IOC) qualification events for Paris, 2024, presented in kg as per the IOC)

Sport	Sex	Weight
Lightweight rowing	Men	≤72.5 kg (team average weight ≤70 kg)
	Women	≤59 kg (team average weight ≤ 57 kg)
Judo	Men	>100 kg >90 kg and up to and including 100 kg >81 kg and up to and including 90 kg >73 kg and up to and including 81 kg >66 kg and up to and including 73 kg >60 kg and up to and including 66 kg ≤60 kg Open, with no weight restriction.
	Women	>78 kg >70 kg and up to and including 78 kg >63 kg and up to and including 70 kg >57 kg and up to and including 63 kg >52 kg and up to and including 57 kg >48 kg and up to and including 52 kg ≤48 kg Open, with no weight restriction.
Boxing (IOC Weight classes in boxing qualification events for Paris, 2024)	Men	51 kg 57 kg 63.5 kg 71 kg 80 kg 92 kg +92 kg
	Women	50 kg 54 kg 57 kg 60 kg 66 kg 75 kg

Source: International Olympic Committee, https://olympics.com/en/olympic-games/paris-2024.

For example, a lightweight rower in great health and achieving personal bests may still have a problem if they weigh in 500 grams (1 pound) over their cut-off, as this means that—regardless of how talented and prepared they are—they cannot compete.

For professional jockeys, there is even more pressure, with failure to meet the weight cut-off for a given race potentially leading to fines and suspensions as well as loss of income. While riding weights around the world range from the set minimum of 51–53 kilograms (113–118 pounds) (which includes the saddle and riding equipment, but not the whip and cap) up to approximately 61–64 kilograms (134–140 pounds), most jockeys strive to be the minimum weight as this increases the number of races they are suitable for/able to race in (based on horse handicapping). For this reason, it is not unusual for weight-making behaviours to occur in these sports.

Common weight-making practices

While making weight may not always lead to problems, extreme weight-making behaviours are problematic. Such weight-making practices include extensive use of saunas to dehydrate the body, use of diuretics, excessive exercise, running dressed in heavy, non-breathable clothing to promote sweating, not eating or drinking, and the use and abuse of diet pills, purging and other such practices.[1] Unfortunately, these more extreme weight-making behaviours have both short-term and long-term health effects and have contributed to the death of athletes in some cases.

It is not unusual to see athletes trying to lose 2–5 kilograms (4–10 pounds) in the days leading up to competition. This will often involve extreme measures, such as cutting/shaving their hair, trimming fingernails and even inducing vomiting or nosebleeds in situations where they are a few grams over the cut-off at weigh-ins.

The potential negative health effects of extreme weight-making include:

- dehydration leading to significant plasma volume loss and increasing risk of heat illness;
- drop in metabolic rate with repeated weight-making practices utilising fasting as a result of muscle loss;
- impaired cognitive functioning, including increased fatigue, confusion, and mood changes;
- lean tissue loss;
- impaired bone synthesis during periods of severe energy restriction, which may make athletes more susceptible to injury and have a long-term impact on bone health.

Managing weight-making

In 2021, The American College of Sports Medicine released an Expert Consensus Statement on Weight Loss in Weight-Category Sports and put forward some important recommendations for safer weight-making practices in weight category sports.[2] There were several that were of relevance for sports nutrition professionals working with athletes in weight category sports, including:

> The selection of a suitable weight category for each athlete, and the timely achievement of true alterations in BM towards the event target should underpin all weight making practices. A suitable weight category is one that can be safely achieved by the athlete without undue physical, nutritional or psychological stress.

The athlete's natural or day-to-day BM should be within reach of their specific weight class, allowing them to achieve their usual training goals while maintaining dietary practices that support adequate energy availability, requirements for all nutrients, and a healthy relationship with food and its contribution to growth, development, and the quality of life.

Hence, when working with athletes in weight category sports, there are two main avenues that can be taken to address weight-making: (1) support the athlete to achieve a 'regular' weight that fits their weight category, thereby removing the need to make weight; or, if this is not possible, (2) support the athlete to 'make weight' in a safe way.

While the first option is obviously desirable from a health perspective and aligns with the abovementioned recommendations, it is not realistic for all athletes, as many prefer to compete at a weight that is far from ideal for their actual body type and shape. Considering that athletes in most weight category sports require significant lean body mass, which increases their overall weight, there arises a conflict between building muscle and being able to compete. It is unfortunately common for coaches to encourage athletes to compete in a lighter weight division than that to which they are naturally best suited, as they are seen as having an advantage over naturally smaller/lighter athletes. While this may be true from a physical strength perspective, an athlete who is severely dehydrated and has not properly eaten is not able to perform at their best.

Weigh-in times in different sports, and even between different levels of competition, vary. Some sports/competitions have athletes weigh in the day before competition, allowing refuelling and rehydration if required, but others have weigh-ins immediately before competition or even, in some cases, before every bout/match, making rehydration challenging for those who have utilised dehydration techniques to make weight. As discussed in Chapter 11, this has a significant impact on performance.

The following section describes some of the approaches athletes may choose to take.

Regular weight = competition weight approach

This is considered the more sensible and healthy approach, as it eliminates the need to 'make weight' and undertake risky diet and/or dehydration behaviours. The approach involves selection of the most appropriate weight category (within 5 per cent of natural weight if possible) for an athlete based on the weight they can attain and maintain while eating appropriately, training well, and performing at a high level. This will involve losing weight for some athletes and gaining weight for others. While this may sound easy and obvious, it is an approach athletes and coaches are often not comfortable with, mostly because once athletes find a place in their 'category' the notion of moving into another category is almost as daunting as changing sports, with changes in the competition and the competitors. It may also be challenging for athletes who do not actually know what their 'normal' non-dieting weight is; this is particularly true for younger athletes who started in a weight category in their late teens and remained in the same category into their twenties despite significant growth in height. These cases can require time to identify the best option—and time is not something that is always easy to find for competitive athletes. Where possible, nutrition professionals can encourage athletes to use the off-season to find a more 'natural' weight. Anthropometric assessment (see Chapter 13 for more details) by a trained professional should be used to help athletes assess the most appropriate weight category in which they should compete.

Where an athlete naturally sits just above a weight class it may not be clear which weight category is best. One option is to encourage the athlete to work on gaining additional muscle mass to gain further strength and get their weight up, closer to the top of the weight category, or alternatively support them to make weight for the lower category in a safe and healthy way in the lead-up to competition.

Safer weight-making practices

From a health perspective, it would be best if athletes did not have to make weight at all; however, this is unfortunately unlikely to be the case where sports remain categorised by weight class. Therefore, it is important to help athletes to make weight in the safest way possible, without compromising short- or long-term health.

This means that athletes need to be encouraged to allow enough time before competition to lose the extra weight. They should avoid dehydration practices or, if they must use them, have adequate time to rehydrate before competition. It should be made clear to athletes that any weight-making strategies are short-term measures—for example, if significant energy or fluid restriction is taking place, it is only for a clearly defined period of time, after which healthy patterns of eating and drinking return. It is easy for athletes to fall into a very restrictive way of eating or disordered eating involving bingeing, purging, or utilising laxatives and/or diuretics as part of their usual routine, compromising their wellbeing and performance. Appropriate strategies for managing weight in weight category athletes are outlined in Box 20.1.

Box 20.1 Examples of advice for weight category athletes aiming for safer weight-making practices

Well ahead of the competition:

- Develop a long-term plan for weight on- and off-season.
- If necessary, consume an appropriate energy-restricted diet aiming for a maximum of 500 grams (1 pound) of weight loss per week (see Chapter 13).

Shortly before competition/weigh-in:

- Avoid high-salt foods that may lead to water retention (for example, processed foods such as deli meat, canned soups/foods, frozen meals, potato chips, soy sauce, pickles, and fast food).
- Aim for a low-residue, low-fibre diet (for example, consume white bread instead of wholegrain, peel fruit and vegetables before cooking/eating, and avoid food made with seeds and nuts).
- Consume appropriate amounts of fluid, making sure that fluid loss does not exceed 2 per cent loss of body weight and is replaced before competition.

Refuelling strategies (if fluid and/or energy restriction was used to make weight):

- Where possible, allow enough time to rehydrate (2–4 days).
- Consume 150 per cent of the fluid loss (for instance, drink 1.5 litres of fluid for each kilogram of weight lost).
- Utilise drinks containing electrolytes and carbohydrate to maximise hydration (see Chapter 11 for more details on optimising rehydration).
- Consume carbohydrates to maximise glycogen stores.

It is important that athletes have an opportunity to consider their options and discuss them with their support team when deciding about the best approach for them. Advice needs to be aligned with the rules of the sport, timing of weigh-ins, and the physiological needs of the athlete. It is strongly recommended that athletes participating in a weight category sport should seek the advice of a qualified sports dietitian to individualise their weight management plan.

Aesthetic Sports

Aesthetic sports are those sports where there is a strong focus on appearance as part of the way performance is assessed. These include dance, gymnastics, aerobics, figure skating, cheerleading, ballet, and diving. In many of these aesthetic sports, how an athlete looks while performing will be a component of how their performance is evaluated. Execution of particular technical movements is important, but so is the grace and beauty of that movement. This is where problems relating to nutrition can arise, as this focus on aesthetics can lead to problems with body image and suboptimal dietary practices to try to control body size or shape. Most commonly, this manifests as disordered eating and energy restriction.[3] Another factor that is not particularly helpful is that athletes often get involved in these sports at a young age, and their bodies continue to grow, develop, and change shape as they age. However, for many athletes these changes can be seen as undesirable; for example, the development of larger breasts and wider hips is not considered desirable for a ballerina. These pressures make teenage girls in aesthetic sports particularly vulnerable to restrictive or disordered eating. More details about disordered eating and the challenges of working with young athletes can be found in Chapters 7 and 23.

Nutrition recommendations for athletes in aesthetic sports need to be particularly mindful of how dietary changes could impact the physical appearance of the individual athlete. While muscle gain is desirable in many sports, for aesthetic athletes, a muscle distribution that is less physically attractive can lead to lower competition scores.

It is important to acknowledge the stereotypical body shapes and physiques found in many aesthetic sports, but also to remind athletes that they are individuals and not everyone is the same. Where possible, it is wise to have some examples of high-performing athletes in their sport with different body shapes from the standard. In gymnastics, a good example is the difference in physique between two top 2008 Beijing Olympic gymnasts, Nastia Liukin and Shawn Johnson (both from the USA team). These two gymnasts have vastly different body shapes; they won both gold and silver medals in the same events, demonstrating that different body shapes can still lead to great outcomes. Simple visual examples can have a significant effect on young, impressionable athletes, and help to encourage even aesthetic sport athletes to focus on optimising their performance more than worrying about the exact size and shape of their bodies. In situations where body-image concerns are present, it is wise to consider the involvement of a sports psychologist to support the athlete.

Summary

This chapter has introduced the nutrition-related challenges faced by athletes competing in weight category and aesthetic sports. Athletes who compete in weight category sports are under extreme pressures to achieve a specific weight to avoid exclusion from competition. Weight-making is a common practice among athletes in weight category sports and can lead to both short- and long-term negative health outcomes; therefore, athletes need professional guidance and support to either attain and compete at a weight that is easily sustainable for the athlete or to support them to make weight in a safer manner. Aesthetic sport athletes are under an additional spotlight in relation to their physical appearance, as how they look when performing is a component of how their performance is evaluated. These athletes are more likely to develop concerns regarding their body image and should be supported to adopt healthy eating practices in line with personalised goals.

Chapter highlights

- Athletes in weight category sports are prone to undertake risky weight-making behaviours.
- Weight category sport athletes should be supported to minimise the need to make weight or do so in a safer manner.
- Aesthetic sport athletes are at higher risk of disordered body image and, hence, disordered eating.
- Aesthetic sport athletes should be supported to focus on their personal goals and performance, rather than on body size or shape.

References

1. Crighton B, Close GL, Morton JP. Alarming weight cutting behaviours in mixed martial arts: A cause for concern and a call for action. *Br J Sports Med.* 2016;50(8):446–447.
2. Burke LM, Slater GJ, Matthews JJ, et al. ACSM expert consensus statement on weight loss in weight-category sports. *Curr Sports Med Reports.* 2021;20(4):199–217.
3. de Bruin AK, Oudejans RR, Bakker FC. Dieting and body image in aesthetic sports: A comparison of Dutch female gymnasts and non-aesthetic sport participants. *Psychol Sport Exerc.* 2007;8(4):507–520.

21 Contemporary sport athletes

Marisa Michael, Aimee Morabito, Kate Gemmell and Adrienne Forsyth

Sports nutrition practice is constantly evolving in response to new evidence and the emergence of new recreational and competitive sports. Funding for sports nutrition is closely linked to sports represented at major international competitions, so sports nutrition professionals may find themselves working with sports newly added to Olympic competition. For the Paris 2024 Olympic Games, this includes breaking (breakdancing), with sport climbing, skateboarding, and surfing having debuted at the Tokyo 2021 Olympic Games.

Learning outcomes

This chapter will:

- outline the premise and competition format of contemporary sports;
- explain the energy systems used in contemporary sports;
- describe training and competition nutrition recommendations for contemporary sports;
- highlight special nutrition considerations for contemporary sports.

Sport climbing

Competition sport climbing is relatively new, with the first formalised competition taking place in Italy in 1985. Since then, it has grown exponentially and debuted as an Olympic sport in the Tokyo 2021 Olympic Games. Competitors include youth climbers and professional/elite climbers. The average age of international elite climbers is 23 years.[1] Formal competitions also often have an adaptive climber/Para climber division.

Competitions take place on an artificial wall, usually indoors, with a point system in place that rewards the climber who can ascend the highest. It includes the disciplines of lead climbing, speed climbing, and bouldering. Lead climbing entails a 15-metre-high wall where the competitor must finish within 6–8 minutes, depending on the competition round, and is often considered "endurance" climbing. Bouldering is climbing without ropes on shorter walls, up to six metres high, and is a more powerful and dynamic style of climbing. Speed climbing matches two climbers side-by-side on two identical routes 15 metres high. They race to the top and whoever is first wins. Current speed climbing times are around 5–6 seconds.

DOI: 10.4324/9781003321286-24

Energy systems

Both aerobic and anaerobic energy systems are used while climbing. Competition routes consist of holds set on artificial walls. These holds vary in shape, size, and distance between each hold. The walls may be straight or overhung at an angle. Both the hold placement and wall angle determine the difficulty of the route and the style of climbing which will be used. Routes that are higher may use more of the aerobic energy system, with a consistent climbing cadence where strength, flexibility, and endurance are tested. Shorter routes for bouldering often demand powerful, quick movements and even jumping or swinging, thus using both aerobic and anaerobic energy systems. Some studies have demonstrated that a greater ability to re-oxygenate muscles after a bout of climbing predicts better climbing performance, and that climbers have a cardiorespiratory fitness similar to other intermittent sport athletes.[2]

Nutrition for training

Training nutrition should include adequate overall energy to support the demands of the sport and prevent relative energy deficiency in sport (REDs). Climbers often have no off-season, so prioritising and periodising nutrition to match the training load is prudent. Allowing for carbohydrate intake to increase with a corresponding increase in training hours may allow for better training outcomes. Youth climbers need to fuel for their training load with additional energy intake to support growth and puberty (Chapter 23).

While evidence-based nutrition guidelines specifically for sport climbing are lacking, sports nutrition professionals can draw on sports of a similar nature, such as intermittent sports, strength-based sports, and sports requiring a high strength-to-weight ratio. As such, it is suggested currently that climbers may need approximately 3–7 g/kg/day of carbohydrates, and 1.3–1.8 g/kg/day of protein. More than these suggested ranges may be needed for intense training loads. Energy intake should be enough to prevent REDs (see Chapter 7), and energy intake must support training loads. Some studies have shown 42–46 kJ/min (10–11 kcal/minute) of active climbing are used, and more energy is often expended if the route is unfamiliar, overhung, or outdoors.[3] Table 21.1 outlines nutrition considerations for a variety of climbing scenarios.

Nutrition for competition

Climbing competition often has several rounds throughout the day and multi-day competitions. Since climbing entails a level of being able to understand which moves would be executed for certain types of routes and holds, climbers are put into isolation prior to climbing the competition route so as to ensure they will not gain an unfair advantage by observing how other climbers are climbing the same route. Climbers should know how long they will be in isolation, how many routes they are climbing, and when they will climb. This will enable them to develop a fuelling and hydration strategy for the duration of the competition.

Fuelling with simple carbohydrates throughout the day at regular intervals will support a climber's energy level without making the stomach too full or heavy to comfortably climb, especially if speed climbing. A general rule of thumb is to aim for about 30 g of carbohydrate per hour, 240 mL of fluids per hour, and protein as needed and tolerated. Avoiding greasy, fatty, or fibrous foods may help support quick digestion and avoid upset stomach. Refer to Table 21.2 for a suggested meal plan for an all-day competition.

Table 21.1 Practical nutrition tips for competitive rock climbing

	Energy expenditure during climb session	Daily carbohydrate intake	Daily protein intake	Fluid intake during climb session	Practical challenges	Practical tips
General training	~10–11 kcal/min	3–7 g/kg BW/day	1.3–1.8 g/kg BW/day; 0.3 g/kg BW per meal or snack, 3–4 times per day	~250 mL/hr water or sports drink	Risk of under-fuelling and under-hydrating with short climbs	Begin training hydrated and fuelled. Use training to test tolerance to foods planned for consumption during competition
Competition speed climbing	Estimated starting point at ~10–11 kcal/min. More research is needed[a]	3–7 g/kg BW/day	1.3–1.8 g/kg BW/day; 0.3 g/kg BW per meal or snack, 3–4 times per day	~250 mL/hr water or sports drink	Risk of over-fuelling and over-hydrating with short climbs	Begin climb hydrated and fuelled. Consume easily digestible foods/beverages after competition to optimise recovery and refuel for subsequent climbs
Competition lead/bouldering	Estimated starting point at ~10–11 kcal/min. More research is needed[a]	3–7 g/kg BW/day; ~20–30 g/hr; recovery meal at end of competition; mouth rinse as required	1.3 g/kg/day; ~10 g/hr between climbs; 0.3 g/kg BW after climbing for recovery	~250 mL/hr water or sports drink	Potential for incomplete recovery between climbs	Eat after competition to optimise recovery and refuel for subsequent climbs. Consume easily digestible foods/beverages
Youth climbers	Fuel for growth and sport	Possibly use less CHO than adults	Follow paediatric guidelines for age group, growth pattern, and activity level	Likely ~250 mL/hr is adequate; monitor for euhydration	Growth pattern needs to be preserved	Track growth patterns and make kcal recommendations accordingly

Source: Michael et al.[4]

[a] ~10–11 kcal/min of active climbing is based on the measured energy expenditure of climbers in a non-competitive situation.[5] More research is needed to determine the actual energy expenditure of competitive climbers.

Table 21.2 Sample meal plan for multi-event, day-long competition*

Event	Time	Time eaten	Food
Breakfast	8 am	Prior to event	Steel cut oats with walnuts, berries, and milk. Orange juice as a beverage
Round 1 climbing	10 am	After event	Pretzels and sports drink
Round 2 climbing	12 pm	After event	Peanut butter and jam sandwich on white bread with apple slices. Chocolate milk as a beverage
Round 3 climbing (isolation)	3 pm	Eat/drink as needed in isolation	Sports gummies and sports drinks. Carbohydrate mouth rinse if well-hydrated
Round 4 climbing	5 pm	Prior to event as required	Raisins and sports drink
Dinner	7 pm	After event	Quinoa bowl with black beans, salsa, cheese, avocado, and ground beef with a fruit and yoghurt smoothie

Source: Michael et al.[4]

* Food and beverage quantities vary based on age, body weight, number of rounds, and discipline.

Special nutrition considerations

Climbing has a culture of promoting weight loss to improve performance. This drive for thinness and optimising strength-to-weight ratio may lead to disordered eating, eating disorders, and REDs. The literature suggests that training hours per week, years of experience, strength, flexibility, endurance, and psychology all play a greater role in climbing performance than weight if the climber is already at an appropriate weight.

Preliminary research attributes between 1.8% and 4% of performance to anthropometric characteristics.[6] Rather than focusing on weight loss for climbing performance, it would likely be more beneficial to support adequate fuelling throughout the training cycle. Sports nutrition professionals should advise climbing athletes to approach weight loss as a performance-enhancing strategy with caution (see Chapter 20). Ensuring the climber is adequately fuelled will help promote performance and prevent REDs.

Surfing

Surfing is one of the most popular lifestyle sports around the world among junior (groms) to senior surfers, with recent advances in competitive surfing seeing the sport debut at the Tokyo 2021 Olympic Games. Surfing is unique in that it is dependent on several environmental conditions including surf break type, swell, tides, and wind. When each of these aligns to produce optimal conditions, surfers can spend several hours surfing, with few, if any breaks.

At a competitive level, 2–4 surfers compete against each other in "heats", generally 20–30 minutes in duration. Within each heat, there is no limit on the number of waves a surfer can catch, within the constraints of the priority rule; however, a surfer's final heat score is the sum of their top two scoring waves. Each wave caught is scored out of 10 points, and is based on commitment, degree of strategy, manoeuvres performed, speed, power, and flow. Surfers with the best score at the end of the heat progress through rounds until they reach finals.

Energy systems

Several activities are incorporated into surfing, requiring both aerobic and anaerobic energy systems. Prolonged periods of endurance paddling accumulate to nearly 50% of total surf time, with the remaining time spent stationary (~40%), paddling at a higher intensity for wave take-off (~5%), and wave riding (<5%).[7,8] These physiological demands are impacted by environmental factors, for example, longer continuous periods of endurance paddling are required at point breaks, compared to beach breaks.

While short (4–5 seconds), high-intensity paddling accounts for a small proportion of surf time, better-performing surfers are able to generate more speed, and ride waves for longer, providing a greater opportunity to perform more manoeuvres. Strength, power, and aerobic capacity are therefore all important requirements for optimal surf performance.

Nutrition for training

Training nutrition for surfing should be individualised to support requirements based on each surfer's level of surfing, training and competition load, cross-training, individual goals, specific requirements to support health, and increased adjustments for growing groms. Surfers may spend several hours per day surfing, limiting their opportunities to eat or drink. When this accumulates over a week, time spent in the water is substantial, increasing surfers' risk of low energy availability. Attention to overall intake is therefore necessary to ensure sufficient energy and carbohydrate availability to support training, minimise early onset of fatigue, and maximise endurance, speed, and power.

Tips

- It is not common practice for surfers to come in from the water during a surf, however, encouraging breaks during prolonged surfing to refuel and rehydrate is one strategy that can assist surf performance and overall energy availability;
- Surfers will often adjust their surfs to accommodate the best wave conditions. Providing surfers with the knowledge and skills to adapt their nutrition intake based on different surf times and durations is important to achieve appropriate fuelling.

Nutrition for competition

During competitions, surfers need to be prepared to surf multiple heats across a single day or consecutive days. Events often start early in the morning, so for surfers competing in early heats, consuming a carbohydrate-rich dinner the night prior, followed by a carbohydrate-rich breakfast will ensure glycogen stores are topped up. Each surfer's preferences and other factors impacting their performance, such as sleep and surf preparation, will influence the timing, type, and amount of food consumed prior to competition.

Duration between heats will vary depending on the event and surf conditions. It is recommended that surfers snack on light, carbohydrate-rich snacks in between heats, particularly if the time between is less than 60 minutes. When there is more than one to two hours between heats, more substantial carbohydrate-rich meals are recommended. Recovery nutrition is particularly important after the final heat of the day and across multi-day competitions.

It is necessary that surfers are aware of how many heats they may need to surf in if they progress to the final, so they can plan their intake throughout, and across days accordingly. However, a consideration in surf competitions is that the time between heats may be impacted by surf conditions. It is not uncommon for heats to be postponed or called off for the day. Therefore, similar to training nutrition, surfers need to be equipped with the knowledge and skills to adapt to late variations in event schedules.

Special nutrition considerations

- Surfers spend much of their surf time in the prone position (lying face down), making gastrointestinal comfort an important consideration. Foods consumed before any surf should be familiar to the surfer, and contain a high amount of easily digestible carbohydrates while being low in fibre and fat content.
- Surf locations may be remote with little, if any, access to food. Surfers need to account for this in their planning and pack snacks, meals, and fluids accordingly – that is food required before, during, and after a surf, and in between heats on competition days.
- Surfers should aim to start their surf well-hydrated, as fluid loss is likely to increase with surf duration, increased air, and water temperatures, and with the addition of neoprene wetsuits.[9] Like refuelling, there is no opportunity to hydrate during a surf.

Skateboarding

Skateboarding was first invented around the 1940s–1950s in California as a way for surfers to practice when the surf was flat. Since the 1940s, skateboarding has grown and flourished into an extreme sport (e.g. skate parks, ramps, big airs, speed skating) as well as a leisure activity and a mode of travel. Skateboarding debuted as an Olympic sport at Tokyo 2021 with the disciplines of street and park in both men's and women's competitions, and featured medalists as young as 12 years old. Street skateboarding involves flat-ground tricks, grinds, slides, and aerials in a street-based environment. Common items found in a suburban street such as bins, stairs, handrails, and picnic tables can be traversed as part of a single trick or a series of tricks known as a line. Park skateboarding takes place in a purpose-built skatepark and involves riding bowls, transitions, verts, and grinds; this usually includes skating lines and flowing through different sections of the park. Park requires the use of a skatepark whereas street can be done on any street with skate obstacles. Park is normally based on building up speed to perform bigger airs and tricks.

Competitions take place outdoors at purpose-built street or park facilities. In the park discipline, 20 athletes compete in a preliminary round of four 45-second heats with five athletes per heat. Five judges score the runs on a 0–10 point scale. The top three scores count and the top eight athletes progress to the finals. In the final, athletes have three 45-second runs and the best score wins.

In the street discipline, 20 athletes compete in a preliminary round of four 45-second heats and five trick attempts with five athletes per heat. Five judges score the run and tricks on a 0–100 point scale. The top eight athletes progress to the final which consists of two runs and five tricks where again, the top score wins.

Energy systems

Given the short nature of competition, mostly anaerobic energy systems are at play. However, in the days leading up to competition, the skateboarders are given pre-competition practice which usually involves the athlete familiarising themselves with the park or street layout and practising their lines and tricks. This practice involves repeating the 45-second run over and over and would likely engage both anaerobic and aerobic energy systems depending on the difficulty of the park layout and time spent out on the course. Skateboarding is an intermittent sport so during practice athletes stop frequently, allowing the energy systems to regenerate ATP and reoxygenate muscles. On competition day, athletes are given a 5-minute warm-up period to practice their tricks before the competition. Given the intermittent nature of this practice and the 45-second competition runs, the entire competition would mostly involve anaerobic energy systems.

Nutrition for training

Skateboarding training is usually unstructured and casual in nature, often involving the athlete grabbing their board and going out for a skate. As the sport has progressed to the Olympic level, athletes now have access to professional support including coaches, physiotherapists, sports doctors, strength and conditioning staff, and sports nutrition professionals. This has changed the training scene for many skateboarding athletes who previously did not have access to these services. Athletes need to make sure they are consuming adequate energy to match their training demands and minimise the risk of REDs. Since many skateboarders are adolescents, growth and development need to be factored into their energy requirements.

As skateboarding is a relatively new sport there is a lack of research into the nutrition requirements specifically for skateboarding. However, like sport climbing, recommendations can be drawn from other intermittent sports (see Table 21.1), with requirements varying based on athletes' age and stage of development as well as school, other sports, work, life, and training demands. Energy intake should be sufficient to prevent REDs and athletes should be monitored to ensure they are consuming adequate intake for their training demands.

Hydration is an important factor during training as athletes are more likely to engage the aerobic energy systems and increase their sweat rates. Skateboarding is also often practised outdoors during warmer atmospheric conditions and in skateparks that are made of concrete which become very hot. Adequate fluid intake is essential to support concentration and performance throughout training. Due to the intermittent nature of training for skateboarding, athletes have ample opportunity to take on foods and fluids and should be adequately fuelled and hydrated.

Nutrition for competition

Skateboarding competitions are relatively short in nature as there is a maximum of five rounds of 45-second runs per athlete, which is less than 4 minutes per athlete in total. Each athlete has ample time in between their runs to re-fuel and rehydrate, if needed. Nutrition is most important in the lead-up to competition where athletes should focus on carbohydrate and fluid intake. Given skateboarding requires short sharp skills and quick reflexes and reactions, anything that affects concentration is going to be crucial. Adequate carbohydrate intake will ensure the brain and working muscles have plenty of fuel at hand. Hydration is particularly important for concentration and reaction times so the athletes will need to be well hydrated and should be monitoring their hydration status in the lead-up to the competition as well as on the day of competition.

Special nutrition considerations

Skateboarding is an extreme sport and with extreme sport comes extreme risk. It is common for skateboarders to fall, lose skin, bleed, bruise, and break bones. For this reason, iron and calcium are of particular importance for skateboarders. The need to support healing and rehabilitation is further compounded by extra nutrient requirements to support the growth and development of younger athletes. See Chapter 16 for more information about nutrition for injury management and rehabilitation and Chapter 23 for more information about the nutrition needs of young athletes.

Another consideration in skateboarding is that competitions and athletes are often sponsored by energy drinks. Athletes can be supplied with generous amounts of energy drinks that they may overconsume, which is particularly problematic for young skateboarders for whom energy drinks are not appropriate. Careful consideration of caffeine intake is required for this group of athletes including the time of day it is consumed, how it impacts other aspects of life, whether the athlete is old enough to understand the effects, caffeine sensitivity, and carbohydrate intake associated with supplements such as energy drinks.

Breaking

Breaking, also known as breakdancing, is a dance style that emerged with hip hop culture in New York in the 1970s. The popular urban dance form has a well-established international competition circuit and is one of the newest additions to the sport list at the Olympic Games, contested in Paris 2024 after first debuting at the Summer Youth Olympic Games Buenos Aires 2018.

Breaking involves combinations of dance elements referred to as top rock, down rock, and freezes. Top rock refers to standing dance moves, down rock refers to moves performed on the ground including spins and power moves, and freezes are isometric holds, often supporting body weight in challenging positions with one or two hands only (Table 21.3). Movements tend to be quick and explosive, combining elements of dance and acrobatics.

In social settings, breakers dance in cyphers where breakers form a circle and take turns dancing within the circle. The competition involves battles that can be performed solo or in crews (teams), where competitors take turns performing before a panel of

Table 21.3 Elements of breaking

Element	Description
Top rock	Standing moves while preparing to go down to the floor
Down rock	Moves in contact with the floor using hands, back or chest *Drops*: movements to transition to the floor *Footwork/legwork*: steps while breaking on the ground *Spins*: turn of at least 360 degrees on the ground or in the air *Power moves*: fast dynamic movements with spinning motion; usually without feet touching the floor *Blow ups*: quick and explosive movement combinations *Air moves*: jumps, flips, and air spins *Transitions*: linking moves to create a cohesive performance
Freezes	A held position usually requiring great balance, flexibility, and strength

Source: Adapted from World Dance Sport Federation Breaking Rules and Regulations Manual.[10]

judges who judge based on six criteria: creativity, personality, technique, variety, performativity, and musicality. Competitions often begin with round robins or showcase rounds from which the top 8 or 16 performers are selected to compete in knock-out battles until a champion is awarded. Battles are typically comprised of three to five sets of 45–90 seconds each (three sets of 60 seconds each for Olympic competition). Battles often run continuously with very few breaks in competition, so competitors have a rest time between battles that is only as long as the duration of other battles and any discretionary time permitted by judges. The number of battles a breaker performs in competition will vary depending on their competitive success.

Energy systems

With improvisation common, and no set requirements for the number and type of elements used in competition, it is difficult to ascertain in advance the specific physiological requirements of competition. Studies of oxygen utilisation suggest that breaking is a higher intensity activity than many other forms of dance but is still considered to be an aerobic sport.[11] Breaking involves multiple short high-intensity intervals, with average VO_2 less than 90% VO_2max but reaching peaks of 90–99% VO_2max.[11]

In competition, breaking will draw on all energy systems to varying degrees depending on the intensity of the performance. Muscle glycogen can be expected to be a significant fuel source but does not risk depletion with a total performance time of less than 30 minutes.

Nutrition for training

Recommendations for nutrition strategies in breaking may be drawn from related sports such as rock climbing, gymnastics, and other genres of dance. Nutrition strategies should be individualised, periodised, and practical for the individual athlete. Energy intake should be adequate to fuel exercise and energy availability but closely monitored to achieve physique goals. Given the importance of physique in the ability to perform some breaking moves and the impact of aesthetics in some elements of judging, practical strategies for attaining a desired physique should be considered. A focus on building lean mass with less emphasis on weight loss and energy restriction, as explained in Chapter 17, maybe a useful strategy to achieve reductions in fat mass while maintaining/gaining lean tissue.

Nutrition for competition

In competition, athletes will need to consider the availability of appropriate and familiar foods and where possible bring their own foods that are convenient to consume between battles. Foods should be trialled in training to ensure they are well tolerated, and breakers should be encouraged to plan their competition day diet in advance.

A small carbohydrate-rich meal/snack may be consumed prior to and between battles to help replenish fuels used and support carbohydrate availability throughout the competition. High-fibre foods should be avoided prior to and during competition to promote gut comfort. Complex movements involving twisting, bending, and inversion may also be less comfortable immediately after drinking or with a full bladder, so the timing and amount of fluid ingestion should be planned to maximise comfort in performance while maintaining hydration for physical capacity and mental acuity, and this should be practised in training to identify an individualised solution.

Special nutrition considerations

Breakers, like other dancers, have been found to have low levels of vitamin D.[12] This is particularly problematic given the high incidence of injuries in breakers.[13] Vitamin D status should be monitored, and calcium and vitamin D supplements considered where recommended by a doctor or sports nutrition professional. Iron status should also be monitored as the high rate of haemolysis[14,15] combined with energy restriction places dancers at high risk of iron deficiency.[16]

While breaking has historically had a strong culture of clean living, supplements such as creatine, caffeine, and whey protein isolates are likely to be of benefit to support training and performance goals and emerging research suggests these are being used in practice by elite breakers.[12] Breaking has only recently been supported by many state and national sporting associations, so breakers may not have had advice from sports nutrition professionals, and be reliant on peers, coaches, and the internet including social media for their training and nutrition advice. Sports nutrition professionals working with breakers will need to be well-versed in popular diets and be prepared to discuss modified versions of these diets to build rapport with clients. Using a supportive client-centred approach may enable sports nutrition professionals to effect positive dietary change for motivated athletes.

Summary

This chapter has introduced contemporary sports – sport climbing, surfing, skateboarding, and breaking, outlined the energy systems used, and described nutrition considerations for training and competition. As new Olympic sports, evidence to support performance nutrition is emerging and sports nutrition professionals may be guided by evidence-based recommendations for similar sports as well as guidance from athletes and their performance teams.

Chapter highlights

- Contemporary sports use a combination of aerobic and anaerobic energy systems and include powerful movements that require muscular strength, power, flexibility, and agility.
- Nutrition for training in contemporary sports should be individualised and periodised to strategically support energy and carbohydrate availability as well as training goals.
- Energy and carbohydrate use during competition is unlikely to deplete glycogen stores; however, adequate hydration and carbohydrate intake will support physical preparedness and mental acuity.
- Gut comfort is important to consider for sports where athletes need to twist, turn, and perform powerful movements.
- It is important to understand the competition structure and physical environment in which training and competitions occur, and plan adaptable nutrition plans accordingly.
- Athletes in sports new to Olympic competition may have had little exposure to high-performance teams and sports nutrition professionals, and there may be limited

evidence-based sport-specific nutrition recommendations, so guidance may be taken from more established sports with similar physiological requirements.

- Contemporary sports typically attract a broad age range of competitors, with Olympians as young as 12 and over 40 competing in sports like skateboarding. Nutrition education and support strategies should be adapted to account for different dietary needs across the lifespan, as well as individual circumstances and preferences.

References

1. IOC Buenos Aires 2018 Youth Olympic Games: Proposal for Additional Sports. (2018, July 18). https://stillmed.olympic.org/media/Document%20Library/OlympicOrg/Games/YOG/Summer-YOG/YOG-Buenos-Aires-2018-Youth-Olympic-Games/ba2018-new-sports-Annex-1-Factsheets.pdf#_ga=2.63287211.520424737.1531853538-2019145073.1485288774
2. Fryer SM, Giles D, Palomino IG, de la O Puerta A, España-Romero V. Hemodynamic and cardiorespiratory predictors of sport rock climbing performance. *J Strength Condition Res.* 2018;32(12):3534–41.
3. Mermier CM, Robergs RA, McMinn SM, Heyward VH. Energy expenditure and physiological responses during indoor rock climbing. *Br J Sports Med.* 1997;31(3):224–8.
4. Michael MK, Witard OC, Joubert L. Physiological demands and nutritional considerations for Olympic-style competitive rock climbing. *Cogent Med.* 2019;6:1667199.
5. Watts PB, Daggett M, Gallagher P, et al. Metabolic response during sport rock climbing and the effects of active versus passive recovery. *Int J Sports Med.* 2000;21:185–190.
6. Mermier CM, Janot JM, Parker DL, et al. Physiological and anthropometric determinants of sport climbing performance. *Br J Sports Med.* 2000;34(5):359–65.
7. Farley ORL, Secomb JL, Raymond E, et al. Workloads for competitive surfing: work-to-relief ratios, surf-break demands, and updated analysis. *J Strength Condition Res.* 2018;32(10):2939–48.
8. Minehan CL, Pierra DJ, Sheehan B, et al. anaerobic energy production during sprint paddling in junior competitive and recreational surfers. *Int J Sports Physiol Perform.* 2016;11(6):810–15.
9. Atencio JK, Armenta RF, Nessler JA, et al. Fluid loss in recreational surfers. *Int J Exerc Sci.* 2021;14(6):423–34.
10. World Dance Sport Federation. World Dance Sport Federation Breaking Rules and Regulations Manual. https://www.worlddancesport.org/Division/Breaking. 2023.
11. Wyon MA, Harris J, Adams F, et al. Cardiorespiratory profile and performance demands of elite hip-hop dancers. *Med Probl Perform Art.* 2018;33(3):198–204.
12. Montalbán-Méndez C, Giménez-Blasi N, García-Rodríguez IA, et al. Body composition and nutritional status of the Spanish national breaking team aspiring to the Paris 2024 Olympic Games. *Nutrients.* 2023;15(5):1218.
13. Tsiouti N, Wyon M. Injury occurrence in break dance: an online cross-sectional cohort study of breakers. *J Dance Med Sci.* 2021;25(1):2–8.
14. Carlson DL, Mawdsley RH. Sports anemia: a review of the literature. *Am J Sports Med.* 1986;14(2):109–112.
15. Peeling P, Dawson B, Goodman C, et al. Athletic induced iron deficiency: new insights into the role of inflammation, cytokines and hormones. *Eur J Appl Physiol.* 2008;103(4):381.
16. Sousa M, Carvalho P, Moreira P. Nutrition and nutritional issues for dancers. *Med Probl Perform Art.* 2013;28(3):aa119–23.

22 Occupational athletes in the military

Bradley Baker

Occupational athletes include military and emergency service professionals who perform roles with extreme physical and/or cognitive demands, often under various physical, physiological, and cognitive stressors. They include a range of military occupations, such as those with front-line ground combat roles, Special Forces soldiers, as well as emergency services professionals (such as firefighters both in the military and general population). The focus of this chapter will be on occupational athletes in the military, with particular emphasis on those in the army. Due to their high demands, occupational athletes, like sports athletes, often seek enhancement of their training adaptations, performance, and competitiveness on the battlefield through nutrition strategies.

Learning outcomes

This chapter will:

- define and identify occupational athletes, including those who perform roles with high demands;
- outline physical, physiological, and cognitive demands placed on occupational athletes in the military according to the role they perform;
- describe the key factors that influence the energy, macronutrient, and micronutrient requirements of occupational athletes in the military;
- outline nutrition-related barriers facing occupational athletes in the military;
- describe nutritional strategies which can enhance the health, performance, and safety of occupational athletes in the military.

Physical, physiological, and cognitive occupational demands

The physical, physiological, and cognitive demands placed on occupational athletes in the military vary depending on the stage of their career or occupation, and are further influenced by a wide range of factors. In the context of the Australian Army, new recruits undertake approximately 6 months of physically and mentally demanding training, known as Initial Training (IT). This begins with Basic Training (BT), which lasts for almost 3 months. Following recruits' successful completion of BT, they graduate to the rank of trainee and then undertake their Initial Employment Training, an almost 4-month course that is tailored to their chosen career pathway (i.e. Infantry, Combat Engineering,

DOI: 10.4324/9781003321286-25

Artillery, Armour, and Transport). The entire duration of Australian Army IT is characterised by the physical, physiological, and cognitive demands of training for supporting and undertaking ground combat. The energy expenditures of male and female Australian Army recruits are approximately 16 MJ (3,825 kcal) and 11.5 MJ (2,750 kcal), respectively.[1,2] Those destined for front-line combat roles, such as Infantry trainees, often display higher energy expenditures. Male and female Infantry trainees can expend up to 19 MJ (4,545 kcal) and 13 MJ (3,110 kcal) per day, respectively. Following their successful completion of IT, all new Army members begin their occupation in their area of speciality, with varying demands depending on the nature of their role.

Army occupations that engage in front-line ground combat have high demands, particularly when undertaking field training and deployment. For example, Infantry/front-line soldiers perform their ground combat roles on foot, for prolonged periods of 8 hours or more, in varying terrain and weather conditions (including heat and cold), often while carrying heavy loads of equipment, ammunition, water, and food (which can total 50 kg or more). They require the endurance to cover varying distances on foot, often under time pressures dictated by the tactical situation. They also require the strength to perform demanding tasks such as moving heavy equipment and performing stretcher and casualty carries. Other front-line Army occupations, such as Combat Engineers, require the endurance and strength to perform tasks such as constructing and destructing battlefield infrastructure (e.g. bridges, roads, bunkers, fortifications, and obstacles) and clearing terrain under arduous conditions. Similar to Infantry soldiers, they may also engage in front-line ground combat, and thus perform their roles under multiple stressors.

All occupational athletes in the military who may be engaged in front-line combat require the cognitive ability to perform complex tasks under various psychological stressors,[3] including the stress of operating in life-threatening situations.[4] Indeed, they often train under, and perform roles involving, intense psychological stress,[3] with six overarching psychological stressor dimensions having been described by Bartone[5]: isolation, ambiguity, powerlessness, boredom (alienation), danger (threat), and workload. Moreover, they may undertake field training and deployment involving prolonged periods of sleep deprivation,[6] all stressors that must be mitigated to enable them to meet their cognitive demands (e.g. alertness, attention, and vigilance) and maintain their overall job safety and performance.[7] Thus, depending on the role they perform, occupational athletes in the military train and work under multiple, superimposed physical and cognitive stressors.[8]

The level of physical and cognitive demands involved in an occupational athlete's role is a major determinant of their energy expenditure. Energy expenditure studies using the doubly labelled water method have shown the average energy expenditure of military personnel to be comparable to that of some sporting athletes, but highly varied depending on their occupation and the nature of the training they are undertaking.[1,2,9] The energy expenditures of 424 male military personnel from various countries were assessed, with their average energy expenditures ranging from 13.0 to 29.8 MJ (3,109–7,131 kcal) per day depending on the occupation being studied. A total of 77 female military personnel, also from various countries, were assessed among the reviewed studies, with their energy expenditures ranging from 9.8 to 23.4 MJ (2,332–5,597 kcal) per day.[9] Personnel with energy expenditures at the lower end of these ranges are typically those with occupations that support front-line combat operations (e.g. those who specialise in communication systems, intelligence, logistics, transport, maintenance, health and catering).

In contrast, those in specialist front-line combat occupations, such as Special Forces soldiers, Naval Clearance Divers, and US Marines, display the highest daily energy expenditures, especially when undertaking field training and deployment.[1,2,10] Exceptionally high daily energy expenditures of 28 MJ (6,695 kcal) and 29.8 MJ (7,130 kcal) have been reported during Australian and US Special Forces field training courses, respectively.[1,2,10] Comparatively, when undertaking their day-to-day training on a military base, Special Forces soldiers typically expend up to 18 MJ (4,300 kcal) per day.[1,9] Other soldiers with physically demanding roles, such as Infantry soldiers and Combat Engineers, typically expend up to 16 MJ (kcal) per day when undertaking day-to-day training on a base.[1,2,9] The day-to-day job of combat soldiers can involve challenging physical training sessions, to maintain and build their fitness commensurate with their job requirements, as well as training and rehearsing combat skills and tactics.

Occupational athletes in the military may have limited time and opportunities to eat and drink when performing their roles, in particular during arduous field training and deployment. For those who perform front-line ground combat roles, such as Infantry soldiers, their ability to eat and drink is often dictated by the tactical situation.[8] Depending on the nature and duration of their mission, a range of other factors may hinder their dietary intakes, such as limited time to prepare and eat food during fast-paced missions, and limited space and capacity to carry sufficient food while also needing to carry several days' supply of other critical supplies such as water, ammunition, and equipment. The multi-stressor environment of combat field training and deployment may also suppress their appetite, particularly during missions involving severe sleep deprivation.[11] Thus, despite their heightened physical and cognitive demands during arduous field training and deployment, they may be in substantial energy deficit, adding further physiological stress.[8] Studies show that substantial daily energy deficits corresponding to ≥40% of daily energy requirements often occur during arduous field training and deployment lasting up to 2 weeks.[1,8,12] Thus, consideration should be given to whether or not occupational athletes' eating opportunities may be limited during their training and/or deployment when determining appropriate and realistic nutrition strategies.

Nutrition strategies to optimise health, performance, and safety

Due to the physical, physiological, and cognitive demands placed on occupational athletes in the military, their nutritional requirements are often far greater than those of the general adult population. Nutrition strategies to optimise their health, performance, and safety should be tailored based on their role, the volume and intensity of physical activity they undertake, and their overall energy, macronutrient, and micronutrient requirements. Therefore, sports nutrition professionals working with them (whether individuals or populations) should ask the following questions:

- What is their role?
- What stage of their career or training are they currently in, and are they currently undertaking a field training course or deployment (that would elevate their nutritional requirements)?
- Do they perform a front-line ground combat role that involves particularly high physical, physiological, and cognitive demands?

- What types of physical activity do they undertake on a day-to-day basis, whether training on base or in the field, both as part of their role and in their own time? For example, strength conditioning, running, swimming, marching (with or without load carriage), fire and movement, carrying heavy equipment and/or completing obstacle courses.
- Approximately how many hours of each type and intensity of physical activity do they undertake per day, both as part of their role and in their own time?
- What literature exists on the energy expenditure and nutritional requirements of this individual or population?
- What is their level of nutrition knowledge and self-efficacy specific to their occupational demands?

Evidence-based military-specific nutrition guidelines should be applied in strategies to improve the self-efficacy, eating behaviours, and dietary intakes of occupational athletes in the military. Many nations have adapted their respective national recommended dietary intake values to meet the needs of their military members, and these should be used as a reference point. For example, the Australian Defence Force (ADF) has adapted the Nutrient Reference Values (NRVs) for Australia and New Zealand into Australian Defence-specific nutritional requirements and criteria.[1,2] Five categories of Military Recommended Dietary Intakes (MRDIs) have been established to account for the varying physical activity levels of Australian Defence Force Members according to their occupation and the stage of their career and training they are in.[1,2] These MRDIs can be used for assessing the adequacy of dietary intakes of Australian occupational athletes in the military. Similar reference documents exist around the world.

Energy

Occupational athletes undertaking arduous combat training and deployment should aim to minimise their overall energy deficit over the duration of their bout of field training or deployment to levels below which performance decrements occur.[12] A meta-analysis by Murphy et al.[12] showed that the losses of body weight that occur during combat training and deployment involving energy deficit are significantly associated with losses of both lower-body power and strength. They found that to prevent small (2%) declines in lower-body performance, the total cumulative energy deficit should not exceed 80 MJ (19,120 calories) over the duration of field training or deployment. Further, they found that minimising total cumulative energy deficits to less than 164–248 MJ (39,196–59,273 calories) can prevent larger losses of lower-body power and strength of 8–10%. Thus, the energy requirements of occupational athletes undertaking arduous field training and deployment should be determined, and their total daily energy intakes should be planned accordingly over the planned duration of their field training/deployment.

Carbohydrate

When undertaking activities involving prolonged and/or intermittent, moderate-to-high intensity physical activity lasting ≥60 minutes, carbohydrate intakes of occupational athletes should be in accordance with the levels required for athletic training and competition.[13] In the instances of army recruits and soldiers in physically demanding occupations who are undertaking day-to-day training on a military base, their carbohydrate intakes should be at least 6 g per kilogram of body weight per day to support their fuel requirements.[13] During more demanding army training courses, and demanding field training, individuals should ideally achieve higher levels of carbohydrate intake, between 8 and 10 g per kilogram of their body weight per day, to support their fuel needs and facilitate the rapid and maximal restoration of glycogen stores between exercise bouts.[13] Occupational athletes who undertake exceptionally high volumes of physical activity, such as members of the Special Forces when they are undertaking particularly arduous field training, should ideally achieve an intake of 10–12 g/kg of carbohydrate.[13] However, it must be acknowledged that occupational athletes in the military may not always be able to achieve their optimal intakes during arduous training and deployment, due to the constraints discussed in this chapter. Depending on the situation, an intake of 6–8 g/kg of carbohydrate may be more achievable for short periods during particularly fast-paced training and deployment, and until rest and recovery can occur. When undertaking any prolonged moderate-to-high intensity activity on-base, such as part of their regular physical training sessions or routine physical fitness assessments, occupational athletes should aim to optimise their pre-training or pre-assessment carbohydrate intakes in accordance with the levels needed during athletic training and competition.[13] During any prolonged moderate-to-high intensity activity, occupational athletes should aim to regularly eat and drink high-carbohydrate foods and fluids, also in accordance with the levels recommended before and during athletic training and competition.[13] During field training and deployment, eating high-carbohydrate foods and fluids whenever the operational situation best allows, as frequently as possible, should be achieved.

Protein

Occupational athletes in the military require protein intakes comparable to those recommended for other types of athletes. Intakes of 1.5–2.0 g/kg per day have been suggested to support their training adaptations, recovery and overall health.[1,2,14,15] Protein distribution across the day should also be advised as discussed in Chapter 9 to optimise lean body mass. Further, more recent data suggests that during periods of unavoidable energy deficit, such as during arduous field training and deployment, this regular and even pattern of protein intake may lead to greater preservation of lean body mass (e.g. skeletal muscle).[15,16]

Micronutrients

Occupational athletes in the military should aim to achieve vitamin and mineral intakes in accordance with their appropriate recommendations or MRDIs where available.[1,2] Failure to achieve recommended micronutrient intakes may impair their health and overall job performance and safety, particularly for key micronutrients such as iron, calcium, and vitamin D.[17] This is particularly pertinent during demanding and prolonged training courses. Females' iron status has been shown to decline during basic training, with decreased iron status associated with decreased running performance in routine fitness tests.[18] Thus, females' iron status should be assessed, particularly during demanding and prolonged training and deployment.[18]

Practical strategies

Occupational athletes often receive Combat Ration Packs (CRPs) or Meal, Ready-to-Eat (MRE) as their sole source of food during field training and deployment when fresh food provision isn't possible (e.g. due to the tactical situation). These ration packs/meals are specially designed to provide significant energy intake (e.g. >16 MJ in Australian CRPs) and nutrients while being suitable for the environments in which they are consumed. They are required to meet a wide range of requirements, such as being sufficiently shelf-stable to withstand high temperatures and durable to be carried and tightly packed into backpacks and pockets. Further, foods must be provided that are convenient to eat while on-the-move, and that are also as lightweight as possible, especially if multiple days' supply of food must be carried. Individuals may also choose to carry extra foods for variety and to supplement their intake according to their personal preferences. For these reasons, examples of suitable foods can include specific varieties of muesli and cereal bars, energy bars, fruit bars, tuna pouches, trail mix, freeze-dried meals, **retort packet** ready meals, instant mash, powdered meal replacement beverages that are forti- fied with essential vitamins and minerals, powdered sports drinks, beef jerky, and confec- tionary (including sports confectionary).

Retort packet

A flexible laminate package in which perishable food items are preserved by physical and/or chemical means.

Summary

This chapter has outlined how occupational athletes in the military can have high physi- cal, physiological, and cognitive occupational demands, and appropriate nutrition is a paramount consideration in enhancing their health, performance, safety, and overall effectiveness on the battlefield. This is particularly important for occupational athletes who undertake training and deployment involving front-line ground combat. Adopting appropriate nutritional strategies, in accordance with evidence-based guidelines, should be promoted to occupational athletes, with practical guidance for meeting these guide- lines through appropriate foods and fluids.

Chapter highlights

- The energy and nutrient requirements of occupational athletes in the military are often far greater than adults in the general population, and are highly varied according to the physical, physiological, and cognitive demands of their chosen occupation.
- Depending on their sex, the stage of their career and their chosen occupation, the energy requirements of occupational athletes in the military vary greatly (between approximately 11.5–29.8 MJ (3,109–7,131 kcal) per day).
- Soldiers who undertake front-line ground combat have particularly high nutrient and energy demands, especially when undertaking field training and deployment.
- Protein and carbohydrate recommendations for occupational athletes in the military are comparable to those of other athletes based on their training and work perfor- mance requirements.
- Over the duration of their bout of field training or deployment, occupational athletes undertaking arduous combat training and deployment should aim to minimise their total cumulative energy deficit in order to prevent performance decrements from occurring.

References

1. Forbes-Ewan C. Australian defence force nutritional requirements in the 21st century (version 1). Defence Science and Technology Organisation, DSTG-GD-0578, Human Protection and Performance Division, Victoria, Australia; 2009.

2. Peterson R, Baker B, Probert B, et al. Australian Defence Force Nutritional Requirements and Criteria: 2022 Updates (Version 2). Defence Science and Technology Group, DSTG-GD-1164, Land Division, ACT (Australia); 2022.

3. Flood A, Keegan RJ. Cognitive resilience to psychological stress in military personnel. *Front Psychol.* 2022;13:809003.

4. Dekel R, Solomon Z, Ginzburg K, et al. Combat exposure, wartime performance, and long-term adjustment among combatants. *Military Psychol.* 2003;15(2):117–131.

5. Bartone PT. Resilience under military operational stress: can leaders influence hardiness? *Military Psychol.* 2006;18(S1):S131–S148.

6. Miller NL, Shattuck LG, Matsangas P. Sleep and fatigue issues in continuous operations: a survey of US Army officers. *Behav Sleep Med.* 2011;9(1):53–65.

7. Lieberman HR. Nutrition, brain function and cognitive performance. *Appetite* 2003;40(3): 245–254.

8. Tassone EC, Baker BA. Body weight and body composition changes during military training and deployment involving the use of combat rations: a systematic literature review. *Br J Nutr.* 2017;117(6):897–910.

9. Tharion WJ, Lieberman HR, Montain SJ, Young AJ, Baker-Fulco CJ, Energy requirements of military personnel. *Appetite.* 2005;44(1):47–65.

10. Hoyt RW, Jones TE, Stein TP, et al. Doubly labeled water measurement of human energy expenditure during strenuous exercise. *J Appl Physiol.* 1991;71(1):16–22.

11. Radcliffe PN, Whitney CC, Fagnant HS, et al. Severe sleep restriction suppresses appetite independent of effects on appetite regulating hormones in healthy young men without obesity. *Physiol & Behavior.* 2021;237:113438.

12. Murphy NE, Carrigan CT, Philip Karl J, et al. Threshold of energy deficit and lower-body performance declines in military personnel: a meta-regression. *Sports Med.* 2018;48:2169–2178.

13. Burke LM, Hawley JA, Wong SH, et al. Carbohydrates for training and competition. *J Sports Sci.* 2011;29(S1):S17–S27.

14. Pasiakos SM, Montain SJ, Young AJ. Protein supplementation in US military personnel. *J Nutr.* 2013;143(11):1815S–1819S.

15. Fonda C, Baker B, McLaughlin T, et al. Australian Combatants' Protein and Amino Acid Requirements and Recommendations for Combat Ration Packs. Defence Science and Technology Group, DSTG-GD-1174, Land Division, ACT (Australia); 2022.

16. Gwin JA, Church DD, Wolfe RR, et al. Muscle protein synthesis and whole-body protein turnover responses to ingesting essential amino acids, intact protein, and protein-containing mixed meals with considerations for energy deficit. *Nutrients.* 2020;12(8):2457.

17. Maughan RJ, Burke LM, Dvorak J, et al. IOC consensus statement: dietary supplements and the high-performance athlete. *Int J Sport Nutr Exerc Metab.* 2018;28(2):104–125.

18. Martin NM, Conlon CA, Smeele RJ, et al. Iron status and associations with physical performance during basic combat training in female New Zealand Army recruits. *Br J Nutr.* 2019; 121(8), 887–893.

23 Young athletes

Helen O'Connor and Bronwen Lundy

Engagement in physical activity has a range of important physical, social, and mental health benefits for young people. Young prepubertal athletes are often engaged in more than one sport, even at a relatively high level. However, as they progress into adolescence and reach national or internationally representative levels, sports participation becomes increasingly specialised, typically focusing on only one sport.

Nutrition is important for young athletes to support overall growth and development as well as optimal sports performance. Engagement in sport has the potential to motivate improved dietary practices to support performance improvement. In developed countries, and increasingly in developing countries, young athletes experience an obesogenic environment and the literature suggests that athletes—even those at elite or professional levels—consume diets that are not consistent with public health or sports nutrition guidelines although there is evidence that the dietary intakes of young athletes are superior to their non-athletic counterparts). Typical food habits in childhood and adolescence—which include a preference for fast foods, inadequate vegetable intake, and high intakes of nutrient-poor discretionary foods and sugar-sweetened beverages—are also reported in young athletes.[1] There is a need for nutrition education which includes skills in shopping and cooking throughout these developmental years. As young athletes may spend much of their spare time training, they often have less time to participate in or observe food preparation skills in the home.

Young athletes can also be at an increased risk of inadequate or inappropriate dietary intake or supplement use. These risks may result from the additional demands of training on their capacity to consume a diet that has sufficient energy and macro- and micronutrients. Additionally, pressure to attain a specific weight or body composition can encourage restrictive eating practices or the use of inappropriate dietary supplements or ergogenic aids, contributing to this risk. Clearly, childhood and adolescence are important life stages for growth and development, as well as an opportunity to establish healthy eating habits, a positive relationship with food and a robust body image.

Learning outcomes

This chapter will:

- describe special nutritional requirements and considerations for young athletes;
- explain the challenges of ensuring young athletes consume sufficient energy and nutrients to sustain growth as well as optimise training adaptations and sports performance;

DOI: 10.4324/9781003321286-26

- describe differences in thermoregulation between young and adult athletes and how this may impact hydration strategies and the risk of exertional heat illness;
- explain how dietary supplements are attractive to young athletes but also the potential risks associated with their use at the early phase of their development and sports career.

The role of nutrition in supporting growth and development of young athletes

During childhood, growth and development are relatively steady and occur at a similar rate in boys and girls. The physical strength and exercise capacity of prepubertal males and females is generally similar at this age stage and, although they often compete separately, many recreational sports permit them to compete together. During puberty, the rate of growth increases until peak height velocity is reached. This more rapid rate of growth is often referred to as the pubertal growth spurt, although it is important to recognise that the onset and growth rate during this 'spurt' varies widely. Females generally commence their growth spurt and reach peak height velocity two years earlier (~12 years) than males.

High-level engagement in sport can sometimes make it more difficult for young athletes to consume sufficient energy to meet the demands of training, especially during the pubertal growth spurt when there are additional energy demands for growth. Inadequate energy intake can result in delayed growth and, sometimes, increased fatigue, poor recovery, and a range of more serious consequences if this is chronic. Although increased physical activity usually increases appetite to a level that helps the young athlete match their energy needs, young athletes will still need specific guidance to help plan their dietary intake around training demands. This can also sometimes be the case when there is a relatively rapid increase in the duration or intensity of training, which can occur when a young athlete is identified for a talented athlete program or if they move up to a new training level.

There are several practical factors that can make it more difficult for young athletes to consume sufficient energy. The demands of busy training schedules, either before or after school, can reduce the time available for food preparation and consumption. Some young athletes avoid food and/or fluid close to or during training sessions due to issues with gastrointestinal (GI) discomfort or the fear of experiencing a 'stitch'. These issues are more common in sports that involve running, jumping, or tumbling, as opposed to swimming and cycling where the torso experiences less impact. Young athletes usually need to consume additional food and fluids during school hours to meet their higher energy demands; preparing and carrying the additional food, or accessing this at school, presents another challenge. Higher intakes can sometimes result in comments from other, less active peers about the volume of food consumed, which can make some feel self-conscious. Fussy eating can also challenge the attainment of sufficient energy and addressing this merely by increasing the volume of a limited range of foods can make the diet monotonous and unappetising. Younger athletes need support and encouragement to widen the range of foods consumed, which is valuable for positive longer-term health and performance outcomes.

Special nutrient requirements of young athletes

Protein

Children and adolescents need additional protein (compared to adults) to support growth with many dietary guidelines recommending in the order of 3–18% more protein per kg body weight for children relative to adults. Adult athletes need additional protein to assist in the growth and/or maintenance of lean body mass and there is some evidence for a similarly increased protein requirement (1.35–1.6 g/kg BM/day) in young athletes, especially in adolescents with high musculature or undergoing heavy training.[2] As young athletes in developed countries typically consume around 1.2–1.6 g/kg BM/day of protein, it is anticipated that almost all would obtain sufficient protein from food and not require a supplement.[3]

Sufficient energy intake is critical to the maintenance of positive **nitrogen balance** in athletes. In practice, inadequate energy is more often a factor limiting muscle gain than inadequate protein; however, younger athletes on restrictive diets may be at risk of both inadequate energy and protein intake. Although the research on protein requirements in athletes focuses on adults, it seems likely that younger athletes would benefit from strategies used by adults to optimise the development and maintenance of muscle, including the distribution of protein over the day and protein intake around the time of training (see Chapter 9).

Nitrogen balance

Nitrogen is a component of amino acids, so changes in nitrogen status are reflective of changes in protein status. A positive nitrogen balance, where nitrogen is accrued, indicates protein gains, while a negative nitrogen balance indicates protein loss.

Carbohydrate

As with protein requirements, there is limited research on how the carbohydrate requirements of young athletes differ from those of adults. Early muscle biopsy studies found that young athletes have greater oxidative enzyme concentration and aerobic capacity, and less adaptation to anaerobic enzyme capacity.[4] They have been reported to rely more on oxidative (aerobic) metabolism during exercise.[5] Other studies have shown no difference in adaptation compared to adults.[6] Taken together, there is little evidence to support major differences in carbohydrate adaptation or fuel utilisation between younger and adult athletes.

Athletes should focus on planning carbohydrate intake around exercise duration and intensity (see Chapter 9 for recommended intake ranges). Young athletes typically have lower training volumes than adults, although this depends on both the sport and the individual athlete. This is usually the case for endurance and team sports, where training loads are built gradually until training loads are similar to those of adults in late adolescence. For this reason, carbohydrate loading is not necessary for young athletes until they undertake longer-duration endurance events in late adolescence.

Micronutrients at risk in young athletes

Young athletes commonly have insufficient intakes of calcium and iron,[3] especially female athletes after menarche when menstrual loss increases iron requirements. Iron loss may also be greater in athletes participating in endurance sports (see Chapter 17). Iron intake is usually lower in athletes restricting energy intake and sometimes in those who are vegetarian or eat less animal protein (see Chapter 5).

Calcium is another key nutrient, given the increased requirement during childhood and adolescence to support bone development. Inadequate calcium intake is often reported during childhood and adolescence in the general population and is also commonly reported in studies of young athletes. This may have a lifelong detriment to bone health. The risk of inadequate intake is increased in those who avoid or restrict dairy products.

Vitamin D is another nutrient which may be lower in athletes who train longer hours indoors or in latitudes where there is less sunlight and foods are not fortified with vitamin D. Sunscreen use, while important to prevent sun damage, does limit the synthesis of vitamin D from the skin, so sun exposure without burning, where possible, is a valuable strategy to support adequate vitamin D levels. Athletes with darker skin and those who wear full-length clothing will produce less vitamin D from sun exposure and may be more reliant on obtaining vitamin D from dietary sources.

It is important to recognise that the use of supplements to treat an existing nutrient deficiency may be warranted. This should be undertaken after a medical diagnosis and in conjunction with professional support from a sports nutrition professional to assist the athlete to improve dietary intake and prevent future deficiency through a balanced intake of whole foods.

Thermoregulation and hydration in young athletes

Historically, it was believed that children were less able to regulate their body temperature than adults, but this has now been disproven. Children's greater surface area-to-mass ratio is actually an advantage for heat loss in most circumstances, except when the environmental temperature is greater than skin temperature (>3°C (37°F)).[7] In practice, younger athletes do not usually train or compete at the same work rates as adults; rather, they exercise at loads commensurate with their age and body size, which protects them from excessive heat storage.[7] Children also have higher skin blood flow during exercise, and this promotes increased convective heat loss. Children do sweat less than adults but this actually helps to reduce the risk of hypohydration. Relative to their body mass, prepubertal athletes have been shown to have better evaporative cooling than young adults. The smaller, more diffuse sweat drops produced in prepubertal children promote better evaporation than larger sweat drops in adults, which tend to join and drip rather than evaporate from the body. The lower body mass in children essentially means they need to produce less sweat than adults to maintain heat balance for the same change in core temperature.[7]

The American Academy of Pediatrics policy statement[8] concluded that young athletes do not have less effective thermoregulatory ability, insufficient cardiovascular capacity, or lower physical exertion tolerance compared with adults during exercise in the heat if adequate hydration is maintained. Aside from inadequate hydration, the primary determinants of reduced performance and exertional heat-illness risk in youth during sports in hot environments include undue physical exertion, insufficient recovery between repeated bouts of exercise, and closely scheduled same-day training sessions or competition rounds. Inappropriate clothing, uniforms, and protective equipment also play a role in excessive heat retention. In practice, serious heat illness in young athletes is infrequently reported in the medical literature, suggesting that such events are rare.[7] In practice, many of the strategies for hydration and competition refuelling used for adults are appropriate for young athletes. Although the volumes of fluid required are less for young athletes, they should still aim to reduce net fluid loss to <2% of body weight (see also Chapter 11).

Risks and challenges associated with optimising physique attributes in young athletes

Physique is an important attribute for success in many sports. Characteristics such as larger stature and arm span are important for shooting and reach in sports such as basketball, swimming, and tennis, while in gymnastics, diving, and figure skating, a shorter, compact frame facilitates the ease of aerial rotation. Other physique characteristics important to many sports include increased muscularity and lower levels of body fat. Although these can be modified by diet and training, they are also under genetic control and so there are limits to the capacity for change. Natural physique attributes are often early influencers of sport selection. Boys who are muscular and tall for their age may be attracted to sports such as rugby union rather than gymnastics.

The timing of the onset of puberty may also influence sport success. In contact football sports such as rugby, there is concern that early pubertal development provides an unfair advantage for talent identification over athletes of the same age who are relatively prepubertal but similarly or more talented than their earlier-developing counterparts. The reverse is also true in some women's sports, where the desired body shape and size are closer to the prepubertal physique. Normal changes that occur during puberty, including an increase in both muscularity and, predominantly in females, acquisition of body fat, may result in some talented athletes developing a physique that is less desirable for their sport.

Restrictive eating, dieting, disordered eating, and energy deficiency in young athletes

Risks of restrictive eating and dieting

Young athletes in sports where leanness is highly desirable (such as gymnastics, ballet, diving, or figure skating) or weight-making sports (such as lightweight rowing, boxing, and martial arts) are at an increased risk of restrictive eating, which can have negative short- and long-term consequences. In the short term, they may consume inadequate energy to train effectively, recover, adapt, and improve performance. Growth may also be compromised. Inadequate carbohydrate intake may result in glycogen depletion, and this can increase fatigue and reduce training capacity and the potential for optimal metabolic adaptation. Inadequate protein intake may compromise growth and lean mass development. When overall food intake is reduced, there is also an increased risk of deficiency of key micronutrients.

Disordered eating and eating disorders

Dieting may develop into disordered eating over time and can happen gradually and without the awareness of the young athlete, coach, or parent. The disordered eating patterns can eventually progress to an eating disorder such as anorexia or bulimia nervosa. Although prevention should always be the primary aim, when disordered eating behaviours develop, early intervention is essential and is associated with significantly better longer-term outcomes. Although disordered eating can be difficult to identify in its early stages, athlete, coach, and parent education can assist with earlier recognition of the problem.[9]

Young athletes should not be encouraged to reduce weight or body fat without serious consideration of the potential negative effects. Weight management in young athletes requires clinical expertise and professional support from a sports nutrition professional. Critical comments about weight or body composition often initiate inappropriate dieting, and this increases the risk of adverse outcomes in young athletes who are vulnerable to misinformation and may seek to rectify their weight 'problems' with 'fad' diets or non-evidence-based approaches. Once disordered eating practices develop they are difficult to reverse and intensive clinical intervention from a psychologist/psychiatrist and a dietitian is required. Medication, family therapy and, sometimes, hospitalisation may be needed. The development of an eating disorder can seriously jeopardise the future sports prospects of the athlete and lead to poorer longer-term physical and mental health. Making the decision about whether a young athlete with disordered eating should continue participating in sport can be challenging. Guidelines for sport exclusion and return to play have been developed on a score-based system and can help coaches and practitioners make objective decisions.[10]

Relative energy deficiency in sport

Relative Energy Deficiency in Sport (REDs) is described in detail in Chapter 7. Whilst all athletes may experience exposure to low energy availability, young athletes may be more at risk due to the needs for growth and pubertal development. For young female athletes, menstrual cycles may be less well-established and more easily disrupted than in mature females. Body image and peer influence may increase the risk of restrictive eating patterns and the influence of REDs on bone health is also more severe at this life stage.

Sports supplement use in young athletes

Young adolescent athletes in sports where larger mass and muscularity are important may be attracted to use supplements to support lean mass gain. While cautious use of supplements, particularly balanced products such as liquid meals, can assist young athletes in meeting energy needs more easily, heavy use of single nutrient supplements, such as protein powders and amino acids, may displace healthy foods and potentially increase the risk of ingestion of substances prohibited for use in sport. Even if the athlete is not yet undergoing drug testing, some of these substances (for example, stimulants and anabolic steroids) are detrimental to health. Stimulant abuse can result in a wide range of negative health consequences, including addiction/dependence, headaches, GI upset, and interrupted sleep patterns. Anabolic steroids can result in increased aggression and liver or heart damage, along with a range of other serious effects.

These substances may be contaminants in the product and not disclosed on the label. There is also evidence that early use of supplements for lean mass gain may later influence the inclination to use substances prohibited by sports drug agencies. For these reasons, a 'food first' approach is recommended for athletes younger than 18, with supplement use limited to sports foods (carbohydrate-electrolyte drinks, gels, sports bars, and liquid meals) rather than ergogenic aids.[11] Young athletes have so much development potential from training, and the use of ergogenic aids at this stage introduces additional risk; performance assistance is best incorporated after optimising young athletes' preparation through a well-designed eating plan, effective training, psychological strategies, and technical development. Supplements are often viewed as the 'magic bullet' and can contribute to a 'win at all costs' mentality. The risks of supplement use often remain poorly understood at this developmental stage.[3]

Summary

This chapter has discussed the special nutrition needs of young athletes to support growth and development as well as training. These mostly revolve around the need for additional energy and for key nutrients such as protein, carbohydrate, iron, and calcium. The additional needs for protein and carbohydrate are generally consistent with adult athletes per unit of body weight, although more research is required. Strategies such as carbohydrate loading are not needed until late adolescence, as the durations and distances of endurance events are shorter for young athletes. At this stage, developing athletes are often conscious of body image and can be vulnerable to restrictive eating, energy, and nutrient deficiency. Support to maintain a positive body image and a healthy diet is crucial to optimal physical and mental health. Where warning signs of RED-S or disordered eating emerge, early professional intervention supports more positive longer-term outcomes. Despite earlier concerns, younger athletes are not at a greater risk of exertional heat illness than adults. Finally, young athletes are often attracted to dietary supplements and ergogenic aids. At this age, a 'food first' approach is recommended with an overarching philosophy of encouraging healthy eating and physical, mental, and technical development over the use of supplements (unless there is a deficiency), particularly ergogenic aids.

Chapter highlights

- Young athletes have special nutrition needs. There is an increased requirement for energy, especially during adolescence, to support the accelerated rate of growth and development, in addition to the needs of training.
- Young athletes may undertake restrictive eating to reduce weight or body fat and this can result in insufficient energy consumption. This not only increases fatigue and compromises training adaptations and performance but also places the young athlete at increased risk of relative energy deficiency in sport (RED-S).
- Young athletes on restrictive diets are at risk for micronutrient deficiency, as requirements for nutrients such as iron and calcium are increased during growth and development.
- Eating disorders, and restrictive eating that progresses to disordered eating, pose a serious risk to both physical and mental health. Disordered eating can be triggered by negative comments about weight or shape or the recommendation to lose weight or fat without support from a qualified health professional. Young athletes are at a vulnerable stage of life and a positive body image must be nurtured.
- Limited research in young athletes indicates that macronutrient requirements per kilogram of body weight are similar to those for adult athletes, although, as they usually train and compete for shorter durations, carbohydrate intake should be periodised to training loads and strategies such as glycogen loading are not needed until late adolescence.

- Although young athletes had initially been reported to thermoregulate less effectively than adults, recent research indicates they are not at significantly greater risk of exertional heat stress when compared to adults. Many of the strategies used for hydration and competition fuelling can also be applied in principle to young athletes.
- Ergogenic aids, while popular at this stage, should generally be avoided and a 'food first' approach encouraged. A key strategy for sports nutrition at this phase of development is to ensure the athlete develops knowledge, skills, and increasing independence in selecting a healthy diet.

References

1. Parnell JA, Wiens KP, Erdman KA. Dietary intakes and supplement use in pre-adolescent and adolescent Canadian athletes. *Nutrients*. 2016;8(9):526.
2. Aerenhouts D, Deriemaeker P, Hebbelinck M, et al. Energy and macronutrient intake in adolescent sprint athletes: A follow-up study. *J Sports Sci*. 2011;29(1):73–82.
3. Desbrow B, Leverrit M. Nutritional issues for young athletes: Children and adolescents. In LM Burke & V Deakin (Eds), *Clinical Sports Nutrition* (5 ed.). McGraw-Hill Education (Australia); 2015.
4. Erickson BO, Saltin B. Muscle metabolism in boys aged 11–16 years. *Acta Pediatrica Belgica*. 1974;28S;257–265.
5. Taylor DJ, Kemp GJ, Thompson CH et al. Ageing: Effects on oxidative function of skeletal muscle in vivo. In Frank Norbert Gellerich, Stephan Zierz (Eds), *Detection of Mitochondrial Diseases. Developments in Molecular and Cellular Biochemistry*, (Vol. 21). Springer; 1997.
6. Haralambie G. Enzyme activities in skeletal muscle of 13–15 years old adolescents. *Bull Eur Physiopathol Respir*. 1982;18(1):65–74.
7. Rowland T. Thermoregulation during exercise in the heat in children: Old concepts revisited. *J Appl Physiol*. 2008;105(2):718–724.
8. American Academy of Pediatrics, Council on Sports Medicine Fitness, Council on School Health, et al. Policy statement-Climatic heat stress and exercising children and adolescents. *Pediatrics*. 2011;128(3):e741–e747.
9. Wells KR, Jeacocke NA, Appaneal R, et al. The Australian Institute of Sport (AIS) and National Eating Disorders Collaboration (NEDC) position statement on disordered eating in high performance sport. *Br J Sports Med*. 2020;54(21):1247–1258.
10. De Souza MJ, Nattiv A, Joy E, et al. 2014 Female Athlete Triad Coalition consensus statement on treatment and return to play of the Female Athlete Triad. *Br J Sports Med*. 2014;48(4):289.
11. Barkoukis V, Lazuras L, Lucidi F, et al. Nutritional supplement and doping use in sport: Possible underlying social cognitive processes. *Scand J Med Sci Sports*. 2015;25(6):e582–e588.

24 Masters athletes

Janelle Gifford and Helen O'Connor

The incidence of chronic conditions such as obesity, type 2 diabetes, cardiovascular disease (CVD) and musculoskeletal disorders increases with age, placing added pressure on health and societal systems for their management and treatment. Adopting or maintaining a healthy lifestyle with attention to good nutrition and physical activity reduces the risk of developing these conditions and may be effective in their management. Older people who participate in competition or systematic training can be defined as masters (older, veteran, senior, mature) athletes. They may have been active all their lives or have become active to improve their health or treat one or more lifestyle-related conditions.[1] As with younger athletes, the nutritional needs of masters athletes vary according to the type, duration, and intensity of activity, but there are changes in the underlying physiological processes with ageing and any health conditions that may be present add complexity to determining needs. Physical activity also has positive effects on the physiology of ageing, which may have beneficial outcomes. Each masters athlete is, therefore, unique in their physiological profile and requirements.

Learning outcomes

This chapter will:

- define the term 'masters athlete';
- describe some of the physiological changes that may affect the nutrition requirements of masters athletes;
- outline general changes to nutrition requirements with age;
- describe how common nutrition-related chronic conditions may affect the nutrition requirements of masters athletes;
- explain the role of supplements in the diet of the masters athlete.

The changing nutrition requirements of the masters athlete

The definition of masters athletes usually varies according to sport; competitions generally include those 35 years of age or older, but there are younger competitors in some sports (e.g., gymnastics and swimming). The broad age range means that basic nutrition requirements can vary widely. There are no formal sports nutrition guidelines for masters athletes, so guidance may be based on sport-specific recommendations for younger

DOI: 10.4324/9781003321286-27

athletes,[2] physiological changes associated with ageing,[3] and general dietary guidelines which vary for specific age groups This section provides a brief overview of the latter two.

The reduction in the metabolically active fat-free mass (FFM), including muscle tissue, that occurs with ageing, along with a potential reduction in activity or training, translates to a decrease in energy requirements for some masters athletes. However, the energy requirements for masters athletes will be higher than for their inactive peers due to their higher activity levels. If the amount of energy they consume is limited (e.g., to achieve a particular physique), it may be more challenging to meet macronutrient requirements for activity, particularly for carbohydrate. For example, a 70 kg (154 lb) male endurance athlete exercising at moderate to high intensity would require 6–10 g/kg BM/day of carbohydrate,[2] equating to 6720–11,200 kJ/day (1600–2680 kcal/day). While carbohydrate uptake may not be affected by age,[3] glycogen storage may be reduced and fat oxidation may be enhanced as athletes age.[4] The change in fuel storage and usage is a consideration for strategies, such as carbohydrate loading, which is often used to optimise performance in endurance events; if used the standard protocol may need to be modified following practice in training.

Similarly, digestion and absorption of protein do not appear to change significantly with age; however, protein requirements increase due to factors such as a decline in anabolic response to protein intake and disease processes (such as insulin resistance).[5] Additionally, any reduction in energy intake may compromise muscle mass, making protein intake particularly important. Masters athletes may need ≥1.2 g/kg BM/day[5] depending on their age, and 35–40 grams of leucine-rich protein following muscle-damaging exercise rather than the 20 grams usually recommended for younger athletes.[6] However, protein intake does need to be lower for those with impaired kidney function (e.g., because of diabetes). As with younger athletes, attention to timing of intake (in relation to resistance training and distribution of intake over the day) and type (e.g., leucine-containing, fast acting) and quality of protein are important considerations in nutrition advice to support exercise for masters athletes (see Chapter 9 and Bauer et al.[5]). Food sources of high biological-value protein, such as lean red meat, fish, eggs, and poultry and dairy foods, are good protein choices for masters athletes.

Changes in gut function can affect the absorption and digestion of some micronutrients, increasing requirements for calcium, iron, zinc, and B vitamins.[3] Following menopause, hormonal changes also impact bone density and subsequent calcium requirements for women, however, iron requirements reduce. Reduced skin capacity to synthesise vitamin D, reduced immune function, change in liver uptake of vitamin A and increased oxidative stress may increase the need for vitamins A, B6, C, D, E, and zinc.[3] Supplementation may occasionally be clinically indicated; however, increased needs can generally be met with a balanced diet, particularly with the increased food intake needed to meet the demands of sport.

Physiological changes that affect fluid needs should be considered in advice on hydration for the older athlete. Masters athletes may have a decreased thirst perception, reduced kidney function, and altered thermoregulatory mechanisms.[3,7] Reduced thirst perception may increase the risk of hypohydration via reduced fluid intake; however, slower water and sodium excretion may increase the risk of hyponatraemia and hypertension in some masters athletes.[7] This latter risk is potentially greater for smaller and slower masters athletes exercising in cool conditions, since these factors lower fluid requirements. For masters athletes, exercising for long durations and/or in the heat, commercial carbohydrate-electrolyte drinks (such as sports drinks) may be a useful fluid-replacement choice.[1] The use of ice 'slushies' may also be useful in some circumstances. However, a fluid-replacement plan developed by a sports nutrition professional and tailored to the fluid and electrolyte losses of the athlete would be optimal for masters athletes, given their potentially altered physiological and health status.

As men and women age, there may be changes in recommendations for different food groups which should be taken into account in nutrition advice given to masters athletes. Foods in the grains group (e.g., wholegrain breads and cereals) may decrease with decreased energy requirements, while serves of dairy foods and alternatives may increase due to changes in bone health and the increased need for calcium, particularly for women. These are important for masters athletes, since they are good sources of carbohydrate, protein, and energy for physical activity and recovery, as well as micronutrients such as B vitamins. When energy intake is more restricted, the quality of the diet is important so energy-dense, nutrient-poor foods (such as cakes, take-out foods, and sugar-sweetened beverages) should be minimised.

Chronic health conditions in older athletes

While the limited research that has been conducted on masters athletes suggests they may be healthier than their non-active counterparts, masters athletes may still need nutrition advice for conditions such as obesity, type 2 diabetes, CVD, and changes in musculoskeletal function that also aligns with performance goals.

The reduction in energy requirements with ageing can lead to weight gain in the form of fat mass (FM). There is no single dietary approach to guarantee weight reduction; however, an energy deficit created by reducing energy intake and/or increasing energy expenditure is necessary to affect a change in FM. Low glycaemic index, higher-fibre carbohydrates (such as wholegrains and fruits and vegetables), and protein foods (such as meat, dairy foods, and nuts) increase the feeling of fullness and can be incorporated into weight management plans. For masters athletes, periodising energy requirements to support the needs of training and competition, and reducing energy intake on rest days or outside of competition, could accommodate both weight reduction and performance goals.

Increased overall and abdominal FM increases the risk of developing type 2 diabetes and CVD. There is a further increased risk of CVD in people with type 2 diabetes. Dietary management of type 2 diabetes usually includes weight reduction, management of carbohydrate intake, and strategies to reduce the risk of or manage concurrent CVD. For many masters athletes, carbohydrate is an important fuel source, particularly for moderate- to high-intensity training and events that last longer than 60–90 minutes.[2] Masters athletes with type 2 diabetes are advised to consume good-quality (low glycaemic index, wholegrain, higher fibre, and unrefined) sources of carbohydrates, such as dairy foods, wholegrains, fruit, and low glycaemic index starchy vegetables (such as legumes) spread over the day and mapped around training and competition needs. In long training sessions or events, there may be a need for more refined carbohydrate sources such as sports (carbohydrate-electrolyte) drinks or gels to assist in the provision of sufficient glucose to maintain energy and blood glucose. Masters athletes who take glucose-lowering medications may need to adjust their dosage with the support of their physician or diabetes educator, as there is a higher risk of hypoglycaemia with exercise.

Reduction in weight, attention to quality of dietary fat and plant sterols, increase in soluble fibre and reduction in sodium are frequently used strategies to manage CVD for those with or without type 2 diabetes. Previous or current relative energy deficiency in sport (REDs) has also been linked to cardiovascular risk factors such as changes in endothelial function and early atherosclerosis.[8] While fat is energy dense, the inclusion of mono- and polyunsaturated fats (MUFAs and PUFAs) and reduction of saturated fats (as in butter, palm oil, and many processed foods) is important to manage blood fats and other CVD risk factors. Sources such as oily fish, nuts, and mono- and polyunsaturated spreads and most vegetable oils are good choices. Changes in endothelial function, including stiffening of artery walls with age, may contribute to hypertension; however, active individuals are more likely to have healthy arterial function. Diets that have plenty of vegetables (such as the Mediterranean or dietary approaches to stop hypertension (DASH) diets) may assist with lowering blood pressure and other cardiovascular risk factors due to their nitrate content, and nitrates may also enhance performance in some sports.[9] Reduction in sodium intake to manage hypertension may conflict with sports nutrition advice to increase sodium intake for optimising fluid balance and should be managed by a sports nutrition professional.

Two common changes in musculoskeletal function with age are a decline in bone mineral density (BMD), leading to osteopenia or osteoporosis, and the development of osteoarthritis (OA). Postmenopausal women may experience a deterioration in bone health leading to an increased fracture risk due to the decline in circulation of the protective hormone, oestrogen. History of amenorrhoea may also contribute to poor bone health in women; however, REDs (which may cause amenorrhea) may also affect hormonal balance and bone health in men.[8] BMD increases with weight-bearing activity (walking, running, resistance training), so masters athletes with a history of participation in cycling and swimming may have lower BMD at certain sites (e.g., the spine) than masters athletes with a history of sports such as running. Weight-bearing exercise and the inclusion of calcium and vitamin D according to population guidelines are recommended for both female and male masters athletes for optimal bone health. With respect to OA, the principal nutrition strategy is weight reduction to reduce the load on affected weight-bearing joints. Supplement use is relatively common for the treatment of OA but is often ineffective.

Finally, the physiological effects of medications taken to treat chronic disorders should be considered when providing nutrition advice for health and performance.

Supplements in older athletes

Supplements can be categorised as medical supplements, specific performance supplements, and sports foods such as sports drinks. Supplement use is common among athletes at all levels; however, types and reasons for use may be different for masters athletes versus their younger counterparts. This section focuses on medical and sports performance supplement use in masters athletes. Masters athletes commonly use supplements for injury or other health reasons, whereas younger athletes are more likely to use supplements for sports performance. This pattern may partly reflect the use of supplements in the general population.

Masters athletes may take medical supplements for a variety of health reasons, either self-prescribed or recommended by a health professional or others. For example, many take omega-3 fatty acids in fish oils in the belief they will have a positive effect on CVD risk factors; however, these are best sourced from foods such as oily fish (as in the Mediterranean diet). Calcium and vitamin D supplementation may be taken, particularly by female masters athletes, to improve bone health; however, dietary sources of these nutrients are also available. Consuming good sources of calcium (dairy foods and calcium-fortified foods), with the dose divided over the day (more in the evening), will help to maximise absorption.[1] Vitamin D can be obtained from wild-caught oily fish, liver, eggs, and fortified foods; however, prudent exposure to sunlight and/or medically supervised supplementation may be necessary to obtain adequate vitamin D.[1] Supplements for OA are some of the most investigated in older populations. Evidence for the use of substances with anti-oxidant activity (vitamins A, C, and E, and selenium), fish oil supplements, glucosamine, and chondroitin sulphate is not consistent or conclusive in relation to the management of OA.[1] Masters athletes might take vitamin and mineral supplements for the health benefits of some nutrients within a restricted energy budget; however, overconsumption of some nutrients could be harmful.

There are few studies specifically on the performance effects of supplements in masters athletes, so benefits for masters athletes are generally inferred from studies in younger athletes. However, physiological changes in nutrient absorption and metabolism in masters athletes may mean some supplements do not have the same effect as for younger athletes. There is always the concern of harm to health or performance. For example, caffeine is known to enhance endurance performance in younger athletes but may acutely affect blood pressure, which could be problematic for masters athletes with hypertension. On the other hand, supplements such as creatine and whey protein may assist functionally in masters athletes, limiting muscle loss and promoting muscle gain in older individuals. Creatine may also potentially enhance cognitive function.[10] Competing masters athletes should be cautious about taking any supplement, as some products may contain substances banned by the World Anti-Doping Agency (WADA) or may interact with medications.[11] While checking the ingredients list of the product may seem a prudent safeguard, ingredients may be omitted from the list or the product may be inadvertently contaminated by substances during manufacture. Quality assurance programs are now available for testing products and some products will carry a logo as proof of testing.

Summary

This chapter has outlined the diversity in masters athletes in terms of age and ageing, general health, and goals for their sport and general physical activity. There are no formal sports guidelines to support masters athletes' performance and health, and blanket guidelines would be a challenge given this diversity. However, nutrition recommendations for the general population can help us to consider the physiological effects of ageing and should be used as a basic framework to map dietary plans of masters athletes. Guidance for specific sporting requirements can be taken from those of younger athletes while considering the physiological changes that occur with age and any underlying chronic nutrition-related conditions. Supplement taking is common in all athletes, however, may be taken in masters athletes more commonly for health reasons. This may put athletes at risk of adverse consequences including over-consumption of nutrients, interactions with medications, and testing positive for banned substances in competition. Advice should be sought from a sports nutrition professional to support masters athletes in planning their diet for health and performance.

Chapter highlights

- The broad age range of masters athletes and differences in general health means that basic requirements can vary widely within this group.

- There are no formal sports nutrition guidelines for masters athletes. Guidance may be inferred from general dietary guidelines for specific age groups, information on physiological changes with ageing and sport-specific recommendations for younger athletes.
- Potential changes in physiology and physiological function in the masters athlete include a reduction in FFM, changes in glycogen storage capacity, reduction in absorption and digestion of some micronutrients, reduced immune function, and increases in oxidative stress.
- General population guidelines consider physiological changes with ageing and can be used as a basic framework for the diet of masters athletes.
- Chronic nutrition-related lifestyle conditions may alter nutrition advice given to athletes; however, a sports nutrition professional can assist in tailoring advice for individual athletes around changes in energy, carbohydrate, protein, and other nutrients to support health and performance.
- Masters athletes may take supplements for health conditions or to improve performance. Most of the information about performance supplements is inferred from studies in younger athletes. Professional guidance from sports nutrition professional who understands individual clinical and sports performance needs would be beneficial to assist masters athletes in considering the use of dietary supplements.

References

1. Gifford J, O'Connor H, Honey A, et al. Nutrients, health and chronic disease in masters athletes. In: Reaburn P, editor. *Nutrition and Performance in Masters Athletes*. Boca Raton, FL: CRC Press; 2015. pp. 213–41.
2. Thomas DT, Erdman KA, Burke LM. American college of sports medicine joint position statement. Nutrition and athletic performance. *Med Sci Sports Exerc*. 2016;48(3):543–68.
3. Reaburn P, Doering TM, Borges NR. Nutrition issues for the masters athlete. In: Burke L, Deakin V, Minehan M, editors. *Clinical Sports Nutrition*. 6th ed. Sydney: McGraw-Hill Education (Australia) Pty Ltd; 2021. pp. 503–25.
4. Dubé JJ, Broskey NT, Despines AA, et al. Muscle characteristics and substrate energetics in lifelong endurance athletes. *Med Sci Sports Exerc*. 2016;48(3):472–80.
5. Bauer J, Biolo G, Cederholm T, et al. Evidence-based recommendations for optimal dietary protein intake in older people: A position paper from the PROT-AGE Study Group. *J Am Med Dir Assoc*. 2013;14(8):542–59.
6. Doering TM, Reaburn PR, Phillips SM, et al. Postexercise dietary protein strategies to maximize skeletal muscle repair and remodeling in masters endurance athletes: A review. *Int J Sport Nutr Exerc Metab*. 2016;26(2):168–78.
7. Soto-Quijano DA. The competitive senior athlete. *Phys Med Rehabil Clin N Am*. 2017;28(4): 767–76.
8. Mountjoy M, Ackerman K, Bailey D, et al. The 2023 International Olympic Committee's (IOC) consensus statement on Relative Energy Deficiency in Sports (REDs). *Br J Sports Med*. 2023. In press.
9. Mills CE, Khatri J, Maskell P, et al. It is rocket science - why dietary nitrate is hard to 'beet'! Part II: Further mechanisms and therapeutic potential of the nitrate-nitrite-NO pathway. *Br J Clin Pharmacol*. 2017;83(1):140–51.
10. Dolan E, Gualano B, Rawson ES. Beyond muscle: The effects of creatine supplementation on brain creatine, cognitive processing, and traumatic brain injury. *Eur J Sport Sci*. 2019;19(1):1–14.
11. Harnett J, Climstein M, Walsh J, et al. The use of medications and dietary supplements by masters athletes — A review. *Curr Nutr Rep*. 2022;2:253–62.

25 Female athletes

Anthea C Clarke and Mikaeli Carmichael

This chapter introduces readers to the unique physiological characteristics of females that influence sport performance, exercise metabolism, and nutrition. A comprehensive overview of the different life stages for female athletes (from puberty to menopause), the menstrual cycle and related influences on sport performance and nutrition needs, and strategies for working with female athletes are included.

Is it important to note here that the term 'female' is used when describing biological factors that differentiate based on sex and the gender-based term 'women' is used when describing aspects affected from a sociological standpoint. Binary terms such as 'female/male' and 'women/men' do not capture the experiences of all individuals, and there are likely additional and different considerations that require further exploration for those individuals. Given the limited research conducted with gender-diverse populations and the recent emphasis on the research community to better understand the needs of female athletes, this chapter will focus on female-specific considerations.

Learning outcomes

This chapter will:

- outline key differences in the hormonal profiles and the subsequent exercise and nutritional needs of females across the life stages of puberty, pregnancy, and menopause;
- describe the menstrual cycle phases and the influence that hormonal contraceptives have on the natural hormonal profile;
- identify what a 'normal' menstrual cycle is as well as common menstrual dysfunctions;
- explain the current research that links the menstrual cycle phase with training and performance requirements;
- outline the recommended screening practices for female athletes and how to implement effective menstrual cycle monitoring.

Female physiology across the lifespan

Both males and females produce androgens (e.g. testosterone), oestrogens, and progesterones; however, at the onset of puberty, the amounts of these hormones differ between sexes with females producing higher quantities of oestrogen and progesterone, and males producing higher amounts of testosterone. The presence of these hormones causes

DOI: 10.4324/9781003321286-28

subsequent changes in female and male physiology across numerous body systems, including musculoskeletal, cardiovascular, and immune systems. As a result of these hormonal differences, adult males typically have greater muscle and bone mass with lower fat mass than females. This results in males having greater absolute and relative strength and power, as well as greater aerobic capacity. However, oestrogen appears to have a protective effect on muscles, potentially resulting in reduced muscle damage following exercise for females, which may influence both training and nutritional demands. While key differences are present between adult females and males, there are additional sex-specific considerations for different life stages (adolescence, pregnancy, and menopause) that are worth bearing in mind as they relate to the exercise and nutritional needs of female athletes.

The hormonal changes as a result of puberty occur at different ages for females and males. Typically, females start puberty between the ages of 9 and 11, while males start puberty later (~11 years of age). However, ethnicity (e.g. black African females typically start puberty earlier than Caucasian white females), body mass index (higher body mass corresponds with earlier onset), environment, and genetics can all contribute to when an individual starts puberty, particularly for females. Differences between males and females become more obvious around 12 years old for females and 13 for males, where both sexes experience growth spurts and males develop more muscle while females develop more fat (particularly around the hips and thighs). For females, their first period typically occurs around 13 years of age. More details about the nutritional needs of youth athletes during this phase can be found in Chapter 23. When working with this adolescent population, it is important to consider the different timing and duration of growth phases between sexes and how to adequately support them nutritionally.

Following the onset of puberty, females may also become pregnant, resulting in various physical, physiological, and hormonal changes to the body. The World Health Organization recommends pregnant and post-natal individuals undertake at least 150 minutes of moderate-intensity aerobic and strengthening-based physical activity a week (the same as when not pregnant). However, the types of exercise may need to be modified (i.e. limiting exercises while lying on the back, avoiding exercises with the risk of falling or contact with the abdomen, and avoiding hot and humid or high altitude environments).[1] In addition, the nutritional requirements for key micronutrients change both during pregnancy and postnatally and need to be accounted for within the diet. While pregnancy and parenthood have historically resulted in many athletes not returning to elite sport, more and more athletes are showing that they can safely return and even reach career-best performances on return from childbirth. To date, recommendations for pre- and post-natal exercise and return to sport recommendations for highly active females have not been developed and more research is required with this population group.[1]

The other key life stage where female hormones noticeably change is during menopause, typically occurring in women between 45 and 60 years of age. This phase is marked by the cessation of monthly periods when the ovaries no longer produce eggs for potential reproduction. Menopause is reached when an individual has gone 12 months without a period, while perimenopause is the period immediately prior to this where menstrual cycle changes start to occur and periods can become less, or more, frequent. As a result of menopause, the ovaries produce less oestrogen and progesterone. This reduction in oestrogen accelerates the rate of bone loss, increasing the risk of osteoporosis in post-menopausal females. The risk of cardiovascular disease also increases following menopause, likely linked to the reduction in oestrogen. Exercise plays a key role in helping to manage menopausal symptoms, minimise bone loss, and promote bone strength and cardiovascular health. Given a sedentary lifestyle and an energy-dense, nutrient-poor diet are also risk factors for cardiovascular disease, regular exercise and a nutritious diet are essential for post-menopausal females. More details about the nutritional needs of older females can be found in Chapter 24.

The menstrual cycle and use of hormonal contraceptives

In premenopausal females, the menstrual cycle occurs regularly in preparation for potential conception and pregnancy. A menstrual cycle is characterised by a series of hormonal fluctuations that are regulated by the hypothalamic-pituitary-ovarian axis causing key menstrual-related events such as menstruation and ovulation (Figure 25.1). Typically, the menstrual cycle (from the onset of menstruation to the day before menstruation starts again) lasts ~29 days, which includes 4 ± 2 days of menstruation during which 5–80 mL of menstrual blood will be lost. Ovulation occurs about halfway through the cycle; however, this can be highly variable and on average occurs 10–14 days prior to the start of the next menstrual bleed. Females are considered eumenorrheic (experiencing a functional

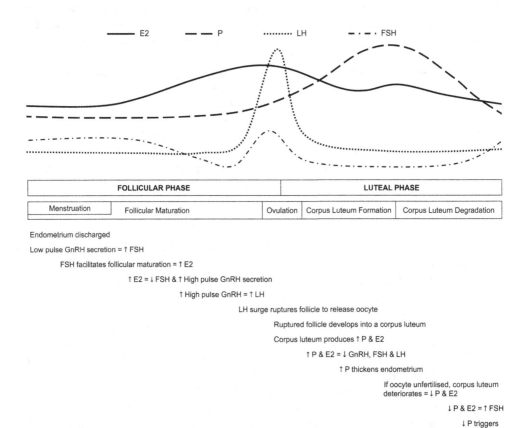

Figure 25.1 Schematic of hormonal fluctuations, phases, and key events within a functional menstrual cycle. Abbreviations: E2, estradiol; P, progesterone; LH, luteinising hormone; FSH, follicle stimulating hormone; GnRH, gonadotropin-releasing hormone.

Table 25.1 Types of menstrual dysfunction

Menstrual Dysfunction	Description
Primary Amenorrhea	An absence of menarche by the age of 15 years
Secondary Amenorrhea	An absence of menstruation for three months in previously menstruating individuals
Polymenorrhea	Menstruation that occurs too frequently (i.e. menstrual cycle duration is less than 21 days)
Oligomenorrhea	Menstruation that occurs infrequently (i.e. menstrual cycle duration is more than 35 days)
Menorrhagia	Heavy menstrual bleeding (i.e. total menstrual blood loss greater than 80 mL)
Metrorrhagia	Uterine bleeding that occurs between periods/menses
Dysmenorrhea	Severe abdominopelvic pain experienced shortly prior to and during menstruation
Premenstrual Syndrome (PMS)	Regularly experiencing at least one physical and/or emotional symptom during the five days prior to menstruation and that dissipates within four days following the onset of menses
Premenstrual Dysphoric Disorder (PMDD)	Regularly experiencing at least five predetermined emotional and behavioural or physical symptoms during the week prior to and following the onset of menstruation, which causes significant distress or disrupts professional, educational, or social activities
Anovulation	An absence of ovulation during the menstrual cycle
Luteal Phase Deficiency	Either an insufficient increase in progesterone (i.e. less than 16 nmol/L) during the luteal phase, or a short luteal phase duration (i.e. less than 10 days)

menstrual cycle) if (1) the menstrual cycle duration is between 21 and 35 days, (2) ovulation occurs, and (3) the peak in progesterone is greater than 16 nmol/L following ovulation.

However, not all females experience a functional menstrual cycle. Menstrual dysfunction refers to a variety of conditions related to abnormal menstrual bleeding or symptoms, or an absence of key events within a menstrual cycle (Table 25.1). Menstrual dysfunction can be underpinned by conditions that affect female reproductive or endocrine systems, such as uterine fibroids, endometriosis, adenomyosis, or polycystic ovarian syndrome. Alternatively, they occur as a result of training and nutrition practices. Some types of menstrual dysfunction, such as amenorrhea, oligomenorrhea, and anovulation, are more prevalent in those frequently engaging in exercise, typically as a result of low energy availability (LEA); therefore, athletes experiencing disordered eating or participating in sports than emphasise aesthetics or leanness are at higher risk of these menstrual dysfunctions, but they can occur in any athlete (see Chapter 23). There is also evidence from various sports that a large proportion of female athletes do not meet their energy or carbohydrate requirements. The presence of these menstrual dysfunctions can also affect fertility and family planning and the formation and resorption of bone (as a result of lower levels of oestrogen and progesterone) which can increase the risk for bone stress fractures. Other types of dysfunctions related to abnormal menstrual symptoms (i.e. premenstrual syndrome (PMS), premenstrual dysphoric disorder (PMDD), dysmenorrhea) can have a substantial impact on an individual's quality of life and affect engagement with work, education, and sport. Heavy menstrual bleeding is also a risk factor for iron deficiency and anaemia (see Chapter 5 and Chapter 17 for more information). It is, therefore, important for athletes to understand what menstrual dysfunction looks like to recognise when to seek medical support.

Contraceptive methods containing exogenous female sex hormones that create a consistent hormonal profile and prevent ovulation are referred to as hormonal contraceptives. The most common form of hormonal contraception currently prescribed is the oral contraceptive pill (OCP), which can vary in the hormones involved (e.g. combined (estradiol and progestin) or progestin-only pills), and in the amount of hormone present across a cycle (e.g. mono-, bi-, or tri-phasic) (Figure 25.2). Other hormonal contraceptive methods include the combined emergency contraceptive pill, an implant (e.g. Implanon), an injection (e.g. Depo Provera), or a hormonal intrauterine device (e.g. Mirena). It is also important to distinguish hormonal contraception from non-hormonal contraception options, such as the copper intrauterine device, as non-hormonal contraceptives do not

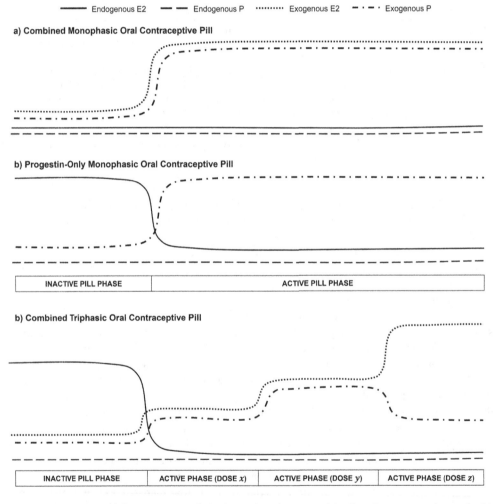

Figure 25.2 Hormonal fluctuations and phases within the a) combined oral contraceptive cycle, b) progestin-only oral contraceptive cycle, and c) combined triphasic oral contraceptive cycle. E2, estradiol; P, progesterone/progestin.

disrupt menstrual patterns with exogenous hormones. Somewhere between 26 and 68% of athletes are currently using some form of hormonal contraceptive, for various reasons such as to avoid pregnancy, manage menstrual symptoms or pain, and to choose when/if bleeding occurs.[2]

Hormonal contraception works by suppressing gonadotropin-releasing hormone, which limits the secretion of follicle-stimulating hormone and luteinising hormone; this downregulation of endogenous female sex hormones prevents follicular development, ovulation, and the fluctuations in endogenous oestrogen and progesterone observed within a functional menstrual cycle. Hormonal contraceptive users, therefore, do not have a menstrual cycle, but OCP users may have an oral contraceptive cycle consisting of an active (consumption of pills containing synthetic estradiol and/or progestin) and inactive (consumption of placebo/sugar pills, which usually results in a withdrawal bleed) pill phase. Some athletes with a history of menstrual irregularity or dysfunction may be more likely to use hormonal contraception and while the withdrawal bleed mimics menstruation it is not indicative of normal menstrual function. As a result, indicators other than the presence/absence of a menstrual bleed must be used for the identification of relative energy deficiency in sport (REDs) or LEA for athletes using hormonal contraceptives.

Hormones, physiology, and performance

In females, the hormonal profile of an individual changes due to life stage (e.g. adolescence, pregnancy, menopause), menstrual cycle phase, as a result of hormonal contraceptive use, or due to health or medical conditions. The hormonal profile can influence an individual's mood, response to exercise, fluid and substrate needs, and ability to thermoregulate. However, due to a current lack of high-quality evidence with female athletes across these various hormonal profiles, training, performance, and nutrition recommendations specific to the menstrual cycle phase are yet to be developed.[3,4]

When oestrogen concentration declines (as typically occurs in the week leading into menstruation) serotonin availability also decreases, which can contribute to low mood states. When oestrogen and progesterone concentrations are relatively low in the early follicular and late luteal phase, females may experience mood disturbances, with some of the most common menstrual symptoms experienced around this time being irritability and low mood. Those with PMS or PMDD (Table 25.1) demonstrate a larger drop in serotonin than those without PMS/PMDD, possibly explaining why these individuals experience more disruptive menstrual symptoms. Additionally, mood disturbances occurring in menopause can be related to declining levels of oestrogen and progesterone. This is why selective serotonin reuptake inhibitors are sometimes used as a pharmacological intervention to increase serotonin availability and manage symptoms of PMS or menopause. While hormonal contraceptives are sometimes prescribed to help manage menstrual-related symptoms, their use does not appear to consistently improve or cause worse mood outcomes in comparison to a natural menstrual cycle.

Given oestrogen has an anabolic effect and progesterone has a catabolic effect, the concept of whether one can train to maximise the phases where these hormones are high and/or low is enticing. Some studies have demonstrated changes in skeletal muscle voluntary activation, short-interval cortical inhibition, motor unit firing rate at recruitment, and maximal voluntary contraction throughout the menstrual cycle. Given the anabolic effect of oestrogen, phases with higher oestrogen may promote hypertrophy by reducing protein degradation, increasing satellite cell activity and production to facilitate muscle repairing, and increasing the secretion of growth hormone. There is some preliminary evidence suggesting that increasing resistance training volume (via increased training frequency) during the follicular phase can produce greater gains in strength and lean mass compared to the increasing volume in the luteal phase or having no phased-based adjustments to training load.[5] However, this is preliminary research that, while exciting as a potential training method, currently has insufficient scientific support for its use. There is also conflicting evidence about the impact that hormonal contraceptive use has on the body's ability to promote protein synthesis and strength development. So, in lieu of sufficient evidence, the use of hormonal contraceptives should be selected based on the medical needs of the individual and in consultation with a medical professional, rather than based on any potential performance outcomes.

Fluctuations in oestrogen and progesterone across the menstrual cycle also have a potential impact on exercise metabolism and fluid balance for female athletes. A detailed review of the mechanisms underpinning menstrual cycle phase differences in exercise metabolism is provided by Oosthuyse et al.[6] Plasma glucose uptake during exercise may be higher during the early follicular compared to mid-luteal phase (particularly during fasted exercise), while oral contraceptive use appears to reduce the rate of plasma glucose uptake during exercise (equating to a decrease of ~5.5 g/h of glucose uptake in a 60 kg (132 lb) woman exercising at 65% VO_2max). However, glycogen sparing has also been seen in the luteal phase, with oestrogen potentially decreasing muscle glycogenolysis and stimulating lipolysis. Whilst there are some conflicting findings regarding substrate utilisation, it appears any difference in fat and CHO oxidation dissipates at higher intensities and if sufficient carbohydrate intake is consumed pre-exercise. Similarly, these differences may not be large enough to result in meaningful changes in performance. The presence of oestrogen also appears to promote fluid retention via increasing thirst stimulation and sodium retention while decreasing the threshold for antidiuretic hormone release. Progesterone may increase aldosterone production, which would also promote fluid retention; however, it compensates by decreasing the reabsorption of sodium, thirst stimulation, and antidiuretic hormone release, limiting fluid intake and retention. Despite these mechanisms and some evidence that plasma volume increases prior to ovulation, there is limited evidence suggesting fluctuating female sex hormones will influence fluid replacement requirements following dehydration or strenuous exercise.[7] Body adiposity measurements via DXA may be affected by these fluctuating hormones,[8] however, and so identification of menstrual phase and/or repeat measurements at a similar phase may be required.

From a physiological perspective, basal body temperature rises during ovulation, and results in higher temperature thresholds for the onset of sweating and vasodilation in the luteal phase. Despite this, gross performance appears to not be affected by this change in temperature regulation during exercise in thermoneutral environments. In hot and humid conditions, however, there may be some impaired exercise performance as a result of physiological or perceptual changes in thermoregulation. Given sufficient hydration and nutrition protocols though, and adjusting to the individual needs of the athlete, it should be possible to limit any changes in performance. It is important to note that while those using an oral contraceptive pill do not ovulate, there still appear to be fluctuations in body temperature across active and non-active pill days. However, this change in body temperature does not appear to influence the sweat response during exercise.

Monitoring menstrual cycles

Menstrual cycle tracking is the practice of systematically recording when menstrual bleeding occurs. At its most basic, menstrual cycle tracking is noting the day menstruation starts. However, menstrual blood flow (i.e. spotting, light, moderate, and heavy), the type and severity of menstrual symptoms, other outcomes such as sleep, stress, and fatigue, and the occurrence of ovulation can also be tracked. Menstrual cycle tracking can be done using a paper-based or digital calendar, smartphone application, or adding relevant outcomes to an athlete monitoring system. Menstrual cycle tracking is a useful tool to gauge an athlete's health by signposting normal development (i.e. menarche by 15 years) and identifying menstrual dysfunction or symptoms of REDs (i.e. amenorrhea, oligomenorrhea, anovulation). It also allows athletes to gain a better understanding of their bodies and how they may be impacted by their cycle. Those using hormonal contraceptives may also track their cycle, which can be useful to identify positive and negative symptoms associated with their use.

It is important to educate athletes, coaches, and other staff about the menstrual cycle, menstrual dysfunction, and why tracking is conducted, especially if athletes are being encouraged to track their cycles. This will enable athletes and staff to know when medical support is required and facilitate conversations with healthcare providers or the referral of athletes to an appropriate healthcare provider. Signs that athletes should seek medical support include the following:

- menstruation is missed;
- menstrual cycle duration changes notably beyond usual;
- menstrual cycle duration is less than 21 or greater than 35 days;
- heavy menstrual bleeding is reported for 3 or more days;
- menstruation continues for 8 or more days;
- menstrual symptoms are severe or disrupt daily life;
- menstrual-cycle-related pain is experienced.

If tracking is conducted in an athlete monitoring system, athletes should be made aware of how their tracking data may be accessed and used, and by whom, given the potential sensitivity of this information. Tracking should remain optional and individualised; for example, for an athlete who feels they have no concerns relating to their menstrual cycle or choice of hormonal contraceptive, forced tracking may create an unnecessary burden for this individual. Similarly, if an athlete does not feel comfortable providing their tracking data this should not be mandatory. However, adequate education relating to the use and potential benefit of this process may help improve the confidence of individuals to be willing to have these conversations. Finally, if using tracking to help identify menstrual dysfunction and REDs, it is important to distinguish menstrual bleeding from withdrawal bleeding (i.e. hormonal contraceptive users may have a withdrawal bleed occurring every 21 days, which is not indicative of menstrual function).

Working with female athletes

Understanding the different life stages of female athletes and the influence that the menstrual cycle or hormonal contraceptive use may have on the training and nutritional demands of athletes is an essential first step when it comes to working with female athletes. These key physiological differences can influence the macro and micronutrient needs of the individual throughout the lifespan. When providing nutritional advice to female athletes, though, it is important to be aware that many of the common nutritional recommendations are based on research undertaken with predominantly male participants. A 2022 audit of 1826 studies observing the use of performance supplements in sport (such as caffeine, beetroot juice, and sodium bicarbonate) observed only 23% of participants were women, with 14% of those studies defining the menstrual status of participants, and only three studies appropriately assessing menstrual phase.[9] Specific to research around carbohydrate intake (undertaken in 2023),[10] only 11% of participants were women (from a total of 937 studies and 11,202 total participants). Despite the potential influence of the cycle phase on carbohydrate metabolism, only 7% of studies that used women as participants adequately controlled for ovarian hormones. Also, fewer than 2% of studies across these two audits were specifically designed to compare sex-based responses. Clearly, there is some way to go in the research to ensure that the evidence base considers sex-based differences, and it is important to remember that what may work for male athletes may not necessarily result in the same outcome for female athletes.

Beyond their sport-specific physiological needs, the nutritional habits of female athletes can also be influenced by their sociocultural environment. Chapter 20 discussed the pressures of conforming to a sport-specific 'ideal' body type and the higher risk in some sports for athletes to have LEA or REDs. Beyond sport expectations, female athletes also deal with societal expectations of what may be considered feminine or appropriate for women. Many female athletes are expected, or at least encouraged, to promote their sport and individual sporting persona through social media platforms (often as a way to generate current or future income). This can place athletes in a position where the general public can scrutinise every aspect of their lives, with a common topic of interest being how female athletes look. This can open athletes up to potentially abusive comments and can affect both the eating habits and mental health of individuals. Similarly, social media can often permeate the idea of what a 'fit' woman looks like, which does not take into account sport-specificity or performance outcomes. As such, athletes come in a variety of 'ideal' body types, and yet these are often very different to what is promoted on social media as being a 'fit and healthy athletic body'. Understanding athletes' engagement with social media and how this may be impacting their mental health are important aspects to be aware of when working with female athletes. Helping athletes build resiliency and an awareness of when to step away from social media is an important component of development and education programs. This is particularly relevant for younger athletes, those with low self-confidence and specifically confidence in themselves as an athlete, or in sports which move away from the traditional 'feminine' body type.

Finally, female athletes may benefit from routine health screening due to their relatively higher prevalence or risk for some disorders and conditions compared to male athletes. These can include yearly screening for disordered eating/eating disorders, LEA, and iron status. Identified 'at risk' athletes (due to test results, history, or sport), may then benefit from additional monitoring beyond this yearly check. Post-menopausal female athletes, or those identified with REDs, may also benefit from periodic bone mineral density screening. Encouraging athletes to track the timing and symptoms related to their menstrual cycle (or hormonal contraceptive use) is also beneficial, particularly when matched with education relating to what is normal and when to seek medical advice. As with all regular monitoring practices though, it is important that this information is routinely monitored and acted upon, with an identified referral system in place should an athlete start to experience menstrual dysfunction. Given discomfort around the topic of 'periods', it is also recommended that athletes have access to a female member(s) of staff whom they can speak with if not comfortable talking to their coaching staff, that parents are involved in the conversation when working with youth athletes, and that cultural sensitivities are recognised and accounted for specific to the group of athletes.

Summary

This chapter has provided an overview of key considerations for female athletes, including females' changing physiology over the lifespan, physiological differences between females and males, what a functional menstrual cycle looks like, the types of menstrual dysfunctions that may be experienced by athletes, and the types of hormonal contraceptives available. This chapter also summarised how hormonal fluctuations with life stage, menstrual cycle phase, and hormonal contraceptive use may relate to female athletes' training, performance, and nutrition. It outlined key practical takeaways for those working with female athletes, including the current state of female-specific research, considerations for menstrual cycle tracking and health screening, and factors influencing female athletes' nutritional habits.

Chapter highlights

- Females typically begin puberty around the ages of 9–11, and this may be affected by ethnicity, body mass index, environment, and genetics.
- Females usually start menstruating around the age of 13 and experience menopause between 45 and 60 years of age.
- A functional menstrual cycle can be identified by a duration between 21 and 35 days, occurrence of ovulation, and progesterone rise greater than 16 nmol/L.
- There are various types of menstrual dysfunction that relate to abnormal menstrual bleeding or symptoms, or the absence of key events observed in a functional menstrual cycle.
- Menstrual dysfunction may be the result of low energy availability or conditions affecting the female reproductive or endocrine systems.
- Menstrual dysfunction can have a significant impact on daily life, including sport, and consequences on fertility, bone health, and iron deficiency.
- There are various types of hormonal contraceptives available.
- Hormonal fluctuations with life stage, menstrual cycle phase, and hormonal contraceptive use can influence mood, exercise responses, fluid and substrate needs, and thermoregulation; although there is generally a lack of high-quality evidence to understand its impact on performance or nutritional requirements.
- Rather than focusing on periodising training or nutrition around the menstrual cycle phase, athletes' dietary adequacy (i.e. consuming sufficient energy and carbohydrates) should be prioritised.
- Menstrual cycle tracking can be performed by noting the day menstruation starts, additional outcomes such as symptoms (menstrual-related or hormonal contraceptive-related), and ovulation. Other wellness measures (i.e. sleep, fatigue, stress) can also be tracked.

- Menstrual cycle tracking can be useful to identify signs of menstrual dysfunction and REDs (note: a withdrawal bleed occurring every 21 days is not indicative of menstrual function, therefore other factors should be considered to assess hormonal contraceptive users' risk of REDs).
- Menstrual cycle tracking in sport should be optional and athletes should consent to how their menstrual cycle tracking data is stored, accessed, and used.
- Female athletes should have access to education surrounding menstrual dysfunction, the uses, and the potential benefits of menstrual cycle tracking.
- Sociocultural factors (e.g. pressures relating to an 'ideal' or 'feminine' body type) can also influence female athletes' nutritional habits and should be considered when working with female athletes.

References

1. Davenport MH, Hayman M. Physical activity during pregnancy: essential steps for maternal and fetal health. *Obstet Med.* 2022;15(3):149–150.
2. Cheng J, Santiago KA, Aburalib Z, et al. Menstrual irregularity, hormonal contraceptive use, and bone stress injuries in collegiate female athletes in the United States. *PM&R.* 2021;13(11): 1201–1313.
3. Elliott-Sale KJ, McNulty KL, Ansdell P, et al. The effects of oral contraceptives on exercise performance in women: a systematic review and meta-analysis. *Sports Med.* 2020;50(10):1785–1812.
4. McNulty KL, Elliott-Sale KJ, Dolan E, et al. The effects of menstrual cycle phase on exercise performance in eumenorrheic women: a systematic review and meta-analysis. *Sports Med.* 2020;50(10), 1813–1827.
5. Thompson B, Almarjawi A, Sculley D. et al. The effect of the menstrual cycle and oral contraceptives on acute responses and chronic adaptations to resistance training: a systematic review of the literature. *Sports Med.* 2020;50(1):171–185.
6. Oosthuyse T, Strauss JA, Hackney AC. Understanding the female athlete: molecular mechanisms underpinning menstrual phase differences in exercise metabolism. *Eur J Appl Physiol.* 2023;123(3), 423–450.
7. Giersch GEW, Charkoudian N, Stearns RL, & et al. Fluid balance and hydration considerations for women: review and future directions. *Sports Med.* 2020;50(2):253–261.
8. Thompson BM, Hillebrandt HL, Sculley DV, et al. The acute effect of the menstrual cycle and oral contraceptive cycle on measures of body composition. *Eur J Appl Physiol.* 2021;121(11): 3051–3059.
9. Smith ES, McKay AKA, Kuikman M, et al. (2022). Auditing the representation of female versus male athletes in sports science and sports medicine research: evidence-based performance supplements. *Nutrients.* 2022; 14(5):953.
10. Kuikman MA, Smith ES, McKay AKA, et al. Fuelling the female athlete: auditing her representation in studies of acute carbohydrate intake for exercise. *Med Sci Sports Exerc.* 2022; 55(3):569–580.

26 Para athletes

Michelle Minehan and Elizabeth Broad

Para athletes compete with physical, vision or intellectual impairments. A classification system allows athletes with similar functional abilities to compete against each other on an even playing field. Since the first Paralympic Games in Rome in 1960, the Para sport movement has developed rapidly. Summer and Winter Paralympic Games now occur every four years and participation is consistently increasing. In 2021, 4400 athletes from 176 countries competed at the Tokyo Paralympic Games.

Working with Para athletes can be challenging due to limited research and potentially complex interplay between athletes' clinical, life and sporting needs. Modern Para athletes train and perform at an elite level with increasingly competitive standards, with some events won by fractions of a second or by a single point. In many cases, the nutritional needs of Para athletes are very similar to able-bodied athletes. In other cases, nutrition recommendations require modification to suit individual circumstances.

Learning outcomes

This chapter will:

- describe the range of physical, vision and intellectual impairments that may affect Para athletes;
- describe key factors driving the need for modification of nutrition recommendations for Para athletes;
- outline how sports nutrition recommendations might need to be modified for some Para athletes.

Classes of para athletes

To compete as a Para athlete, at least one of the impairments in Table 26.1 must be present. Some sports cater for only one type of impairment, while others have classes for all impairments. For example, goalball is played exclusively by athletes who are vision impaired, whereas athletics offers a full spectrum of events. Within each sport, athletes are classified based on their level of impairment. For example, the T42 category in athletics is for track athletes with a 'lower limb competing without prosthesis affected by limb deficiency, leg length difference, impaired muscle power or impaired passive range of movement'. The goal of classification is to create an even playing field for competition.

DOI: 10.4324/9781003321286-29

Table 26.1 Impairments in Paralympic Sports

Impairment	Explanation
Impaired muscle power	A health condition that either reduces or eliminates the ability to voluntarily contract muscles in order to move or to generate force.
Impaired passive range of movement	Restriction or a lack of passive movement in one or more joints.
Limb deficiency	Total or partial absence of bones or joints as a consequence of trauma (for example, traumatic amputation), illness (for example, amputation due to bone cancer) or congenital limb deficiency (for example, dysmelia).
Leg length difference	Difference in the length of legs as a result of a disturbance of limb growth or as a result of trauma.
Short stature	Reduced length in the bones of the upper limbs, lower limbs and/or trunk.
Hypertonia	Increase in muscle tension and a reduced ability of a muscle to stretch caused by damage to the central nervous system.
Ataxia	Uncoordinated movements caused by damage to the central nervous system.
Athetosis	Continual slow involuntary movements.
Vision impairment	Reduced, or no vision caused by damage to the eye structure, optical nerves or optical pathways, or visual cortex of the brain.
Intellectual impairment	Restriction in intellectual functioning and adaptive behaviour which affects conceptual, social and practical adaptive skills required for everyday life. This impairment must be present before the age of 18.

Source: Adapted from www.paralympic.org/classification (accessed October 2022).

Table 26.2 Sports contested at Paralympic Games

Summer Paralympic Sports			Winter Paralympic Sports
Archery	Judo	Wheelchair basketball	Alpine skiing
Athletics	Powerlifting	Wheelchair fencing	Biathlon
Badminton	Rowing	Wheelchair rugby	Cross-country skiing
Blind Football	Shooting Para sport	Wheelchair tennis	Para ice hockey
Boccia	Sitting volleyball		Snowboard
Canoe	Swimming		Wheelchair curling
Cycling	Table tennis		
Equestrian	Taekwondo		
Goalball	Triathlon		

Source: Adapted from www.paralympic.org/sports (accessed October 2022).

Athletes with a physical or cognitive impairment are termed Para athletes, and those who have competed at the Paralympic Games may be called Paralympians.

Para sports vary from traditional events such as athletics to modified events such as boccia and goalball. Table 26.2 summarises the mix of sports contested at summer and winter Paralympic games.

Research challenges

In 1993, the International Paralympic Committee (IPC) established a Sports Science Committee to advance knowledge of Paralympic sport across five central themes: (1) involving the academic world, (2) athlete health and safety, (3) classification, (4) socio-economic determinants of participation and success and (5) Paralympic athlete, trainer and coach education. Research activity is increasing; however, understanding of nutritional issues for Para athletes remains limited. Challenges to conducting research include the following:

- large variation in the functional capacity of athletes;
- athletes dispersed over large geographical distances;
- medical contraindications to participation in experimental research (for example, use of particular medications);
- small athlete pool, which makes it difficult to set up designs with randomisation and control groups;
- small number of scientists actively researching Para athlete issues;
- national focus, with many scientists working with Paralympic athletes having a mandate to help athletes from their own countries win medals, limiting opportunities for collaboration and sharing;
- limited funding opportunities for sport-related research, especially Para sport.

In the absence of a large Para sport-specific research base, it is necessary to extrapolate knowledge gleaned from studies of able-bodied athletes. Budding researchers are encouraged to consider projects with Para athlete populations.

Training age

Para athletes compete across a wide age range. The youngest athlete at the Tokyo Paralympics in 2021 was 14 years old, while the oldest was 51. Many Paralympic athletes follow a traditional sports career path, playing a sport from a young age and gradually improving until they compete at an elite level. Others take up Para sport later in life, after acquiring a disability due to traumatic injury or disease progression.

It is also relatively common for Para athletes to cross over between and within Para sports. The events offered at major events such as world championships and major games can change from event to event. This might require a 400-metre runner to switch to 1500 metres or a javelin thrower to convert to shotput in order to gain a spot on a national team. As new competition opportunities arise, some athletes transfer to new sports. For example, the Para-Triathlon was contested at the Paralympic Games for the first time in 2016, enticing athletes to swap from sports such as athletics, cycling and swimming. Dylan Alcott competed in both wheelchair basketball and wheelchair tennis at different Paralympic Games. There are also athletes who compete in both summer and winter events within the same year, such as Oksana Masters (Nordic ski and cycling) and Kendall Gretsch (Nordic ski and triathlon).

Consequently, athletes can compete at major events with relatively few years of sports-specific training under their belt. It is important to consider the training 'age' of an athlete as well as their chronological age. Nutritional needs can be different for an athlete with a long training history compared to an athlete rapidly adapting to a training stimulus. Altering body composition might be a lower priority while an athlete focuses on building up sufficient strength and stamina to cope with training. It can be easy to assume that older athletes have acquired significant knowledge about how to manage their nutrition intake for their sport, but in reality, they might be on a rapid learning trajectory.

Energy needs

Estimating energy expenditure is a challenge when working with Para athletes. The physiological demands of most Para sports are unmeasured and predictive equations have limited applicability to many Para athletes. Direct measurement of resting metabolic rate (RMR) via indirect calorimetry is useful but not easily accessible for all athletes. In general, predictive equations based on muscle mass (for example, the Cunningham equation) are more useful than equations based solely on height and weight (such as the Harris–Benedict equation). A trial-and-error process based on estimated energy intake and weight changes may be needed to fully understand individual energy requirements.

Athletes with conditions such as spina bifida and cerebral palsy might have proportionally higher energy requirements due to inefficient ambulation and conditions such as athetosis (involuntary movements). Some individuals who walk with a prosthesis might have a higher energy expenditure due to the inefficiency of movement caused by gait asymmetry. In most cases, this additional energy cost is small and possibly offset by factors such as reduced muscle and reduced daily activity.

Energy expenditure of individuals who use a wheelchair is typically reduced compared with able-bodied individuals. as daily movements use a smaller muscle mass. RMR is typically lower (up to 25 per cent) in athletes with spinal cord injuries (SCIs) due to non-functioning muscle and subsequent muscle wasting. The impact is greater the higher the injury to the spinal cord but can vary according to how complete the injury to the spinal cord is and whether the individual experiences involuntary muscle spasms.

Like able-bodied athletes, many Para athletes strive to keep their physique lean. A reduced RMR means they can have a limited energy budget and have to prioritise nutrient density. It can be a fine balance between supporting performance goals while achieving a suitable physique.

Energy availability

Low energy availability (LEA) has emerged as an important issue for athletes (see Chapter 7). Energy availability refers to the amount of energy available to support bodily functions once the cost of training has been met. If energy availability is low, metabolism can slow, leading to negative hormonal changes and reduced bone density.[1] This can put athletes at risk of injury, illness and suboptimal body composition. It has been suggested that Para athletes are at greater risk of LEA compared to their able-bodied counterparts, but it is difficult to determine whether performance decrements are due to LEA or the athlete's impairment.[2] Specific criteria for different types of Para athletes are currently unavailable. However, there is reason to suspect that many Para athletes could be affected, as LEA can arise from both intentional (restricting intake to maintain a lean physique) and unintentional (insufficient opportunity to eat all required food or lack of understanding of total energy requirements) under-eating.

Athletes who do not weight-bear typically have reduced bone density. The primary cause is reduced skeletal loading which may be related to their sport (for example, swimming, cycling) and/or their disability (for example, SCI, amputation). However, the influence of LEA should also be considered.

Macronutrient and micronutrient needs

Carbohydrate requirements are primarily influenced by training load) (see Chapter 9). Rates of glucose utilisation in arm cycling and wheelchair events are largely unknown.

However, the capacity to store glycogen in the arms is less than in the large muscles of the legs. Athletes competing in long-duration arm cycling and wheelchair events might have a higher need for carbohydrate replacement during sessions to compensate for reduced storage capacity. This can prove challenging as athletes with SCI typically do not like to eat or drink while exercising. Studies of athletes with SCI typically indicate that, relatively, daily carbohydrate intakes are at the lower limits of sports nutrition guidelines for able-bodied athletes.[3] The specific protein needs of Para athletes is unclear. However, it is widely accepted that able-bodied athletes require more protein for repair, recovery and muscle growth than sedentary individuals. In general, the same is expected for Para athletes. Athletes with less functional muscle (SCI, amputees) require lower absolute amounts of protein than able-bodied athletes but likely the same intake relative to functional muscle mass. In the absence of clinical trials, a recent review suggests a minimum protein requirement of 1.2 g/kg body mass for athletes with SCI.[4] Some Para athletes with SCI or congenital defects have altered kidney function, which may require modifications to protein recommendations. Timing and spread of high-quality protein is as important for Para athletes as for other athletes and, as such, optimal intakes need to be tailored to each individual.

Requirements for micronutrients are generally expected to be similar for Para athletes. Athletes with restricted intakes due to low energy budgets might have difficulty meeting needs from food alone. Athletes with SCI might be at increased risk of vitamin D insufficiency due to inadequate diet, anticonvulsant medication and reduced sunlight exposure. Supplementation might be warranted in some circumstances. In these instances, vitamin D levels should be monitored and supplementation discussed with a doctor or dietitian.

Hydration and heat regulation

In general, Paralympic athletes are encouraged to start exercise sessions in a euhydrated state and to match fluid intake to sweat losses during exercise. Fluid balance monitoring (weighing before and after exercise) is useful for tracking fluid losses and planning for individualised fluid replacement (see Chapter 11).

Fluid requirements for athletes with SCI need additional consideration. The ability of the brain to control body temperature through dilation of blood vessels and increased sweating is altered in athletes with SCI if the injury is at or above the T8 vertebrae (top half of the spinal column). The extent of the impact depends on the severity and level of the damage to the spinal cord. The higher the lesion, the greater the impairment to thermoregulation. Furthermore, some medications (diuretics, thyroid medication, muscle relaxants) can hamper thermoregulation. Reduced sweating means fluid losses are often less for athletes with SCI but it also means that the capacity to cool is impaired; hence, messages around hydrating effectively may need to be modified, with more focus on external cooling strategies.

Acclimatisation is important when athletes are competing in the heat.[5] Generally, 7–14 days are required for adaptation to exercise in the heat. However, some Para athletes with coexisting medical conditions might require longer. Para athletes need to schedule travel to allow sufficient time for acclimatisation before competing or to implement acclimatisation strategies such as the use of heat chambers before departure. The potential for acclimatisation in athletes with high-level SCI is undocumented. These athletes might consider limiting their exposure to hot environments prior to competition.

Various cooling strategies, such as water immersion, cooling jackets, ice slushies and water sprays, have been tested in athlete populations. Current evidence is mixed as to the effectiveness of these strategies for Para athletes.[6] Athletes with SCI can also have impaired shivering mechanisms and hence have difficulty warming the body when required. A balance needs to be found to deliver the optimal level of cooling.

Many athletes with SCI have disrupted signals from the brain to the bladder and require catheterisation to manage bladder function. It is common for athletes to time fluid intake carefully around competition and travel to manage catheterisation around events. Some athletes may limit fluid intake to avoid having to empty catheter bags or devices. Catheterisation practices need to be considered when planning fluid intake strategies and conducting hydration assessments. Measures such as morning urine specific gravity (USG) and fluid balance might require modification in some circumstances. It may be important to trial new strategies, including the use of electrolytes, to find the optimal balance between appropriate hydration (especially for travel) to minimise the risk of developing a urinary tract infection (UTI) and better support training and recovery.

Injury and illness

Some evidence suggests injury rates are higher in Para sports. This may be due to Para athletes being more likely to have coexisting medical conditions, biomechanical inefficiencies that increase susceptibility to injury, or exposure to high training loads before they are physically ready. Poor nutrition and LEA may also increase susceptibility to injuries and illness.

Athletes who use catheterisation to manage bladder function are more susceptible to UTIs. Recurrent UTI can result in a significant loss of training days over a season. Key measures to prevent UTI include maintenance of good hygiene when using catheters, frequent emptying of catheters (every 3–4 hours) and sufficient fluid intake.[7] Cranberry juice is a popular preventative measure for UTIs, although evidence for efficacy is inconsistent.

Body composition assessment

Many athletes find it useful to monitor body composition over time as it provides useful feedback on the effectiveness of training and nutritional regimes. Surface anthropometry (skinfolds) and dual energy X-ray absorptiometry (DXA) are the most common methods for assessing body composition in athletes. However, other methods are also available and it is important to understand the assumptions and limitations that influence their validity. It is often necessary to modify techniques for Para athletes. For example, according to the International Society for Advancement of Kinanthropometry (ISAK), skinfolds are routinely taken on the right side of the body. However, it is more relevant to measure the left side if an athlete has hemiplegia (weakness) or is missing a limb on the right side. The standard ISAK skinfold protocol involves measures at seven or eight body sites. However, for athletes with SCI, measures are often limited to the biceps, triceps and subscapular and abdominal sites due to muscle atrophy and inability to landmark appropriately.

DXA is useful for measuring body fat and lean tissue changes over time in athletes with a variety of physical impairments. It is often necessary to adjust standard positioning to obtain the most useful information for Para athletes. For example, some Para athletes are unable to lie on their backs in a standard anatomical position with legs straight and arms alongside the body. While it is possible to customise the positioning and analysis of DXA scans, these adjustments are yet to be validated.

Gastrointestinal issues

Athletes with SCI, congenital abnormalities of the gastrointestinal (GI) tract, a history of GI injury or medication use are more likely to experience GI issues than other Para athletes. Some athletes have altered transit time (for example, SCI) while others have various food intolerances or food aversions. Many athletes who compete in wheelchairs avoid eating before training or competing as the bent position in the chair is uncomfortable when the stomach is full. As such, it is important to work with Para athletes to gain a full understanding of GI issues when providing dietary advice. The timing of food and fluid intake around sessions typically needs to be adjusted according to individual tolerance. Some athletes need to focus on eating more in the later part of the day to compensate for restricted intake in the earlier part of the day; this is contradictory to most nutrition guidelines. Experimentation with quickly absorbed forms of carbohydrate such as gels and confectionery is often needed. This can be challenging when the energy budget is limited.

Medical issues and medication

Many Para athletes have coexisting medical conditions such as epilepsy, high blood pressure, kidney impairment, osteoporosis, reflux, diabetes and heart conditions.[8] Many are also managing significant pain. Some athletes require multiple medications. The impact of medical conditions and medications needs to be considered when providing nutrition advice. Some Para athletes have a very poor understanding of their medical conditions, so it is useful to work closely with other support staff—doctors, dietitians, physiologists and physiotherapists—to gain an accurate understanding.

Supplements

A report utilising data from 399 athletes from 21 different nationalities and 28 different sports indicated that the frequency of supplement use is similar in Para and able-bodied athlete populations.[9] Para athletes in this survey identified using a range of products, including nutritional supplements (vitamins, minerals) sports foods (gels, protein powders, sports drinks) and ergogenic aids (such as caffeine and bicarbonate).

All athletes, including Para athletes, are encouraged to meet their nutrient requirements from food. However, there might be circumstances in which nutritional supplementation is warranted. For example, some athletes might need to supplement key micronutrients (such as iron) if their energy budget does not allow for all nutrients to be consumed from food choices.

Minimal research has been conducted on the effect of ergogenic aids on Para athletes. However, it is reasonable to assume that, in the absence of contradictory medical conditions or functionality, similar ergogenic effects are likely. When advising on the use of supplements, potential interaction with any medication and health conditions needs to be considered. Timing and doses might need to be adjusted if GI function is altered or muscle mass is significantly lower than in able-bodied athletes. It is wise to test individual tolerance and response during training sessions before use in competition.

Travel

Travel is an inevitable and uncomfortable experience for all athletes (see Chapter 27). However, some Para athletes face additional challenges. Airlines typically ask people with impaired mobility to board planes first and exit planes last. This can substantially increase the time spent sitting on the plane. Additionally, some athletes choose to limit fluid intake to avoid having to use the toilet or empty a catheter during a flight. It is useful to prepare a fluid intake plan for flights to minimise dehydration.

Large events such as Paralympic Games and World Championships typically cater well for athletes with myriad disabilities. However, modification might be needed when eating at venues unfamiliar with Para athletes. Trays are useful for athletes in wheelchairs when eating buffet-style, although they are not always available. Food serveries are typically at an inconvenient height for people in wheelchairs; this might cause some athletes to avoid dishes towards the back of the servery. Support staff need to look out for challenges and request modifications if required (for example, a temporary servery set up on a lower table, or pre-plated meals). As some Para athletes need to modify eating times according to their GI tolerance, the provision of takeaway containers is useful to allow flexibility for when meals are consumed.

Summary

This chapter has described how Para athletes compete in a wide range of events and with wide-ranging functionality. Some Para athletes have very similar needs to athletes competing in corresponding able-bodied events. Others require bespoke modifications to suit their individual characteristics. As research regarding the nutritional requirements of Para athletes is limited, an individual approach to nutrition planning should be used along with a trial and modification process to determine optimal nutrition support.

Chapter highlights

- Para athletes compete in a diverse mix of sports and have diverse physiological requirements—there are no generic nutrition recommendations for Para athletes.
- Limited research is available regarding nutritional requirements for Para athletes.
- Energy, macronutrient and micronutrient needs are affected by some types of impairments and require individualised modification.
- Athletes with SCI are more likely to have altered heat regulation, GI tolerance, and increased illness risk compared to other Para athletes.
- Body composition protocols need to be modified for some Para athletes.
- Theoretically, ergogenic aids should have similar effects for Para athletes; however, individual testing and adjustment are needed.
- Sports nutrition professionals working with Para athletes need to work closely with other support staff (medicine, physiotherapy, physiology) to fully understand the requirements of each individual.

References

1. Blauwet CA, Brook EM, Tenforde AS, et al. Low energy availability, menstrual dysfunction, and low bone mineral density in individuals with a disability: implications for the Para athlete population. *Sports Med.* 2017;47(9):1697–1708.

2. Jonvik KL, Vardardottir B, Broad E. How do we assess energy availability and RED-S risk factors in Para athletes? *Nutrients*. 2022;14(5):1068.

3. Ruettimann B, Perret C, Parnell JA, et al. Carbohydrate Considerations for Athletes with a Spinal Cord Injury. *Nutrients*. 2021;13(7):2177.

4. Flueck JL, Parnell JA. Protein considerations for athletes with a spinal cord injury. *Front Nutr*. 2021; 8:652441.

5. Stephenson BT, Tolfrey K, Goosey-Tolfrey VL. Mixed active and passive, heart rate-controlled heat acclimation is effective for Paralympic and able-bodied triathletes. *Front Physiol*. 2019;10: 1214.

6. O'Brien TJ, Lunt KM, Stephenson BT, et al. The effect of pre-cooling or per-cooling in athletes with a spinal cord injury: A systematic review and meta-analysis. *J Sci Med Sport*. 2022;25(7): 606–614.

7. Compton S, Trease L, Cunningham C, et al. Australian Institute of Sport and the Australian Paralympic Committee position statement: urinary tract infection in spinal cord injured athletes. *Br J Sports Med*. 2015;49(19):1236–1240.

8. Johnson BF, Mushett CA, Richter K, Peacock G. *Sport for athletes with physical disabilities: injuries and medical issues*. BlazeSports America. 2004.

9. Graham T, Perret C, Crosland J, et al. Nutritional Supplement Habits and Perceptions of Disabled Athletes [Review of Nutritional Supplement Habits and Perceptions of Disabled Athletes]. WADA; World Anti-Doping Agency; 2014.

27 Travelling athletes

Shona L Halson, Georgia Romyn, Michelle Cort and Matthew Driller

Most athletes are required to undertake significant travel for competition. This can have consequences for both physiological and psychological status and has the potential to impair performance. Nutrition is one aspect of travel which requires careful planning to minimise the risk of illness and to ensure nutritional goals are met. Obtaining adequate sleep when travelling (especially if crossing multiple time zones) can also be problematic for many athletes, and there is emerging evidence that nutrition may influence sleep quality and quantity and, therefore, may be important to consider for the travelling athlete. Carbohydrate, protein (tryptophan), alcohol and caffeine may influence sleep and jet lag in athletes. This chapter will discuss the key nutrition-related considerations for travel, including jet lag, training and competition schedule, accommodation and meal arrangements, availability of food and drink at destination, hygiene issues, climate and venue facilities.

> **Learning outcomes**
>
> **This chapter will:**
>
> - describe the causes and consequences of jet lag;
> - outline strategies to minimise travel fatigue and jet lag;
> - explain how to plan, prepare and execute effective travel nutrition;
> - identify some of the nutritional issues athletes face when travelling;
> - explain why sleep is important to athletes;
> - describe how nutrition may influence sleep.

Jet lag and the impact of travel on performance

The competition and training schedules of elite athletes often require them to undertake frequent long-haul air travel that negatively affects the **sleep–wake cycle**. Accordingly, air travel can interrupt training schedules and increase the physiological and perceptual loads of athletes prior to competition.[1] With performance often required within days of arrival in a new time zone, it is important to develop a plan to combat the detrimental effects of sleep disruption, **circadian process desynchronisation** and travel fatigue so athletes can return to optimal performance as soon as possible. This will reduce the days

DOI: 10.4324/9781003321286-30

lost to training following travel and may help to optimise competition readiness and performance.

Sleep–wake cycle

Also known as circadian rhythm, a daily pattern that determines when it is time to sleep and when it is time to be awake.

Circadian process desynchronisation

A misalignment between the body's circadian system and the light–dark cycle (external environment).

Jet lag is associated with rapid eastward or westward travel across three or more time zones resulting in temporary impairment in circadian processes (e.g., sleep and wakefulness). Circadian processes influence the physiological, mental and behavioural changes that occur daily on approximately 24-hour cycles. When circadian processes do not correspond with the external environment jet lag symptoms occur, the severity of jet lag increases with the number of time zones crossed.[2] The primary symptoms of jet lag are difficulty initiating and maintaining sleep at night, daytime sleepiness, impaired physical and mental performance, poor mood, appetite suppression and gastrointestinal complaints.[3]

Jet lag

Temporary impairment of biological functions when circadian processes do not correspond with the new external environment.

Jet lag is not experienced with north-to-south or south-to-north long-haul travel as no time zones are crossed. However, this travel still involves exposure to mild **hypoxia**, cabin noise and cramped and uncomfortable conditions; some athletes may also experience anxiety.[4] This leads to **travel fatigue** and sleep disruption, contributing to decreases in aerobic performance, reaction time, concentration, alertness, skill acquisition, mood, immune function, tissue regeneration and appetite regulation.[4] A study of northbound long-haul travel on sleep quality and subjective jet lag in professional soccer players found that sleep was disrupted due to flight and competition scheduling, causing travel fatigue.[5]

Hypoxia

Deficiency in the amount of oxygen reaching the tissues.

Travel fatigue

The perceived tiredness that accompanies extended journeys, be it trans-latitudinal travel (north-south/south-north) or transmeridian travel. It results from a combination of physical, physiological and psychological factors that build up during the course of a trip and can even accumulate over an entire competition season in athletes.

Minimising travel stress

Jet lag and travel fatigue are of concern to athletes as they can compromise physical and cognitive performance. Sleep hygiene recommendations before, during and after the flight may help alleviate the negative effects of travel on sleep. Under normal circumstances, internal circadian processes respond to external cues from the outside environment. These cues are called **zeitgebers** and the most influential are sunlight and the light–dark cycle. Food, exercise, sleep and pharmacological interventions that mimic hormones involved in circadian processes are also zeitgebers but are generally weaker than sunlight.[2]

Zeitgebers

External or environmental cues which synchronise an individual's biological rhythms to the Earth's 24-hour light–dark cycle.

One commonly used strategy to minimise jet lag is to optimise light exposure and avoidance techniques to adapt when arriving at a new destination. While natural sunlight has powerful phase-shifting properties, some laboratory-based research suggests that correct timing of artificial/indoor light exposure and avoidance may also be used to facilitate adaptation to a new time zone.[1] More research on the impact of scheduled artificial bright light exposure and avoidance on circadian process resynchronisation following long-haul aeroplane travel is required.

Melatonin is a hormone produced by the body at night, or under dark conditions, that signals night-time to the body. In normal circumstances, melatonin is secreted into the bloodstream between about 9 p.m. and 7 a.m.,[3] in line with the timing of the innate drive to sleep. Melatonin has several effects on the body, including dilation of blood vessels on the skin, which increases heat loss from the body, subsequently causing the drop in core body temperature required for sleep.[3] In the absence of melatonin, heat loss and the subsequent drop in core body temperature are affected and sleep onset and quality will be negatively impacted. Normally, melatonin is released in the body approximately two hours before bedtime, provided there is limited light exposure at this time. When circadian processes are desynchronised with the external environment, melatonin secretion is incorrectly timed; this is one of the primary reasons for sleep disruption when jet-lagged. Therefore, melatonin may be used to treat jet lag, although the timing of ingestion is highly specific and individual. The dose of melatonin is also highly individual and, if the dose is too high, melatonin may remain in the bloodstream too long and act at the wrong time. Additionally, melatonin should be administered with caution in athletes as it is considered a medication, can only be prescribed by a doctor, is not readily available and, in many cases, must be provided by a compound pharmacist.

It has been found that exercise lasting 1–3 hours can induce significant circadian phase shifts. The time of day at which exercise is completed, intensity of exercise, lighting conditions and age and gender of participants are confounding factors. Furthermore, most previous research in this area has been conducted on elderly patients, a population vastly different to elite athletes. However, since athletes are highly likely to engage in training before and after travel, there is potential to schedule this training at the times most likely to correctly adjust circadian processes.

The strategies in Box 27.1 may be used to minimise travel fatigue and jet lag.

Box 27.1 Nutrition-related strategies to minimise travel fatigue and jet lag

Before Travel

- fill water bottles (after boarding) and drink enough water to stay hydrated;
- pack personal food for the flight and for the duration of the trip if travel food does not meet nutritional needs. Choose foods that fit with the nutrition plan for the current phase of training and competition; be mindful of carbohydrate and protein foods to maintain requirements;
- plan catering options at the destination before departure.

During Travel

- ask when meals will be served to plan when to sleep and ensure meals are received;
- drink enough fluid to stay hydrated. If possible, eat meals at the time they will be consumed at the destination. To help avoid disruption to sleep, avoid large amounts of caffeine (<1 cup of coffee per four hours) and stop drinking coffee, cola and other caffeinated beverages in the 6–8 hours before bedtime;
- avoid alcohol;
- be aware of food hygiene—wash hands regularly and ensure hot foods are hot and cold foods are cold.

After Travel

- avoid caffeine in the afternoon and evening as it may interrupt sleep;
- if constipated on arrival, consume more fluid and fibre-rich foods as well as natural laxatives (prunes, chia seeds, kiwi fruit, apples, nuts);
- eat meals at the usual time of day (of the destination).

Nutrition and travel

Travel can heighten the risk of an athlete being unable to meet their nutrition goals or developing an illness. Unfortunately, this is often at a time when the outcomes of training preparation and competition performance are of the greatest importance. Athletes should seek personalised advice, as nutrition recommendations vary and will be specific to each destination and athlete.

Planning

Preparation prior to departure can mitigate many of these risks to performance and health. One strategy that is useful for athletes and support staff to undertake well in advance of departure is a travel nutrition 'risk management audit'.

Several questions must be answered within this audit, the first being, what are the risks to successful performance at the destination? Each 'risk' then needs to be further explored and a risk management strategy put in place. Table 27.1 shows an example of the audit process.

It is often useful to talk to other athletes, staff and coaches who have travelled to the destination previously. Their experiences can highlight issues that need to be considered during planning.

A timeline for strategy development and execution, along with the allocation of roles and responsibilities, then needs to be developed.

Considerations that should be incorporated into the planning process include the following:

- itinerary;
- training and competition schedule;
- type of accommodation and meal arrangements;
- familiarity with the destination—food and drink availability, hygiene issues, climate;
- local dietary habits (e.g., timing of meals);
- food and fluids provided by competition management/organisers;
- distance between accommodation and training/competition venue(s);
- venue facilities (safe water supply, refrigerators, etc.).

An athlete's specific nutrition goals need to be central to all planning. While some adaptability will be needed, a nutrition action plan for training and competition days should be made before departure so that major issues are avoided.

Common travel nutrition issues

Many of the common nutrition-related issues experienced by athletes who travel are presented in the following section, along with suggestions for how these issues could be mitigated.

Table 27.1 An example of a travel nutrition risk management audit

Risk	Risk management strategy in place?	Further strategy development required?	Level of risk?	Level of risk with strategy in place?
Example: Unknown food supply on flight	Call the airline and discuss the food provided.	Plan to take your own snacks on board if the airline cannot provide a special meal.	Moderate	Low

Box 27.2   Strategies for managing nutrition-related challenges during travel

Flights

A number of stresses can take place in transit that are independent of the time zones crossed. Dry, pressurised air in the cabin of an airplane results in a need for increased fluid intake during flight. This is especially the case for long-haul flights, where significant dehydration could occur.

- carry an empty water bottle and use the onboard taps (located near the flight attendant stations) to refill;
- request additional fluids beyond those provided at meal services (these are invariably very small containers);
- alcohol can contribute to dehydration and avoidance should be considered;
- caffeine-containing fluids are a suitable choice to add to fluid balance if they are a regular part of an athlete's diet (avoid late afternoon and night if caffeine interferes with sleep).

Food supplied by airlines does not always meet the nutrition requirements of an athlete.

- airlines tend to provide a limited range of foods. Special requests can be made, but airlines may not be able to meet an athlete's requirements;
- special meal requests to airlines should be made well in advance of flights;
- athletes should take their own snacks on board. These are useful if the food provided does not meet requirements, or if unexpected delays occur;
- if an athlete's energy requirements are high, they should take high-energy snacks onboard to snack on, such as trail mix, muesli or energy bars;
- alternatively, if the athlete has low energy needs they will need to be wary of snacking due to boredom. Taking some sugar-free chewing gum and drinking low-energy fluids, such as water, can be a useful strategy to overcome this temptation.

Travel by road

If travelling via car or bus it is advisable to pack a small cooler or lunchbox with meals or snacks and fluids to ensure appropriate items are on hand. This will also be a more economical option than relying on overpriced service station items.

Illness

Gastrointestinal infections related to travelling are frequent among athletes and are often food- and fluid-borne.

- education of athletes and support staff before travel is required;
- many infections can be prevented by taking care with food and fluid choices, along with personal hygiene;

- avoiding the local water supply in countries where potential pathogens could be consumed in this manner is essential. Care should be taken to avoid ice in drinks and to avoid brushing teeth with local water. Drinks should be consumed from sealed containers only;
- beware that salads and peeled fruit may have been washed in local, contaminated water and are best avoided unless confident that they are safe;
- unpasteurised dairy products should be avoided;
- care should be taken to only eat meals that are either served very hot or cold;
- using probiotics and prebiotics both prior to departure and during the travel period can help minimise the risk of certain infections.

Additional food supplies

Packing a supply of food and sports foods from home will be useful if the food supply (type, quality, safety) is unknown, the athlete is a fussy eater, or if they rely on specific products around training sessions and competitions. Always check ahead with customs/quarantine authorities to identify what foods are restricted.

Environment

An athlete's nutrition needs may be different at the destination due to the environment (e.g., due to altitude or heat; see Chapter 14). Develop a plan to counter any negative effects of these changes before leaving home.

Eating out

Eating out can be tricky in terms of meeting nutrition requirements.

- try to check out menus online before selecting a restaurant;
- special dietary needs should be organised ahead of time;
- if travelling with large groups of athletes, calling ahead and arranging for a certain number of specific meals to be ready to serve can help reduce wait times.

Buffets

Buffets offer a large variety of foods and it is easy to eat more than required in this setting.

- it is important that the athlete is familiar with their own nutrition goals;
- athletes should be encouraged to do 'a lap' of the buffet or dining hall to gauge what is on the menu before plating their own meal;
- the athlete should be selective with their choices rather than taking some of everything on offer;
- leaving the dining area as soon as the meal has been consumed helps to prevent the temptation to go back for more.

Self-catering

Staying in accommodation that has access to cooking facilities allows for flexibility in meal times and food options.

- using an online shopping service can be useful if ordering large quantities (e.g., when cooking or ordering for a whole squad);
- having 'go-to' recipes that require few ingredients and minimal cooking equipment (often sparse in rented accommodation) is suggested.

Hydration

Monitoring hydration using morning body weight or with urine-specific gravity testing is advisable, especially after long-haul flights or in hot climates.

- in hot and humid countries and sporting venues, sweat rates can be significant;
- regular body weights of individual athletes before and after exercise sessions are useful to determine hydration status;
- drinking large volumes of water, especially during hard exercise, may lead to hyponatraemia. The use of a sports drink or electrolyte drink can help to address this problem.

Sleep

Sleep is increasingly recognised as one of the critical foundations of an athlete's training program. Sleep is considered the best recovery strategy available to athletes due to its physical and psychological restorative effects. Getting adequate sleep can decrease injury risk, improve reaction time, coordination, concentration, memory, learning, motivation, mood and immunity and increase performance. Sleep also aids the repair and regeneration of muscles and tissues due to important hormonal release (growth hormone in particular) that occurs during sleep.[6]

Nutrition and sleep

Although evidence for how nutrition impacts sleep is still emerging, it is an area of growing interest to researchers and athletes alike. Some nutrition strategies are known to impact both sleep onset and quality and can be manipulated by athletes to achieve improved sleep outcomes.

Several brain neurotransmitters are associated with the sleep–wake cycle. Specific nutrition interventions can act on these neurotransmitters to influence sleep.[6] The rate of synthesis and function of the neurotransmitter 5-HT (which in turn stimulates the production of melatonin), is influenced by the availability of its precursor tryptophan.[7] Tryptophan is an amino acid found in foods such as eggs, meat, poultry and dairy products.

Tryptophan must be transported across the blood–brain barrier for it to have its sleep-inducing impact and carbohydrate is needed to support this process. Therefore, a drink, snack or meal that contains both tryptophan and carbohydrate could help induce sleep. Popular sleep-inducing tryptophan-rich snack options include milk, yoghurt, tuna, crackers, cheese and crackers.

Recent studies evaluating a 'food first' approach to improving athlete sleep and recovery have returned positive findings for the consumption of kiwifruit. Kiwifruit contains melatonin, which as discussed, plays a role in circadian rhythm regulation. A study with 15 elite athletes showed that consumption of two kiwifruit (*Actinidia deliciosa*) one hour before bed over four weeks led to improvements in sleep quality, recovery–stress balance, total sleep time, sleep efficiency, number of awakenings and wake after sleep onset.[8] While these initial findings are promising, further research on the benefits of kiwifruit and other promising food-based strategies including tart cherry juice is required.

There has been recent commercial interest in nutritional supplements for sleep. Athletes should use caution regarding unsubstantiated claims about sleep-enhancing products.[9] Athletes should also understand the risks of a doping violation for supplement products not assessed by an established third-party quality assurance programme.[10]

Alcohol may also help a person feel sleepy and fall asleep more quickly. However, once alcohol levels in the blood fall, sleep is disrupted and the amount of quality sleep is reduced.[11] Athletes should be made aware of this so that an informed choice around alcohol consumption can be made.

Caffeine has a role in the performance plan of many athletes, as well as being a regular feature in many athletes' habitual eating plans. Given caffeine can delay an athlete's natural signals to go to sleep, its use as an ergogenic aid in sport needs to be carefully planned. The athlete should identify the dose and timing of caffeine required to maximise performance and minimise sleep disturbances by trialling caffeine intake strategies in training (see Chapter 12).

Summary

This chapter has described how effective planning and preparation for travel in elite athletes is essential to optimise performance and reduce the risk of illness. Reducing the symptoms of jet lag can aid in reducing training days lost due to travel. Through careful planning and execution of travel, nutrition and sleep strategies, it is possible to minimise some of the negative influences of travel on athletes. This may have a positive influence on health, wellbeing, mood and, importantly, performance.

Chapter highlights

- Jet lag can result in physiological and psychological symptoms that may impair performance.
- Light, exercise, caffeine and melatonin may be used to manage jet lag, although these need to be used with caution.
- Strategies such as sleep, planning, nutrition, exercise and compression garments can be used before and during travel to manage travel fatigue and jet lag.
- Nutritional considerations such as nutrition provisions in transit, food and fluid safety (hygiene), meal availability at the destination, and food and fluid provided by the training or competition venue are important.
- Destination eating options (eating out, buffets and self-catering) have issues that need to be planned for prior to travel.
- Monitoring hydration after travel is recommended.
- The role of nutrition in enhancing sleep is likely to become an important area of future focus.

Nutrition and travel

Prior to departure:

- develop a 'travel nutrition risk management audit' as part of preparation well in advance of the planned travel;
- take familiar foods from home to supplement the food available at the destination.

In transit:

- take extra snacks on board the flight(s) to ensure nutrition needs will be met;
- drink small amounts of fluid regularly;
- caffeinated drinks are fine to consume (before late afternoon/evening) if they are usually part of a usual daily routine.

At the destination:

- pay attention to individual nutrition goals and requirements—don't become distracted by other athletes' nutrition plans or intake;
- ensure that the type of meal provision (buffet, self-catering, restaurant) caters for each individual athlete's needs;
- consider hydration monitoring to help ensure performance is not reduced by dehydration.

Nutrition and sleep

- research into nutrition and sleep is in its infancy and therefore specific strategies are difficult to define;
- alcohol intake can reduce the amount of quality sleep;
- caffeine can impact sleep onset and quality. If athletes are interested in using caffeine as an ergogenic aid, they should trial it well in advance of the competition.

References

1. Fowler P, Duffield R, Howle K. Effects of northbound long-haul international air travel on sleep quality and subjective jet lag and wellness in professional Australian soccer players. *Int J Sports Physiol Perform*. 2014;10(2):648–654.
2. Janse van Rensburg DC, Jansen van Rensburg A, Fowler PM, et al. Managing travel fatigue and jet lag in athletes: a review and consensus statement. *Sports Med*. 2021;51(10):2029–2050.
3. Waterhouse AJ, Reilly T, Edwards B. The stress of travel. *J Sport Sci*. 2004;22(10):946–966.
4. Youngstedt SD, O'Connor PJ. The influence of air travel on athletic performance. *Sports Med*. 1999;28(3):197–207.
5. Fowler P, Duffield R, Morrow I. Effects of sleep hygiene and artificial bright light interventions on recovery from simulated international air travel. *Eur J Appl Physiol*. 2015;115(3):541–553.
6. Halson SL. Sleep in elite athletes and nutritional interventions to enhance sleep. *Sports Med*. 2014;44(S1):S13–S23.
7. Grimmett A, Sillence MN. Calmatives for the excitable horse: A review of L-tryptophan. *Vet J*. 2005;170(1):24–32.
8. Doherty R, Madigan S, Nevill A, et al. The impact of kiwifruit consumption on the sleep and recovery of elite athletes. *Nutrients*. 2023;15(10):2274.

9. Walsh NP, Halson SL, Sargent C, et al. Sleep and the athlete: Narrative review and 2021 expert consensus recommendations. *Br J Sports Med.* 2021:55(7):356–368.

10. Maughan RJ, Burke LM, Dvorak J et al. IOC consensus statement: Dietary supplements and the high-performance athlete. *Br J Sports Med.* 2018:52:439–455.

11. Ebrahim IO, Shapiro CM, Williams AJ. Alcohol and sleep I: Effects on normal sleep. *Alcohol Clin Exp Res.* 2013;37(4):539–549.

28 The art of sports nutrition practice

Evangeline Mantzioris and Case Study Contributors: Alan McCubbin, Anthony Meade, Erin Colebatch, Gregory Cox, Rachel Stentiford, Rebecca Hall, Regina Belski, Ryan Tam, Sarah L Jenner, Stephanie K Gaskell and Stephen Smith

The previous chapters have detailed the science of sports nutrition, and this is perhaps the easy part where we can calculate the type, quantity, and timing of macronutrients to fuel performance. The challenge lies in translating this into practice for athletes; that is the art of sports nutrition practice where the theoretical knowledge must be translated to food to enable fuelling strategies. These strategies need to consider individual taste and food preferences, current health problems and the lifespan stage of the athletes. Furthermore, sports nutrition professionals need to be aware of the cultural, religious, and belief values of the athlete. Additionally, the practicality of food provision needs to be considered – how easily can food be carried and consumed by the athlete during competition, the ease of transport by the support teams to venues and feeding stations, and, of course, micro-biological safety when refrigeration is not available. The sports nutrition professional also requires a good understanding of the athletes' sport, training, and competition contexts and feeding opportunities within the rules of that sport. Finally, they need to know how the environmental conditions will affect fuelling needs and impact food choices, as well as the availability of foods for purchase at the location.

Central to all of this is the need for excellent communication skills for assessing athletes' diets and training and competition requirements, and for counselling and education so athletes can implement fuelling strategies. Additionally, the ability to communicate complex scientific nutrition information in practical lay language with the sports science team is imperative to maximise success.

In this chapter, sports nutrition professionals describe how they navigate the complexities that arise with different athletes, across different sports, and environmental conditions.

Learning outcomes

This chapter will:

- describe strategies for translating scientific messages to the athletes and multi-disciplinary sports teams supporting the athletes;
- highlight the importance of being aware of the cultural differences of athletes and how this translates into nutrition practice;

DOI: 10.4324/9781003321286-31

- describe how to translate the fuelling requirements into fuelling strategies that can easily be adapted by the athletes and using race plans;
- highlight fuelling across the lifespan, and in emerging sports such as skateboarding;
- discuss how to fuel for extreme environments;
- outline fuelling strategies for teams of athletes;
- describe how to cater for large international sport events for multiple different athletes and teams of athletes.

Communication for assessment, planning, and education

Sports nutrition professionals are highly trained in delivering nutrition education and dietary advice for athletes. High-level communication skills are critical for building rapport with the athlete, as well as for detailed nutrition assessment that is required to develop plans that can be implemented, and for involving other members of the athlete support team in these processes.

> Not every conversation with athletes will be a formal consult in a consultation room. While appointments generally make life easier to perform more detailed assessments and provide education, with teams of athletes it is equally important to be visible and to 'float' around to be available to ask questions. Being at training, or key positions such as recovery stations, often leads to conversations that develop rapport and allow you to demonstrate what you do in a more 'public' space. Sometimes overhearing player conversations (or players overhearing your conversations) encourages other individual or group discussions, initiated by the players or the dietitian.
>
> (Anthony Meade)

It is important for the sports nutrition professional to get accurate dietary information from the athletes across their entire diet.

> When taking a dietary recall specific to a day of training, it's important to establish the athlete's typical dietary intake for a rest or non-exercise day and then understand the foods/fluids they have strategically added to accommodate for the additional training.
>
> (Gregory Cox)

The sports nutrition professional needs to maintain good communication with the athlete (and their support team) even after assessment of the athlete and developing their nutrition care plan.

> The sports nutrition professional should continue to work closely with the athlete, coach, and other support team members to fine tune daily dietary intake and modify according to changes in daily training loads throughout the week. Sports nutrition advice is not static and should be modified alongside the annual training plan. This is particularly important for endurance athletes as daily training varies considerably throughout the year.
>
> (Gregory Cox)

Cultural considerations

Athletes often travel abroad for training and competition. Their usual dietary habits and eating plans may be affected when they face new environments with different cultures. Additionally, with globalisation and the ease of international travel, many countries now have teams that are composed of athletes with different ethnic, cultural, and religious backgrounds, as well as different philosophical approaches to choosing food. Although the principles of healthy dietary intake and the nutrition goals for sports performance are similar across different cultures, there is an infinite variety of food combinations that athletes may choose to meet their nutritional goals. An understanding of different cultural perspectives is important for athletes and the sports nutrition professionals who work with them to appreciate how foods from different countries of the world may contribute to their dietary plans for exercise and performance.

Many religions have a set of guidelines for eating; for some religions, they are prescriptive, while for others they are recommendations. Just how closely individuals choose to adhere to the guidelines will be determined by their devotion to their religion, as well as cultural and family influences. As culture strongly influences the foods we consume, it is important to be aware of an athlete's cultural background and personal philosophy before translating sport-specific nutritional guidelines into food-based dietary advice for exercise performance. Some religions also have prescribed or recommended dietary restrictions or fasting periods which require careful consideration.

Vegetarianism features in many religions, and it is important to understand that there are several types of vegetarianism and that athletes may choose a vegetarian diet based on any number of religious or philosophical beliefs. Hence, it is important to ask the athlete what they choose to include in their diet – this could vary along the spectrum from vegans who consume no animal products at all to vegetarians who include both dairy and eggs. Different religions set dietary laws that can affect the type of foods that are consumed, as well as the timing of food consumption. This timing can vary within one religion from day to day and week to week in accordance with religious festivals (i.e., Hindu, Moslem, Eastern Orthodox, Roman Catholic). While taking these factors into account when translating the fuelling requirements into food will be straightforward for individual athletes, it becomes more complex when working with a team who have a variety of different cultural, religious, and philosophical dietary requirements.

Practical fuelling strategies

Developing fuelling strategies for athletes requires consideration of the type and amount of food as well as how it will be delivered to the athlete at the appropriate time. While some sports provide opportunities for fuelling during designated breaks in play, other sports require fuelling while competing which could be while running, swimming (long-distance), cycling, or skiing. In these cases, athletes will need to be able to easily open the food/drink and get the food to their mouth.

> Making food easier to open for the athletes is critical, wrapping the food in foil rather than plastic wrap makes a big difference to opening the food, using flip top drink bottles rather than capped bottles. Reminders for cyclists to fuel by placing masking tape on bike bar with indications of times to consume or setting smart watch alarms to remind athletes of fuelling requirements. Messages can also be sent to them during the race if conditions change their fuelling requirements (if allowed within the rules of the game).
> (Regina Belski)

Elite athletes need to be well prepared for training and competition; it is the role of the sports nutrition professional to educate them and train them to be able to translate their fuelling requirements into food.

> Elite triathletes need to be well organised to meet daily energy, carbohydrate and nutrient needs to maintain training performance, health, and well-being. Timing appropriate snacks around training and including nutritious foods at meals that provide antioxidants in addition to carbohydrate, protein and healthy fats will assist training performance and recovery.
>
> (Gregory Cox)

Race plans for competition days are critical in planning for the event so that the athlete knows exactly what to expect and what they must do to prepare. The race plan should also be very specific about exactly what fuelling is needed at which time point and (if relevant) at which station it will be collected. These are very typical considerations for marathon, cycling, and triathlon. Athletes may carry their fuelling plans as a piece of paper, digitally on smartwatches, or write it on masking tape and stick it on the frame of their bike. Sports nutrition professionals also need to find ways of ensuring athletes consume the food at the appropriate time, which needs to be written into their race plan, as this can be easily forgotten if the athletes are focussing on the competition strategy.

> Endurance athletes should have race plans. It indicates when they need to fuel, and what will be available for them at each feed station. With the availability of high-level accurate weather forecasts, the ambient temperature will also be known which will determine fuelling and hydration needs. Good race plans include shopping lists – for this the sports nutrition professional needs to know what is available from the neighbouring food stores and what the athlete needs to pack. Below is an example of a race plan I developed in collaboration with an athlete., It includes all of these considerations for a Masters' athlete competing in a 50km run in the Blue Mountains, Australia.
>
> (Erin Colebatch)

This race plan is very detailed, with an included shopping plan so that the athlete knows what they must bring from home, and what they can buy on location. To develop these plans, the sports nutrition professional needs to have detailed knowledge of the availability of products in overseas countries and remote locations. The sports foods and supplements listed in this plan are available for athletes in Australia, but may not be available in other parts of the world.

Box 28.1   UTA 50 km race plan

Shopping Lists
Includes carb loading, pre-race fueling & race nutrition

Home
Sports nutrition

- 14 scoops isotonic carbohydrate formula (Infinit brand) (recommend travel with unopened, fully sealed bag)
- 3 energy bars (TORQ brand)

- 8 sports gels (Gu brand)
- 2 hydrogels (no caffeine) (Maurten brand)
- 3 × 100 mg caffeine energy strips (Revvies brand)
- 3 × 70 ml Beetroot juice (Beet It Brand) – may be beneficial to take 1 × 70 ml shot 4 hourly during the race also – if so, add 1 shot

Blue Mountains
Ready meals

- 2 ready meals at least 60 g carbohydrate, for example, fried rice (if not cooking dinners from scratch)

Dairy

- 1 L low fat milk
- 2 × liquid breakfast tetra pack (Up & Go Brand)
- 1 × 600 ml flavoured milk (low fat)

Bakery

- 1 loaf sourdough
- 2 large sweet bakery items, for example, finger bun
- 1 loaf of fruit cake

Fruit and vegetables

- 1 banana
- Salad filling for lunch sandwich/roll
- Mixed vegetables (if cooking dinners from scratch)

Meat/meat alternatives

- Sliced meat filling for lunch sandwich/roll
- 500 g beef/chicken/seafood (if cooking dinners from scratch)

Pantry items

- 1 small jar of jam
- 1 small jar of peanut butter
- 1 packet of small muesli bars
- 500 g Jasmine rice (if cooking dinners from scratch)
- 1 × 40 second rice pot
- 2 × 420 g creamed rice
- Hot chocolate powder
- Oil for cooking
- Coffee
- 1 small box of snap-lock bags

Snack foods

- 1 packet marshmallows
- 1 small packet of lollies/candies/sweets of choice
- 1 small packet of ginger lollies/crystallised ginger

Drinks

- 2 × 375 ml of cola-based sugar soft drink
- 2 × liquid breakfast tetra pack (Up & Go Energize Brand)

Sports nutrition

- 5 × 600 ml sports drink (or purchase powder and make up yourself)

Additionally, information is provided on extra items that the athletes will need to pack with them specifically for the race, in addition to the mandatory race pack gear. In this case, the schedule of the event has also been listed so that the plan contains all the necessary information.

Box 28.2   Packing list

Add any extra items you need

- Sports nutrition as per home shopping list
- Race pack
- 5 soft flasks
- 1.5 L bladder
- Mandatory gear (see race pack list)
- Soft, collapsible cup

Event schedule

Add any extra info you need

Date	Time	Activity	Location
Tuesday			
Wednesday		Shopping	
Thursday	7:30–11:00 am	Race check-in 11 km	KCC Auditorium
	11:00 am	11 km start	Scenic World
	4:30 pm	11 km presentations	Scenic World
	1:00–8:00 pm	Race check-in 50 km	KCC Auditorium
Friday	9 am	Mandatory gear announcement	Facebook/app/website
		Pack finish drop bag & race pack	
	10 am–5 pm & 5:30–7 pm	Race check-in 50 km	KCC Auditorium
	5:30–6:15 pm	Race briefing	KCC Auditorium

Date	Time	Activity	Location
Saturday	6:32–8:02 am	50 km start	Scenic World
	From 10:45 am	50 km finish	Scenic World
	10:32 pm	50 km cut off	Scenic World
Sunday	10:30–11:30 am	50 race presentations	Scenic World

Weather

Katoomba average weather May: low 6°C, high 14°C, relative humidity 77%

One of the most important features of the race plan is to provide the exact details on what is to be consumed before, during and after the race. In the following tables, details include the time to consume the products, and with the amount of carbohydrates, in case the athlete needs to find a replacement product. In the actual race day plans, the sports nutrition professional has advised the athlete to drink to thirst, this would be a reflection of previous discussions about the athlete's hydration status during events – allowing for flexibility according to environmental conditions at the time. Back-up plans are also given if the athlete experiences gastrointestinal distress or if they start cramping. There are also details about what to pack each day for the race and the topography of the racecourse.

Box 28.3   Thursday UTA 11 km & carbohydrate loading

Meal/Snack	Food/Drinks	Carbohydrate (g)
7 am Breakfast	2 thick slices sourdough with 1 tbsp jam spread + peanut butter on each 600 ml Sports drink Milk coffee + Start sipping 2nd 600 ml sports drink after BF	171
9 am Morning tea	Finish 300 ml from the second bottle of sports drink 1 handful lollies/candies + 1 finger bun 1 Beet It shot	90
11 am Run	500 ml Infinit + 500 ml water	60
12:30 pm Recovery	2 × Up & Go Energize + TORQ bar	97
3 pm Afternoon tea	Frozen fried rice microwaved + 600 ml sports drink	96
6:30 pm Dinner	Rice dish – in or out (aim for 1.5 cups cooked) + 1 can of cola soft drink	147
Supper	1 × 420 g of tin creamed rice	78
Drinks	1 × Beet It shot (any time of day) Water to thirst	18
TOTAL		757 (12.4 g/kg)

- Avoid high fat foods, wholegrain breads and cereals, heavy nuts and/or dried fruit, legumes, skins/seeds/stalks of fruit and vegetables, spicy foods, excessive onion and/or garlic
- Suggest using the Easy Diet Diary app to track daily carbohydrate intake to ensure meeting target

Friday – Carbohydrate loading

Meal/Snack	Food/Drinks	Carbohydrate (g)
Breakfast	2 thick slices sourdough with 1 tbsp jam spread on each Milk coffee 600 ml sports drink – sip through the morning	117
Morning tea	1 TORQ bar OR 1 large bakery item, for example, fruit scroll/finger bun/ date scone	43–60
Lunch	1 large focaccia/Turkish bread/2 white bread sandwiches with a small amount of salad and sliced meat 600 ml sports drink – sip through the afternoon	96
Afternoon tea	600 ml low fat flavoured milk OR 1 large slice of fruit cake	60

Dinner	Stir fry with 1.5 cups cooked Jasmine rice + 100 g beef/
	  chicken/seafood
	+1/2 cup cooked (1 cup raw) bok choy, spring onion tips,
	  capsicum, & broccoli florets
	OR
	1.5 cups cooked cous cous + max 1 cup bolognese/
	  chicken sauce
	OR
	Pre-made supermarket meal, (Choose higher carb, lower
	  fibre options) + 1 cup pre-cooked rice packet
	1 can of cola soft drink
		140–170

Supper	1 × 420 g of tin creamed rice OR Hot chocolate with 250 ml low fat milk, 1 tbsp choc powder + 2 marshmallows	45–78
Drinks	Total ~1.5 L high carbohydrate fluid across the day (include as above, or swap around) 1 × Beet It shot (any time of day) Water to thirst	
TOTAL		520–600 g (8.5–10g/kg)

- Avoid high fat foods, wholegrain breads and cereals, heavy nuts and/or dried fruit, legumes, skins/seeds/stalks of fruit and vegetables, spicy foods, excessive onion and/or garlic
- Suggest using the Easy Diet Diary app to track daily carbohydrate intake to ensure meeting target

Saturday, UTA 50 km

Bring finish drop bag to start line & drop at the CMS Building

Meal/Snack	Food/Drinks	Carb (g)	Pro (g)	Fluid (ml)	Caffeine (mg)	Sodium (mg)
Pre-race breakfast 5:00 am	2 thick slices white sourdough toast with 1 tbsp jam spread on each + 1 banana Milk coffee 70 ml Beet It + up to 250 ml water if thirsty or dark urine on waking	111	8	320–570 ml	~100 mg	-
Pre-race top up 6:45 am	1 handful lollies (30 g) 1 Revvies Sips of water	30	-	Sips	100 mg	-
During race Start: 7:00 am **Est. race time**: 6.75–8.5 hrs	See *detailed race plan*	55–75 g/hr	-	235 –295ml/hr Infinit (2 scoops per 500 ml) Drink water to thirst Plan has you carrying enough for total 590–740 ml/hr Drink extra water at checkpoints if you are thirsty	1 × 100 mg	410 mg/L (if all fluid on plan is consumed)
Recovery	Any combination you like!	>50	35–40	As desired	-	As desired
Back up plans	• If GI distress: Back off food and fluid • Mouth rinse sports drink • Slow down until you can take in nutrition again • Ginger (crystallised/lollies/ginger beer) for nausea If cramp: • Stretch • Slow pace					

Race pack UTA 11 km *(italics = mandatory gear)*

In front part of pack:

- Flask 1: Infinit (2 scoops in 500 ml water)
- Flask 2: Water
- *Whistle*

In back part of pack:

- *Long sleeve thermal top (polypropylene, wool)*
- *Waterproof and breathable jacket with fully taped waterproof seams and hood*
- *Beanie, balaclava or buff*
- *Small back up light*
- *Mobile/Cell phone – battery fully charged*
- *Space blanket*
- *1 × compression bandage (minimum dimensions 7.5 cm wide × 2.3 m long unstretched)*
- *Participants emergency instructions card*
- *Race number*
- *Timing tag for backpack*

Course Profile – UTA 11 km

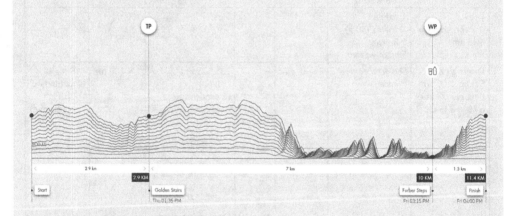

Race pack UTA 50 km

In front part of pack:

- Flask 1 & 2: Infinit (2 scoops in 500 ml water)
- 8 Gu gels
- 1 Revvies – pack carefully so you don't lose it!
- 1 soft/collapsible cup (for drinking at checkpoints if needed)
- *Whistle*

In back part of pack:

- Bladder: 1500 ml water
- Flask 3 & 4: Infinit (2 scoops, no water)
- <u>Emergency pack:</u> 1 × 2 Scoops Infinit in soft flask (no water), 2 × Maurten gel, 1 handful ginger lollies (in Glad bag), 1 Revvies
- *Long sleeve thermal top (polypropylene, wool)*
- *Waterproof and breathable jacket with fully taped waterproof seams and hood*
- *Beanie, balaclava or buff*
- *Hi-visibility safety vest*
- *Headlamp*
- *Small back up light*
- *Mobile/Cell phone – battery fully charged*
- *Compass*
- *Space blanket*
- *1 × compression bandage (minimum dimensions 7.5 cm wide × 2.3 m long unstretched)*
- *Lightweight dry sack or zip lock bags*
- *Ziplock bag for rubbish*
- *Waterproof map case (can be in zip lock bag)*
- *Course map & course descriptions*
- *Participants emergency instructions card*
- *Race number*
- *Timing tag for backpack*

<u>Additional items to consider:</u> body lubricant, sunscreen, hat, spare socks, spare headlight batteries, spare headlamp, additional first aid items (e.g., sterile dressings, strapping tape, blister care items, antiseptic wipes, medications), external phone battery charger.

UTA 50 race plan (6.75–8.5 hours)

ETA	Leg	Leg km	Race km	+/−	Pace (min/km)	Leg time	Carb reqt (g)	Fluid	Food	Notes
Start: 0700 0850–0925	Start-CP1 (Fairmont)	16.8	16.8		6.30–8.30	1'50–2'25	135–180	1000 ml I 1500 ml W	2–3 Gu gels	Undulating then steep descent 9–10 km. Stepped climb out to 11 km. Undulating to CP **Toilets**: 5.9 km (Scenic World), 8.5 km (Echo Point), 12 km (Leura Cascades Carpark), 14 km (Gordon Falls Reserve) **Provisions**: Water, NAAK Electrolyte (pre-mixed), NAAK Bars & Waffles, Winners gels, chocolates, bakery goods, fruit, salt, chips, soup and lollies will be available. Hot water, tea, and coffee available. **Eat**: 1 big handful of lollies **Take**: 1 big handful of lollies in zip lock bag

ETA	Leg	Leg km	Race km	+/−	Pace (min/km)	Leg time	Carb reqt (g)	Fluid	Food	Notes
1005–1105	CP1–CP2 (QV Hospital)	11.4	28.2		6.30–8.30	1'15–1'40	95–125		1 handful lollies	Undulating with a couple of steep descents and ascents. **Toilets**: 21.8 km (Conservation Hut), 23 km (Wentworth Fall Picnic Area) **Provisions**: Water, NAAK Electrolyte (pre-mixed), NAAK Bars & Waffles, Winners gels, chocolates, bakery goods, fruit, salt, chips, soup and lollies, hot water, tea and coffee **Eat**: 1 waffle + 1 Revvies **Fill**: Water and Infinit
1150–1320	CP2–Emerg Aid Station	12.8	41		8.00–10.00	1'45–2'10	130–165	1000 ml I 1500 ml W	1 bar 1–2 Gu gels	Descent down Kedumba Pass to 36 km and then two climbs out and short downhill to EAS **Toilet**: 41.2 km (EAS) **Provisions**: Water, NAAK Electrolyte (pre-mixed), salt, lollies. **Eat**: 1 big handful of lollies
1340–1535	EAS–Fin	9	50		12.00–15.00	1'50–2'15	95–135		2–3 Gu gels	Climbing all the way, including Furber Stairs **Recovery provisions**: water, electrolyte, fruit

A carbohydrate serve-ready reckoner is also provided to educate and give the athlete flexibility so that they can adopt their eating plan as needed, for example, if food products are unavailable.

Box 28.4 Carb serves calculator

Food/fluid	Serve size	Carbohydrate (g)	Sodium (mg)	Caffeine
Infinit	500 ml (2 scoops + 500 ml water)	60	400	-
NAAK electrolyte	500 ml (2 scoops + 500 ml water)	55	400	-
NAAK waffle	1 waffle	17	140	-
TORQ bar	1 bar	43	74	-
NAAK bar (caffeinated)	1 bar	28	180	65 mg
Gu gel	1 gel	23	55	
Maurten gel	1 gel	25	34	
Winners' gels	1 gel	30	36	-
Lollies	30 g lollies (1 large handful)	30	0	-
Potato crisps	1 snack pack (2 handfuls)	8	179	-
Banana	1 large banana	22	0	-
Orange	1 orange	15	0	-
Watermelon	1 medium slice	5	0	-
Bakery good – sweet	1 large item	40–60	200–400	
Bakery good – savoury	1 large item	40–60	200–450	-
Soup	250 ml	0–20	500–900	-
Chocolate	1 mini bar	10	18	neg
Coke	250 ml	25	44	25
Revvies	1 tablet	-	-	100

Fuelling across the lifespan

While traditionally, elite athletes might be regarded as being between 18 and 30 years of age, this is being challenged by younger athletes performing in the world circuit in new sports, and by masters athletes training and performing at highly competitive levels. Each age group presents its own challenges to the sports nutrition professional with the youth still growing and developing and the masters' athletes being at increased risk of developing chronic hereditary and lifestyle diseases. While teenagers have always been involved in sports and competition, the introduction of emerging sports such as skateboarding to the professional elite level has led to a greater number of adolescents competing, beyond the traditional sports of ballet, diving, and gymnastics.

Skateboarding is a new Olympic sport with no universal minimum age to compete at the Olympics. This has resulted in many talented skateboarders (as young as 13) with increased incentive to travel the world on the Pro skateboarding circuit and compete at events to accrue points for selection onto national Olympic teams. Skateboarders will often spend long days at the skatepark, and while focused on skateboarding, can forget to eat, or don't pack adequate nutrition and hydration for the day. You need to talk to them about suitable options, for example to pack a snack box with options that don't need refrigeration and having multiple drink bottles. The young age of many professional skateboarders and nature of the sport presents some unique challenges from a nutrition point of view, to elicit intrinsic motivation within these athletes to prioritise time to develop their nutrition knowledge, appreciation of the impact nutrition can have on health and performance, and how to apply this in their training and competition environments.

A creative nutrition education program to teach adolescent skateboarders, their caregivers and coaches is essential, including information about the importance of total energy, protein, carbohydrates, and micronutrients for training, health, and robustness, and how they can achieve this. Focusing on practical information and infographic resources are effective. Highlighting the positive impact that good nutrition can have on energy and performance at the skatepark and recovery can help get them on board, as often food and hydration is an afterthought; they just love skateboarding. Practical information is key: ready to grab snacks, (long-life milk drinks, roasted chickpeas or fava beans, trail mixes, fruit, peanut butter sandwiches, yogurt pouches), having an insulated lunch bag, and suitable options from the corner shop when needed. Also encouraging practical fluid intake strategies, to have a drink bottle (preferably more than one) that is see through, so they are aware of how much they are drinking, placing their drink bottle and snacks in clear sight at the skatepark, and getting the coach and parents involved to give hydration and fuelling reminders.

(Rachel Stentiford)

Masters athletes

Masters athletes (>35 years) need to be supported in their training to ensure adequate fuelling for their events. In addition, they may have chronic health problems which also need to be managed.

A 63-year-old female from Australia, is a recreational endurance athlete. She trains 15-25 hours per week and has achieved national age-category wins. She has recently been diagnosed with elevated blood lipids, and has a family history of cardiovascular disease.

She sought assistance to improve body composition and performance for ultramarathons. She weighs 58.2 kg (BMI: 21.1kg/m²) and aims for an ideal race weight of 56-57kg. DXA scan results indicate 18% body fat and normal bone density. Her usual 24hr diet history showed she includes 200-350g of carbohydrates (3.5-6g/kg) and 120-165g of protein (2.1-2.8g/kg). She consumed low amounts of bread, cereals, and dairy foods, only fuelled prior to training >2hrs, and did not include carbohydrates with lunch or snacks. Her carbohydrate loading strategy achieved 4-5g carbohydrates/kg and during long training and races she consumed 45-60g carbohydrate/hr. She supplemented with fish oil, glucosamine and chondroitin, vitamin D, calcium, greens powder, whey protein isolate, colostrum, collagen powder, sports bars, gels, and drinks.

With no signs of disordered eating or low energy availability, she was supported in her goal of improving power-to-weight ratio for performance. We agreed to maintain her ideal race weight briefly before key events, allowing her weight to return to normal during recovery to prevent fatigue, injury, or illness. Skin fold measurements were taken every 4-12 weeks based on her training stage.

It was important to prioritise optimising training nutrition and hydration rather than solely focusing on racing. We focused on ensuring adequate intake of energy, macro- and micronutrients at the right times with a structured training meal plan. This involved pre-fuelling before intense morning and long training sessions and increasing carbohydrates at lunch and snacks. Protein portions were reduced at dinner, with a focus on lean protein sources (particularly chicken and fish), and the use of protein supplements were ceased. She was encouraged to stop all supplements (except fish oil) with no evidence of benefit and posing a risk of banned substances.

Over 1-2 months, she increased fuelling during long training to 75g carbohydrates per hour, including glucose and fructose. She often reported she didn't have time or forgot to do sweat rate testing. Nonetheless, a drink to thirst strategy supported her performance without formal assessment. Carbohydrate loading targeted 8-10g/kg body weight, requiring careful planning due to limited food availability during travel for events. For multi-day events, we focused on optimising recovery with simple strategies such as a liquid breakfast drinks, fruit and sports drinks. She tested caffeine and nitrates in training which she found supported her performance.

She has completed three 50km runs and three multi-day events, with podium finishes in her age category. Her best performance aligns with her ideal race weight and lower skin fold measurements. She is able to develop draft race plans, which we fine-tune and formalise during our sessions. Her blood lipids have also fallen to within normal clinical range.

(Erin Colebatch)

Exercise-associated gastrointestinal symptoms in athletes

Exercise-associated gastrointestinal symptoms (Ex-GIS) affect many athletes; in ultra-endurance events up to 85% of athletes may be impacted (Chapter 15). It is important that an experienced sports nutrition professional takes a thorough clinical assessment of the athlete's presenting Ex-GIS including athlete characteristics, type of symptoms, onset of symptoms, environmental conditions that prompted Ex-GIS, and eating and drinking habits.

Not all athletes experience the same GIS and/or experience GIS in the same conditions. Some athletes may be more prone to experiencing symptoms in certain environmental conditions i.e., heat vs temperate ambient conditions or only experience GIS further into the duration of an event (i.e., >3h) whereas other athlete's symptoms may be more sporadic in nature. Some athletes suffer severe GIS during nocturnal exercise but have no problems during diurnal exercise. In addition, each athlete tends to have varying levels of feeding tolerance which means gut training practices need to be tailored to the athlete. As can be seen, there is no one-size fits all approach for managing Ex-GIS. Once an assessment is made and the probable causal and triggering factor(s) identified a prevention and management plan can be put into place for the athlete to implement.

A common causal pathway of Ex-GIS in many athletes is the neuroendocrine-gastrointestinal pathway and it therefore makes sense that if the sports nutrition professional is unable to undertake an exercise GI assessment on the athlete, nutrition management strategies should probably focus on targeting this pathway. Common nutrition strategies that have been shown to be effective in helping alleviate symptoms triggered by this pathway include short-term (24-48h) low FODMAP, low fibre and residue dietary intake; gut training (i.e., challenging the GI tract with target amounts of food and/or fluid repeatedly and consecutively during training); small and frequent intake of carbohydrate during exercise and possibly pharmacotherapy intervention.

(Stephanie Gaskell)

Fuelling strategies in extreme environments

Extreme environments such as cold, heat, and high altitude require special consideration not only on how nutrition requirements may change but also on how to ensure the athlete has access to foods.

Extreme cold

Aerial skiing in Australia is a talent transfer program for athletes with a background in gymnastics or diving. This transfer happens around 15-18 years of age, with most of these athletes having never skied before. Therefore, in the first few years of their development in the sport, these athletes chase winter around the world to maximise time on snow to refine their skiing skills, while complimenting their skiing with sports specific dryland training.

Fuelling and hydration on snow presents challenges such as: limited access to/higher cost of food once on the mountain, limited access to bathrooms when on ski runs, food and fluids freezing unless stored appropriately, reduced appetite and thirst at altitude, and increased energy expenditure and glycogen utilisation at altitude.

Nutrition tips and strategies to help address this include: carbohydrate-rich snacks (dried fruit, fruit straps, pretzels, muesli bars) decanted and stored in zip-lock bags which makes access easier and stored within an inside pocket for body warmth to prevent freezing while skiing, snacks with higher fat content (e.g. energy bars with coconut oil) to minimise freezing, juice pop tops with a pinch of salt for hydration that fit in the ski jacket pocket, maximising small and frequent intake of fluid and fuel while on ski-lifts, insulated drink bottles at the base of runs with carbohydrate-containing and possibly warm fluid (sports drink, blackcurrant juice, sweetened tea), an insulated container to store snacks and drink bottles at the base of runs, carbohydrate-rich main meals (preferably warm, like chicken soup and bread or a toasted sandwich and hot chocolate), and grocery shopping in larger towns when possible where the costs are often lower.

A combination of the above strategies results in having regular access to suitable fuelling options to maintain energy levels for training performance, concentration, and health. Athletes will continue to refine their nutrition as they progress through the pathway and build their knowledge and confidence in fuelling appropriately for the work being done.

(Rachel Stentiford)

Similarly snowboarding presents similar problems for the sports nutrition professional.

Acute changes in weather can also delay or postpone training or competition and subsequently put a halt to fuelling plans. A sudden drop in temperature may also increase an athlete's energy expenditure due to shivering (to keep warm) and/or start to freeze the options they brought with them to consume if without a warm pot to store them.

There can also be hesitation from snowboarding athletes to adequately rehydrate between runs/heats due to the sometimes large time demands of travelling to and from a bathroom. Exposure to cold mountain air also increases fluid losses through respiration and can compound inadequate rehydration practices. Employ strategies to ensure the athlete is starting the day of training well-hydrated. It is important to consider hydration options for on snow that also contain electrolytes and or fluids consumed with food (which already contains electrolytes) to encourage retention and reduce the need for a bathroom stop during training. Make use of a thermos/insulated drink bottles and start with slightly warmed fluids. The coach and athlete should schedule bathroom stops into long training sessions. Encourage incorporation of higher fluid containing foods as part of a rehydration and recovery strategy from long training days (soups, casseroles/stews, yoghurts, fresh fruits etc.

(Rebecca Hall)

Any nutrition plan for a snowboarding athlete needs to be tailored to the individual athlete's goals and needs to be adaptable in the event of training cancellations and changes due to weather/environmental conditions.

Providing education and counselling is critical so that the athletes understand the rationale for fuelling plans and can adapt as the conditions and environment change.

Ultimately, the sports nutrition professional needs to work with the athlete to understand fuelling for the work required on any given training day. This may mean educating an athlete on how to calculate the amount of physical work they are completing versus the amount of time they are spending on snow. For example, a snowboarder may spend 3.5 hours in training but only one hour of that 3.5 hours is snowboarding and/or doing physical work. The remainder of the time may be spent catching the chairlift back to the top, speaking to the coach, waiting for the course to clear, or waiting for the weather to change. Providing nutrition recommendations and examples based on the amount of physical work done versus time on snow, enables a snowboarder to be more adaptable day-to-day with the unpredictable nature of training in a challenging environment.

(Rebecca Hall)

Extreme heat

Athletes are also having to increasingly train and compete in extreme heat and humidity conditions; the predicted future climate change is likely to extend this trend. Motor racing is one sport which, regardless of the weather, places athletes under great heat stress.

Heat stress is a big one with motor sports like motocross and Moto GP, desert racing like the Dakar Rally, and Formula One. These athletes can't lose heat from sweat evaporation due to their protective equipment, so that heat is retained. When experiencing heat stress their perception of effort is a lot higher. There's a reduced ability to train or compete at the intensity they want to, and a reduction in mental focus and decision making.

We heat acclimate the endurance athletes if we know they're going to be competing in the heat. We test sweat rates, and practice hydration strategies in training. The motorsport guys I think are already heat acclimated, because they're always wearing the protective gear that traps the heat in. They're also quite restricted in terms of what they can do hydration-wise. Moto GP and other elite motorsports can take on fluids during the race, but it's only a very small amount, more to help reduce thirst. We also use pre-cooling strategies like ice slushies throughout the day. We work closely with catering at the races. We create our own ice lollies from smoothies or fruit juice, which the athletes really like.

(Alan McCubbin in conversation with Stephen Smith)

Recreational athletes must ensure they stay well hydrated without the backing of support teams – this means they need education and counselling to be able to determine their own fluid balance and manage their hydration.

A 24-year-old recreational road cyclist planning to participate in the 'Tour Down Under' sought the support of a sports nutrition professional. The 'Tour Down Under' is a 160km ride held in late January in the Australian summer. This is a hot climate with previous average temperatures of approximately 33°C when the event concludes at around midday.

The athlete is concerned about hydration as on her weekly long ride, which is first thing Sunday morning, she often feels a bit dizzy towards the end of the 3-hour session. She expects The Tour Down Under to take approximately 5 to 6 hours. She doesn't feel like she 'hits the wall' with energy during the ride but will feel sluggish and lethargic for the rest of the day afterwards. On her long rides, she consumes only a mix of coconut water and plain water.

The athlete and the sports nutrition professional work together to put several strategies in place. First, they identify strategies to minimise her total fluid loss to less than 2% of her total body weight. She conducts a fluid balance test to understand her approximate sweat rate in different warm/humid conditions, and finds this is between 400-800ml/hr of fluid. This information is used to inform her training and race-day hydration plan. While sweat testing is not necessary for an athlete at a recreational level, it is worth having the athlete consider whether she is a 'salty sweater' by trying to observe any salt deposits on her clothing post-exercise. She is advised to swap coconut water for a commercial or homemade sports drink, as coconut water contains insufficient sodium and carbohydrate to meet her fuel and hydration needs during exercise. A sports drink contains approximately 10-30 mmol/L (230-690mg/L) of sodium and 6-8% carbohydrate.

She is also encouraged to check her morning urine colour on waking, aiming for a pale yellow or straw colour prior to commencing her long ride. This would include consuming approximately 5-10 ml/kg BW of fluid in the 2-4 hours before exercising. For her early rides where this drinking over 2-4 hours before the ride is not practical, it is recommended that she goes to sleep well hydrated to minimise the risk of dehydration on waking. It takes some trial and error to minimise bathroom-related disruptions to sleep. A salty snack (e.g., crackers) prior to sleep could assist with topping up muscle glycogen stores and fluid retention overnight.

Finally, they discuss the importance of adjusting her fluid intake to changes in weather, with more fluid needed before, during, and after exercise in hot conditions.

(Ryan Tam)

Altitude

Training at altitude requires special focus on iron for all athletes due to the increased synthesis of haemoglobin, leading to increased requirements of iron to facilitate altitude adjustments and maintain iron balance. Prevention of iron deficiency is critical for health and performance outcomes and planning for it must occur prior to the training period at altitude.

> With altitude training we pay a lot more attention to iron intake and carbohydrate as well. We want to prevent iron deficiency in the lead-up to training camps, so we test the blood to make sure they're not deficient. If they are, we commence iron supplements. We also pay more attention to the hydration, to combat some of the reduced thirst they report. We plan fluid intakes more so they're not just relying on thirst. We utilize syrups, cordials, or flavoured electrolytes, not so much for the electrolyte content, but for the taste.
>
> (Alan McCubbin in conversation with Stephen Smith)

Working in extreme environments can be quite testing and back-up plans are needed. Again, it is important that athletes understand the rationale for fuelling strategies so that they can make decisions under pressure in challenging circumstances.

> It's important to remember these environments are often out in the wilderness. It's not knowledge limiting our ability to optimise nutrition, it's the delivery. That's where the wins are made, focusing on how you can deliver these nutrition interventions in these environments. Sometimes athletes are living in remote villages and the food you want isn't available, or in a hotel where the quality might not be great. I coach the athletes to prepare and take some food, like freeze-dried meals. If everything else doesn't work, at least they've got something to fall back on. Planning is where the biggest gains are to be made, you don't want to be reactive to situations. For the alpinists it's life-and-death, so we discuss things like 'if you arrive and can't get this sort of food, what can you do?' Sometimes athletes really want to eat what we'd say is optimal, but those provisions are just not available. So, we teach them 'maybe it's not optimal, but here's what you can do in that situation.
>
> (Alan McCubbin in conversation with Stephen Smith)

Working with teams

When working with teams the sports nutrition professional has to find a way to provide nutrition support for a team that has a variety of different nutrition needs. This becomes more complicated when the players on a team have quite different requirements and body sizes depending on their positions, such as in professional rugby. Sports nutrition professional, Sarah Jenner, highlights the challenges and solutions she has used with professional rugby teams.

> The nutrition demands of professional rugby athletes, will be largely dependent on their training and competition demands, as well as individual athlete goals (e.g., body composition, positional demands i.e., tight head vs scrum half). Given the intermittent nature, as well as the demands of collision-based movements, there is a requirement

for athletes to consume adequate carbohydrate intake matched to training and competition needs, as well as adequate total protein, and meet overall energy requirements.

During competition season, a professional rugby union team will follow a periodised training plan to prioritise an athlete's preparation leading into competition and reduce the risk of overtraining and any negative effects on match-day performance. A training week may include high-load volume sessions early in the week, and taper volumes towards the end to optimise recovery leading into games.

Therefore, if we take into consideration the science behind the 'fuel for the work required' whereby an athlete's carbohydrate intake is adjusted according to the day-by-day fuelling demands across a training week, as well as the desired outcome of the training session (e.g., achieving high-intensity exercise) we can aim to introduce practical carbohydrate intake strategies to guide athletes on their fuelling needs over a training week. We do need to acknowledge that such strategies as 'fuel for the work required' were developed within endurance sports, however there is need in many team sports such as rugby union to find practical ways to maximise an athletes' dietary intake around training sessions from a fuelling and recovery perspective.

(Sarah Jenner)

Sarah Jenner outlines the importance of a sports nutrition professional targeting the nutrition advice to the training undertaken by the athlete and the role that the multi-disciplinary team play in this:

Sports nutrition professionals are one cog in a very large wheel, and the importance of cross-pollination between professionals in the multi-disciplinary team is essential. To tailor dietary intake to training demands, sports nutrition professionals must work in collaboration with strength and conditioning coaches, sport scientists and coaches, to understand the typical weekly training volume and positional needs of athletes.

(Sarah Jenner)

And then, the art of nutrition practice comes into play, where the sports nutrition professional must bring it all together for the team.

Building an environment around athletes that promotes high performance dietary behaviours is essential in team sport. Strategies can be creative and do not always have to be based around group presentations. Examples of practical group education strategies that have been useful include:

- adapting the weekly catering menu to training demands (i.e. meals and snacks);
- building food-based infographics that align with key nutrition messages (i.e. portion plates);
- using social media to provide recipes and snack ideas;
- including senior players in the delivery of messages (e.g. players to present at team meetings).

(Sarah Jenner)

Games event preparation

Athletes and teams come from a variety of cultural backgrounds which affect food choices. Preparing nutrition plans for numerous different teams at an international games event with athletes that have individual nutrition requirements can be a challenge. Here, sports nutrition professional, Rebecca Hall, who prepared catering for a national contingent at a large international sports event, outlines the problems she encountered and the solutions she developed.

One of the major problems we have is how to meet the nutrition needs of 60 different individual athletes from across many different sports with limited cooking facilities and in the context of a major competition event in a foreign country. How do you provide meal and snack options that are food safe, nutrient dense, varied, meet the athletes' nutrition requirements and can be available on a flexible schedule?

(Rebecca Hall)

The sports nutrition professional must take many factors into consideration to start the planning process for catering. These are some of the questions the sports nutrition professional Rebecca Hall considered in this scenario.

- What do your individual athletes need from a nutrition perspective? This will require speaking with other sports dietitians that work with these athletes as well.
- Any dietary requirements: allergies, intolerances, dietary beliefs, strong food preferences?
- Any specific requests as part of competition preparation? What are the non-negotiables in terms of foods for the different sports/individuals? Any culturally important foods that need to be included/excluded?
- What times do athletes want to eat around competition? Will anyone need special mealtimes (late/early)? How will you store their meal in a food safe way?
- Will athletes need to prepare food to take with them for consumption during competition?
- What do athletes across different sports need in terms of preparation for competition versus recovery etc.? Higher carbohydrate, lower fat needs for endurance-based sports etc. Differences in food volume as well between athletes. How much will you need to cook on any given day? Will you have a way to utilise leftovers etc.?
- What do you have access to in terms of cooking facilities, food supplies, meal preparation, cooking and food serving support?
- How do you avoid meal repetition and flavour fatigue?

Focussing on these questions allows you to begin the planning process and get everything in order. I consulted all athletes and their coaches regarding the nutrition needs well in advance of the event to cater accordingly.

A multi-pronged approach in providing nutrition choice was needed, there was self-service food space in the dining room for 'make-your-own' snacks and simple meals. Facilities that were available to athletes included fridge, microwave, toaster, sandwich press, chopping boards, knives, bowls & cutlery. Food options available included sachets of ready to eat rice/pasta, hard boiled eggs, ham, tins of tuna, flavoured beans, yoghurt, milk, cheese, fruits, fresh vegetables, fresh breads, dried chickpeas. These were checked every few hours for restocking and cleaning purposes.

During meal services, the carbohydrate and protein options were separated so that athletes could select appropriate amounts to meet their fuelling and recovery requirements. It is important to make the meal menu nutritionally diverse each day. Example dinner meals that were provide included; vegetable-based soups, grilled herb chicken, roasted root vegetables including potatoes, fresh bread, garlic & herb bread, garden salads, herb-marinated fish, baked tofu, and for dessert yoghurt, mixed berries, and apple crumble. Again, all components served separately so each athlete can build the meal to their unique requirements.

We also offered a special request service – requests must be made 24 hours prior and in the context of pre or during competition. Take-away meal options were provided to enable food provision for athletes who needed to travel a long way to their event and/or were likely to be out well beyond mealtimes. Food safe storage was provided with take-away options.

Catering for many athletes is always a challenge however the number one goal is to understand in detail the needs of the athlete cohort and from there consider the most efficient way you can meet those individual needs but also still provide athletes with choice.

(Rebecca Hall)

Summary

This chapter has presented practical insights and experiences of sports nutrition professionals who have mastered the art of practising sports nutrition. They have gone beyond the science (macronutrients, micronutrients, and hydration protocols) and made it an art – they have developed their skills over time to craft personalised nutritional strategies. The scenarios presented highlight how sports nutrition professionals understand individual athletes and their training and competition requirements and contexts to ensure that the athlete is able to fuel successfully, even when unexpected situations and setbacks are encountered.

Index

Pages in *italics* refer to figures and pages in **bold** refer to tables.

Printed in the United States
by Baker & Taylor Publisher Services